Cancer Drug Discovery and Development

Series Editor
Beverly A. Teicher
Bethesda, Maryland, USA

Cancer Drug Discovery and Development, the Springer series headed by Beverly A. Teicher, is the definitive book series in cancer research and oncology. Volumes cover the process of drug discovery, preclinical models in cancer research, specific drug target groups, and experimental and approved therapeutic agents. The volumes are current and timely, anticipating areas where experimental agents are reaching FDA approval. Each volume is edited by an expert in the field covered, and chapters are authored by renowned scientists and physicians in their fields of interest.

More information about this series at http://www.springer.com/series/7625

Philip J. Tofilon • Kevin Camphausen
Editors

Increasing the Therapeutic Ratio of Radiotherapy

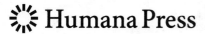 Humana Press

Editors
Philip J. Tofilon
Radiation Oncology Branch
National Cancer Institute
Bethesda, MD, USA

Kevin Camphausen
Radiation Oncology Branch
National Cancer Institute
Bethesda, MD, USA

ISSN 2196-9906   ISSN 2196-9914   (electronic)
Cancer Drug Discovery and Development
ISBN 978-3-319-82201-3   ISBN 978-3-319-40854-5   (eBook)
DOI 10.1007/978-3-319-40854-5

Printed on acid-free paper

This Humana Press imprint is published by Springer Nature
The registered company is Springer International Publishing AG
The registered company address is: Gewerbestrasse 11, 6330 Cham, Switzerland

Contents

Contributors

Mary Helen Barcellos-Hoff Department of Radiation Oncology, Helen Diller Family Comprehensive Cancer Center, University of California, San Francisco, CA, USA

Christopher A. Barker Department of Radiation Oncology, Memorial Sloan Kettering Cancer Center, New York, NY, USA

Sadna Budhu Ludwig Collaborative and Swim Across America Laboratory, Department of Medicine, Memorial Sloan Kettering Cancer Center, New York, NY, USA

Kevin Camphausen Radiation Oncology Branch, National Cancer Institute, Bethesda, MD, USA

Ross Carruthers Translational Radiation Biology, Institute of Cancer Sciences, Wolfson Wohl Cancer Research Centre, University of Glasgow, Glasgow, UK

Anthony J. Chalmers Translational Radiation Biology, Institute of Cancer Sciences, Wolfson Wohl Cancer Research Centre, University of Glasgow, Glasgow, UK

Eun Joo Chung Section of Translational Radiation Oncology, Radiation Oncology Branch, National Cancer Institute, Bethesda, MD, USA

Su I. Chung Section of Translational Radiation Oncology, Radiation Oncology Branch, National Cancer Institute, Bethesda, MD, USA

Deborah E. Citrin Section of Translational Radiation Oncology, Radiation Oncology Branch, National Cancer Institute, Bethesda, MD, USA

Joseph N. Contessa Department of Therapeutic Radiology, Yale University School of Medicine, New Haven, CT, USA

David Cormode Department of Radiation Oncology, Perelman School of Medicine, University of Pennsylvania, Philadelphia, PA, USA

Jay F. Dorsey Department of Radiation Oncology, Perelman School of Medicine, University of Pennsylvania, Philadelphia, PA, USA

Michael R. Folkert Department of Radiation Oncology, Simmons Comprehensive Cancer Center, UT Southwestern Medical Center, Dallas, TX, USA

Adam Gladwish Princess Margaret Cancer Centre, Department of Radiation Oncology, University of Toronto, Toronto, ON, Canada

Kathy Han Princess Margaret Cancer Centre, Department of Radiation Oncology, University of Toronto, Toronto, ON, Canada

Thomas J. Hayman Department of Therapeutic Radiology, Yale University School of Medicine, New Haven, CT, USA

Murali C. Krishna Radiation Biology Branch, Center for Cancer Research, National Cancer Institute, National Institutes of Health, Bethesda, MD, USA

Aaron M. Laine Department of Radiation Oncology, Simmons Comprehensive Cancer Center, UT Southwestern Medical Center, Dallas, TX, USA

Taha Mergoub Ludwig Collaborative and Swim Across America Laboratory, Department of Medicine, Memorial Sloan Kettering Cancer Center, New York, NY, USA

James B. Mitchell Radiation Biology Branch, Center for Cancer Research, National Cancer Institute, National Institutes of Health, Bethesda, MD, USA

Sarwat Naz Radiation Biology Branch, Center for Cancer Research, National Cancer Institute, National Institutes of Health, Bethesda, MD, USA

Robert M. Samstein Department of Radiation Oncology, Memorial Sloan Kettering Cancer Center, New York, NY, USA

DeeDee K. Smart Section of Translational Radiation Oncology, Radiation Oncology Branch, National Cancer Institute, Bethesda, MD, USA

Elizabeth I. Spehalski Radiation Oncology Branch, National Cancer Institute, Bethesda, MD, USA

Robert D. Timmerman Department of Radiation Oncology, Simmons Comprehensive Cancer Center, UT Southwestern Medical Center, Dallas, TX, USA

Departments of Radiation Oncology and Neurological Surgery, Simmons Comprehensive Cancer Center, UT Southwestern Medical Center, Dallas, TX, USA

Philip J. Tofilon Radiation Oncology Branch, National Cancer Institute, Bethesda, MD, USA

Andrew Tsourkas Department of Bioengineering, University of Pennsylvania, Philadelphia, PA, USA

Zabi Wardak Department of Radiation Oncology, Simmons Comprehensive Cancer Center, UT Southwestern Medical Center, Dallas, TX, USA

Ajlan Al Zaki George Washington University, School of Medicine and Health Sciences, Washington, DC, USA

Chapter 1
Improving the Therapeutic Ratio of Radiotherapy by Targeting the DNA Damage Response

Ross Carruthers and Anthony J. Chalmers

Abstract In recent decades, technological advances in radiotherapy delivery have allowed dose escalation or reduction of toxicity for radiotherapy regimens used to treat several major tumour sites. However, tumour radioresistance remains a significant clinical problem. Although it is well established that the major biological effects of ionising radiation are mediated through DNA damage, our knowledge of the biological processes influencing tumour response to radiation is still relatively basic. It is known that tumour cells repair the vast majority of potentially lethal DNA damage inflicted by ionising radiation and that the cellular response to DNA damage is a major determinant of tumour radiosensitivity. Manipulation of tumour DNA damage repair mechanisms to modify the radiobiological response of malignant cells is therefore a very appealing idea with the potential to greatly amplify the therapeutic effects of radiation therapy.

Keywords DNA damage response • Radiotherapy • Poly(ADP-ribose) polymerase • Ataxia telangiectasia mutated • Cell cycle checkpoints • Radiosensitizers

Introduction

In recent decades, technological advances in radiotherapy delivery have allowed dose escalation or reduction of toxicity for radiotherapy regimens used to treat several major tumour sites. However, tumour radioresistance remains a significant clinical problem. Although it is well established that the major biological effects of ionising radiation are mediated through DNA damage, our knowledge of the biological processes influencing tumour response to radiation is still relatively basic.

R. Carruthers • A.J. Chalmers (✉)
Translational Radiation Biology, Institute of Cancer Sciences, Wolfson Wohl Cancer Research Centre, University of Glasgow, Garscube Estate, Glasgow G61 1QH, UK
e-mail: Anthony.Chalmers@glasgow.ac.uk

© Springer International Publishing Switzerland 2017
P.J. Tofilon, K. Camphausen (eds.), *Increasing the Therapeutic Ratio of Radiotherapy*, Cancer Drug Discovery and Development, DOI 10.1007/978-3-319-40854-5_1

It is known that tumour cells repair the vast majority of potentially lethal DNA damage inflicted by ionising radiation and that the cellular response to DNA damage is a major determinant of tumour radiosensitivity. Manipulation of tumour DNA damage repair mechanisms to modify the radiobiological response of malignant cells is therefore a very appealing idea with the potential to greatly amplify the therapeutic effects of radiation therapy.

The components and mechanisms of DNA repair and cell cycle control pathways in normal mammalian cells have now been defined in some detail, and the potential to target and inhibit specific components of DNA damage response pathways is now a reality with the development in recent decades of small molecule inhibitors of some of the key components of these pathways. The current challenge facing radiation oncology is to integrate this knowledge in a manner which will allow specific manipulation of tumour radiobiological response in order to provide clinically useful, tumour-specific radiosensitisation. This chapter will summarise briefly the DNA damage response of cancer cells to ionising radiation and then describe various strategies to manipulate tumour radiobiology by inhibition of key DNA damage response proteins.

The DNA Damage Response (DDR)

Upon encountering DNA damage of any variety, the normal response of mammalian cells, whether malignant or otherwise, is to attempt repair. Cells accomplish this via a complex network of protein signalling cascades and pathways. The term 'DNA damage response' (DDR) will be used to refer to this cellular repair network. There are multiple pathways involved in DDR, often with huge complexity and some redundancy in function. However in general the cellular response to DNA damage can be summarised by two processes: (1) activation of cell cycle checkpoints and (2) initiation and execution of DNA repair. These two processes are complementary; activation of cell cycle checkpoints provides time for the cell to repair damaged DNA before either replicating it or attempting it to undergo mitosis. If repair of DNA damage is successful, the cell will survive and retain reproductive integrity. If unsuccessful, the cell may die via apoptosis, mitotic catastrophe or an alternative cell death mechanism. This is summarised in Fig. 1.1. A brief overview of the cellular DDR to ionising radiation follows.

Detection of Radiation-Induced DNA Damage and Initiation of DDR

Efficient DDR relies upon rapid detection of DNA damage and subsequent escalation of appropriate DDR pathways. The MRN complex consisting of MRE-11, NBS-1 and Rad50 proteins represents the major DNA DSB detector within mammalian cells. Ku70/Ku80 proteins, which are key effectors of the non-homologous

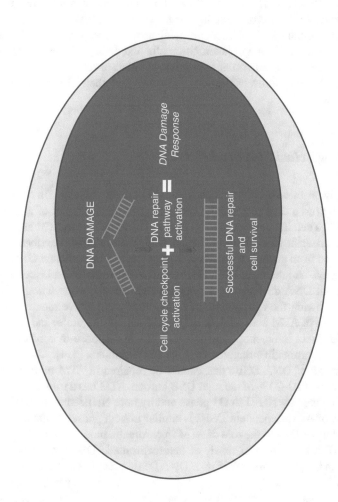

Fig. 1.1 Responses of mammalian cells to DNA DSBs induced by gamma irradiation following induction of DNA DSBs by ionising radiation, a DNA damage response consisting of cell cycle checkpoint activation and DNA repair is generated. If successful, this will result in DNA repair and cell survival

end joining (NHEJ) pathway, also bind directly to DNA DSBs facilitating early repair of most DNA DSBs. Following detection of DNA damage, this signal must be amplified and coordinated in order to facilitate a cellular environment conducive to DNA repair. This is achieved by the actions of three apical DDR proteins: ataxia telangiectasia mutated (ATM), ataxia telangiectasia and Rad 3 related (ATR) and DNA-dependent protein kinase (DNAPK) which are phosphatidylinositol 3-kinase-related kinases (PIKKs). The apical PIKKs phosphorylate a repertoire of DNA repair and checkpoint control proteins ensuring timely activation of cell cycle checkpoints and initiation of DNA repair mechanisms appropriate to DNA lesion stimuli and allow modification of heterochromatin and other more general intracellular environmental features in order to promote cellular survival. Apical PIKKs are appealing targets for radiosensitisation strategies and their functions and are described below.

Ataxia Telangiectasia Mutated (ATM)

ATM is a highly prolific kinase which phosphorylates many substrates in response to DNA DSBs and has a dual role in both cell cycle control and repair of a subset of DNA DSBs. For a detailed review, see Shiloh et al. [1]. Mutations in ATM are responsible for the radiosensitivity syndrome 'ataxia telangiectasia', first described in 1975 [2]. Cells derived from patients with ataxia telangiectasia show deficient G1/S, S and G2/M checkpoints and deficient DNA DSB repair. ATM exists as an inactive dimer or multimer until DNA damage occurs, upon which autophosphorylation at serine 1981 occurs, allowing the dissociation of ATM dimers into active monomers. The exact mechanism of ATM activation is debated in current literature, and activation may occur via direct interaction with DNA DSBs, in response to conformational changes in heterochromatin structure or via the MRN complex [3, 4].

The proportion of DNA DSBs that cannot be repaired in ATM-mutant cells is estimated at around 10–20 % of the total DSB burden. ATM has a role in promoting DSB repair executed by NHEJ in G1 phase and by both NHEJ and HR in G2, and the proportion of ATM-dependent DSBs is similar in both phases of the cell cycle. Goodarzi et al. investigated the role of ATM in chromatin modification and demonstrated that ATM has a role in repair of heterochromatic DSBs [5]. This model proposes that in G1 phase, around 75 % of DNA DSBs occur in euchromatin regions and that ATM is not required for the repair of these lesions. However, in heterochromatic regions, nucleosome flexibility is constrained by factors such as KAP-1, which severely limits DSB repair. In this model, DSBs in heterochromatin are responsible for the slow phase of DSB repair, since the cell needs to execute additional steps to rejoin DSBs occurring in this relatively inaccessible chromatin context. ATM is able to phosphorylate KAP-1, thereby generating sufficient elasticity in DNA tertiary structure to allow repair. It has previously been suggested that ATM's primary role is to deal with complex DNA DSB lesions, since Artemis and ATM defects create epistatic DNA repair defects and Artemis has a vital role in end resection for facilitation of NHEJ [6]. However, the proportion of ATM-dependent DNA DSBs appears not to increase following irradiation with high LET radiation types which cause more complex DSBs, which implies that ATM-dependent repair is not necessarily associated with complex DNA DSBs.

Nevertheless, ATM is also known to have roles in specialised DSB repair mechanisms that are not related to heterochromatin such as VDJ class switching and meiotic recombination. Alvarez-Quilon et al. demonstrated that ATM is necessary for the repair of DNA DSBs with blocked ends and that this requirement is independent of chromatin status [7]. The authors speculated that ATM could promote nucleolytic activity to eliminate blockage at DNA ends via the MRN complex, CtIP or Artemis or it could restrict excessive nucleolytic degradation of DNA ends by inhibiting these same nucleases or by phosphorylation of H2AX. These two models are not necessarily conflicting, since ATM may have roles in both complex DNA lesion repair and modification of chromatin.

Ataxia Telangiectasia and Rad 3 Related (ATR)

ATR has a critical role in the DDR by protecting cells from replication stress. Replication stress can be defined as the slowing or stalling of replication forks during duplication of DNA and is characterised by the presence of single-stranded DNA (ssDNA) within the nucleus. Cancers in general are known to exhibit high levels of replication stress, which is thought to be induced primarily by oncogene activation, leading to upregulation and increased dependence upon the ATR-Chk1 pathway [8]. Furthermore, the DNA damage induced by ionising radiation (both SSBs and DSBs) is a significant source of replicative stress in the irradiated cell. The role of ATR in the DDR is reviewed in Marechal et al. [9]. ATR has an essential role in the survival of proliferating cells, and its deletion leads to embryonic lethality in mice and lethality in human cells [10]. ATM and ATR share many phosphorylation substrates; however, they have distinct roles in DDR and cannot be viewed as redundant in function. ATR is activated by RPA-coated ssDNA; hence, any situation leading to the formation of ssDNA will result in the activation of ATR. ATR phosphorylates Chk1 which leads to G2/M checkpoint activation, allowing time for damage repair. However, both ATR and Chk1 have additional important functions in maintaining the integrity of replication forks. Replication fork collapse is characterised by the dissociation of replisome contents and may result in generation of a DSB. This process is still poorly understood and may be the result of replisome dissociation/migration, nuclease digestion of a reversed fork or replication runoff [11]. ATR is activated by ssDNA generated at stalled replication forks and acts to stabilise the fork and initiate cell cycle checkpoint activation and inhibition of DNA replication origin firing on a global scale throughout the cell nucleus. ATR activation inhibits origin firing via the phosphorylation of the lysine methyltransferase MLL, which alters chromatin structure around replication origins [12]. In this manner, the stalled fork can then be restarted when the replication stress stimulus has been resolved.

DNA-Dependent Protein Kinase (DNA-PK)

DNA-PK has a critical role in DDR via its function in NHEJ, as discussed below. It phosphorylates a smaller number of substrates in comparison to ATR and ATM. However, DNA-PK is able to phosphorylate some substrates of ATM in ATM-defective cells, allowing a degree of functional redundancy. In particular, DNA-PK is able to phosphorylate histone H2AX in the absence of ATM [13].

Activation of the apical DDR PIKKs results in cell cycle checkpoint initiation and attempted DNA repair. These processes will be considered separately as follows.

Cell Cycle Checkpoint Control

Mammalian cells have three main cell cycle checkpoints that are activated following DNA damage: G1, intra-S and G2/M. These are shown in Fig. 1.2. The checkpoints regulate progression through the cell cycle, preventing a cell from progressing into the next phase of the cell cycle prior to satisfying the requirements of the previous phase.

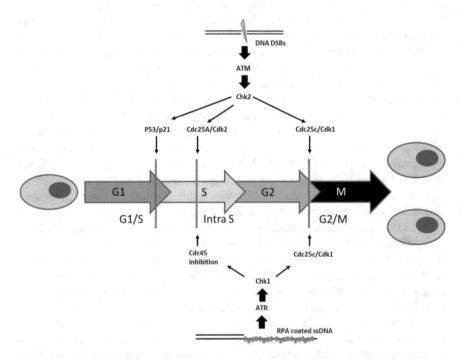

Fig. 1.2 Cell cycle control in response to DNA damage. Simplified diagram of cell cycle control following activation of the upstream PIKKs ATR and ATM. ATM is activated by DNA DSBs and influences all three major checkpoints, whereas ATR is activated by RPA-coated ssDNA and has its major roles in the intra-S checkpoint and maintenance of the G2/M checkpoint

Progression through the cell cycle is controlled by cyclin-dependent kinases (CDKs) and cyclins, the names alluding to their cyclical accumulation and destruction through the cell cycle. These proteins form cyclin-CDK complexes whose activity ultimately regulates the machinery responsible for cycle progression. For a review of the cellular machinery controlling cell cycle checkpoints, see Lukas et al. [14].

The G1 checkpoint is usually very robust in eukaryotic cells; however, in malignant cells, the G1 checkpoint is frequently absent due to mutations affecting the p53 pathway. For example, glioblastoma and other cancer cells frequently fail to initiate a G1 checkpoint response to irradiation. Normal G1 checkpoint function requires functioning p53, which is phosphorylated in response to DNA damage by both ATM and Chk2 proteins. This leads to a reduction in the binding of MDM2 to p53, and subsequent p53 activation, resulting in its nuclear accumulation and stabilisation. Increased levels of p53 protein stimulate increased transcription of p21, which binds and inhibits CDK2-cyclin E activity, preventing the cell from entering S phase. The G1/S checkpoint is highly sensitive, but limited by the time required for p21 upregulation [15]. Alternative activation of the G1/S checkpoint is mediated via phosphorylation of Cdc25A, again by ATM and Chk2, which then targets Cdc25A for proteasomal degradation. Cdc25A removes inhibitory phosphate groups on CDK2, allowing progression into S phase [16].

The intra-S checkpoint is activated in response to replication stress or other difficulties encountered by the cell during S phase. It operates to slow DNA replication rather than stop it entirely and is p53 independent. The components of the S phase checkpoint suppress origin firing and slow replication fork progression to reduce the rate of DNA replication. Abnormalities in S phase checkpoints result in the radioresistant DNA synthesis (RDS) phenotype, i.e. cells are unable to stop or delay the synthesis of DNA following induction of DNA damage by radiation.

Cancer cells frequently demonstrate an increased dependency upon G2/M checkpoint activation to allow repair of DNA damage prior to entering mitosis, since the G1/S phase checkpoint is often dysfunctional in malignant cells due to deficiencies in the p53 pathway. Progression through the G2/M checkpoint with unrepaired DNA damage can result in cell death, and therefore it is essential that control of the G2/M checkpoint is maintained. Activation of the G2/M checkpoint occurs via ATM and ATR which phosphorylate Chk1 and Chk2, leading to phosphorylation of Cdc25 phosphatases. The G2/M checkpoint has a defined threshold of sensitivity, with activation and maintenance of G2/M arrest appearing to require 10–15 DSBs [17]. The G2/M cell cycle checkpoint arrests heavily damaged cells in G2 to provide time for repair of DSBs, and it is proposed that this may be important for slow phase repair in G2 via homologous recombination. However, the G2/M checkpoint is inherently insensitive and allows cells to enter mitosis carrying a measurable number of unrepaired DSB [18].

DNA Repair Processes

Exposure to a 2Gy dose of radiation will produce on average around 2000 SSBs and 80 DSBs. DNA DSBs are much more difficult for cells to repair and have long been considered the lesions responsible for lethality following irradiation.

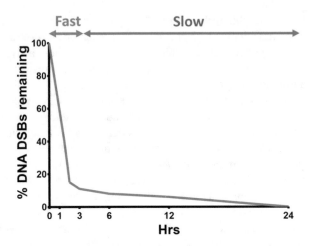

Fig. 1.3 Illustrative schematic of kinetics of DNA DSB repair following irradiation in mammalian cells. The majority of DSBs are repaired a short time after irradiation in the 'fast' phase of DNA DSB repair via NHEJ. However, a subset of DNA DSBs requires much more time for repair, due to complexity and/or chromatin context, and is represented by a 'slow' phase tail on the above illustration. Slow phase repair is achieved via NHEJ in G1 phase and HR repair in G2 phase. Adapted from [19]

Figure 1.3 illustrates DNA DSB repair kinetics in mammalian cells following gamma radiation adapted from Goodarzi et al. [19]. There is an initial fast phase of repair lasting 1–3 h which represents DNA DSBs that can be efficiently repaired by the cell. In addition to the fast phase of repair, there is a longer 'tail' which is termed the slow phase of DNA DSB repair and can extend past 24 h. Both slow phase and fast phase repair occur simultaneously. If left unrepaired, even a single DNA DSB can result in loss of genetic information and cell death [20] so it is unsurprising that mammalian cells have developed complex and highly efficient systems for their repair. DNA DSBs are repaired predominantly by two pathways, homologous recombination (HR) and non-homologous end joining (NHEJ), although back up pathways such as microhomology-mediated end joining (MMEJ) also exist. For a review of DNA DSB repair, see Shibata and Jeggo [21].

Non-homologous End Joining (NHEJ)

The bulk of DNA DSB repair in mammalian cells is undertaken by NHEJ, exclusively so in G1 cell cycle phase where cells have a diploid DNA content. NHEJ is involved in both fast phase repair and slow phase repair in G1 cells and in the fast phase of repair in G2 cells [6]. NHEJ involves the processing of broken DNA termini to form compatible ends which can then be ligated back together. NHEJ is a relatively simple, rapid and efficient method of DNA DSB repair but is error prone and associated with loss of genetic information. The mechanisms of NHEJ can be simplified into three steps: (for a comprehensive review, see Weterings et al. [22]) (1) capture of both ends of the broken DNA molecule, (2) bridging of the two broken DNA ends and (3) religation of the broken DNA molecule. NHEJ is thought to make the first attempt at rejoining the majority of DNA DSBs, even in G2 phase where HR is competent, due partly to the cellular abundance of Ku70 and Ku80 and their high affinity for DNA termini [23, 24]. NHEJ and its major protein components are summarised in simplified form in Fig. 1.4.

An alternative mechanism of NHEJ is thought to occur via microhomology-mediated end joining (MMEJ) [25, 26]. For a detailed review, see McVey et al. [27]. MMEJ has a requirement for limited MRN-dependent end resection and relies upon homologous matching of 5–25 base pairs on both strands in order to correctly align the DNA DSB ends. Any overhanging or mismatched bases are removed and missing bases inserted. The process is particularly error prone, since it does not identify sequences lost around the DSB. MMEJ appears to act as a reserve DSB repair pathway but can also repair DSBs generated at collapse of replication forks. The process is dependent upon ATM, PARP-1, MRE-11, CtIP and DNA ligase IV but operates independently of Ku or DNA-PKcs [27]. The extent to which MMEJ contributes to DSB repair in normal cells is unknown, but it has been shown to assume importance in cancer cells bearing defects in other DSB repair pathways [28].

Homologous Recombination (HR)

The homologous recombination (HR) pathway represents a more complex and sophisticated mechanism of DNA DSB repair. Although NHEJ repairs the majority of DNA DSBs, HR contributes to the repair of DSBs in specific circumstances, such as the one-ended DSB created by the collapse of DNA replication forks and a subset of DNA DSBs in G2 that are repaired with slow kinetics [23, 29, 30]. HR is conventionally considered to be limited to S and G2 phases of the cell cycle, since it relies upon homologous DNA sequences (in the form of the duplicated DNA strand of a sister chromatid) to effect repair. Because of this, however, it is highly accurate. For a more detailed review of the process, see Filippo et al. [31], Li et al. [32] and Krejci et al. [33]. In brief, HR is initiated by resection of the 5' DNA end of the DSB in order to create 3' SS DNA which can then invade a partner chromosome. End processing creates 3' ends following resection of nucleotides from the 5' break ends. Extension of resection is tightly regulated by the repositioning of 53BP1 via a BRCA 1-dependent process (9 Jeggo 2014 review). Resected 3' ends are then quickly bound by replication protein A (RPA), which protects ssDNA and removes DNA secondary structure in order to facilitate formation of a 'presynaptic filament' consisting of Rad51-coated ssDNA [34, 35]. Rad51 is a recombinase, i.e. an enzyme which facilitates genetic recombination and forms a helical filament on ssDNA which holds it in an extended conformation to aid the search for homology. BRCA 2 has an essential role in the loading of Rad51 onto ssDNA.

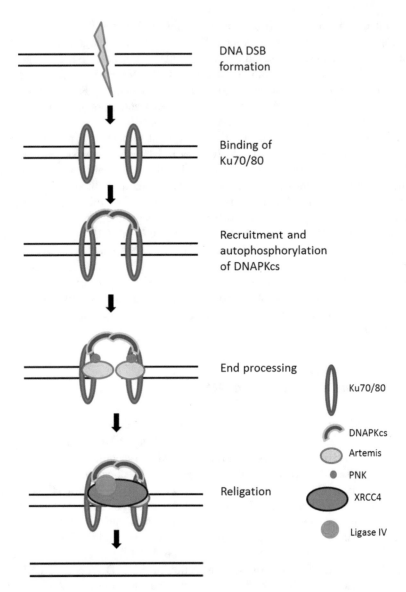

Fig. 1.4 Schematic diagram of non-homologous end joining (NHEJ) repair. NHEJ is initiated by the binding of Ku70/Ku80, followed by the recruitment of DNA-PKcs and its subsequent autophosphorylation. End processing is achieved via Artemis, and additional factors before the broken DNA ends are ligated

Once assembled, the presynaptic filament captures a duplex DNA molecule and begins its search for the homologous sequence. Rad51 facilitates the physical connection between the invading DNA strand and the DNA duplex structure leading to the formation of heteroduplex DNA ('D loop') with a Holliday junction (HJ), as described in Fig. 1.5. Synthesis of DNA and repair of the DSB lesion then occurs

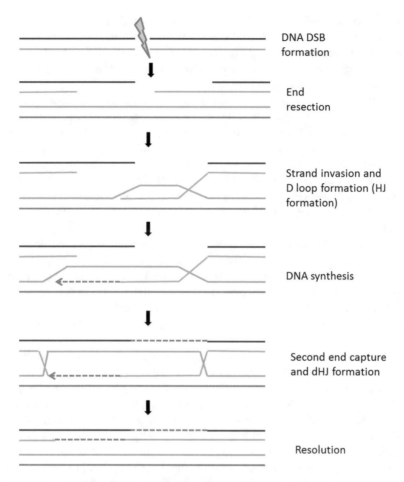

DNA DSB
formation

End
resection

Strand invasion and
D loop formation (HJ
formation)

DNA synthesis

Second end capture
and dHJ formation

Resolution

Fig. 1.5 Schematic diagrams of homologous recombination (HR) repair. HR repair is initiated by end resection and coating of ssDNA by RPA and subsequently Rad51. The search for a homologous sequence on the sister chromatid is initiated by strand invasion and subsequent Holliday junction formation. Synthesis of new complementary DNA sequence and Holliday junction resolution results in successful DNA DSB repair

using the undamaged DNA strand of the heteroduplex DNA molecule as a template. Following successful repair, resolution of the heteroduplex DNA molecule occurs, generating crossover or non-crossover products.

Poly (ADP-Ribose) Polymerases (PARPs)

Whilst the main features of the DDR to DNA DSB have been explored, it should not be forgotten that responses to single-strand DNA breaks also influence the eventual outcome of radiation-induced DNA damage. Gamma or X-radiation induces around 25-fold more SSBs than DSBs, but these are usually repaired promptly. If SSBs are not resolved efficiently, however, they can have significant effects on cell survival via the generation of DSBs. The PARP family of proteins is known to facilitate base excision repair (BER) which is one of the main cellular single-strand break repair pathways.

PARPs form a large protein family with diverse cellular functions including DNA repair, mitotic segregation, telomere homeostasis and cell death. PARPs are characterised by their catalytic function, which is poly(ADP-ribosylation). There are 18 reported family members; however, not all have definite poly(ADP-ribose) catalytic function, and only PARPs 1–3 have well-characterised roles in DNA repair. For an in-depth review of PARP function, see D'Amours and Burkle [36, 37]. PARP-1 is the most abundant and best understood family member, so the term 'PARP' will be used to refer to the actions of PARP-1 for the rest of this chapter.

Activated PARP modifies its substrates via covalent, sequential addition of ADP-ribose molecules that form branching poly(ADP-ribose) (PAR) polymers on its targets. The substrate from which PAR is formed is nicotinamide adenine dinucleotide (NAD+). Poly(ADP-ribosylation) is a commonly occurring post-translational modification in the cell. It creates negative charge on target proteins altering their three-dimensional structure and regulating interactions with other proteins and with DNA [38].

PARP is an efficient sensor of DNA damage and its rapid binding to damaged DNA results in its activation (Fig. 1.6). PARP can bind to a variety of DNA damage structures including SSBs and DSBs [39–42] and plays a major role in PAR synthesis following DNA damage: approximately 90 % of PAR production is attributable to PARP-1 in this context [43]. DNA-bound PARP undergoes automodification via the addition of long, negatively charged PAR polymers [36]. This autoPARylation promotes dissociation of PARP from the DNA molecule, allowing access of other DNA repair components to the damaged DNA [44–46] and facilitating their recruitment to the damaged sites. The list of substrates of PARP is extensive, and their DDR function can be modified both by PARylation and by direct interaction with PARP.

Although the precise role of PARP in DNA repair is still being elucidated, an important contribution to the repair of SSB lesions is well documented. Rather than being essential for SSB repair, however, PARP appears to increase the efficiency and kinetics of this process [47–49]. Activation of PARP promotes recruitment of the scaffold protein XRCC1 to damages sites [50]; PARP modifies and interacts directly with XRCC1 during this process. Lesions then undergo end processing before being repaired by either short patch or long patch mechanisms. PARP is known to interact with and modulate many SSB repair proteins, including DNA Lig III, DNA Pol Beta and others, whilst playing a clear role in base excision repair (BER) does not appear to be an absolute requirement for the function of this pathway [49]. The radiosensitising effects of PARP inhibition will be discussed below.

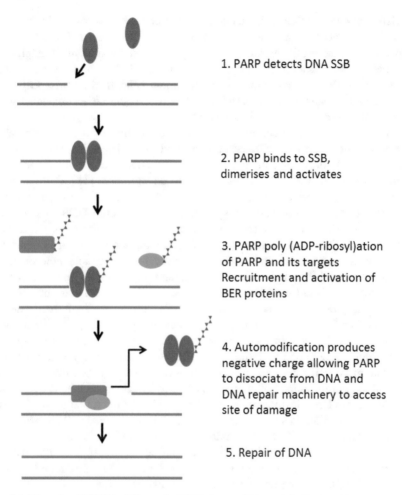

1. PARP detects DNA SSB

2. PARP binds to SSB,
dimerises and activates

3. PARP poly (ADP-ribosyl)ation
of PARP and its targets
Recruitment and activation of
BER proteins

4. Automodification produces
negative charge allowing PARP
to dissociate from DNA and
DNA repair machinery to access
site of damage

5. Repair of DNA

Fig. 1.6 The role of PARP in SSB repair. PARP detects SSBs and facilitates efficient repair via interactions with a variety of base excision repair (BER) factors. Automodification of PARP facilitates its dissociation from the damaged site

DNA Damage Response as a Therapeutic Target

From the discussion above, it can be predicted that targeting of the tumour cell DDR will lead to radiosensitisation via two distinct mechanisms. Inhibition of cellular checkpoint activation will promote transit of malignant cells into mitosis before DNA damage can be completed, thus increasing the probability of cell death, whilst inhibition of DNA repair will increase the incidence and persistence of unrepaired DNA breaks, thus enhancing the lethal effects of irradiation. Some of the key DDR effectors (e.g. ATM) are involved in both of these processes.

Exploitation of DDR as a therapeutic target often raises understandable concerns regarding toxicity to normal tissues. The concept of 'tumour specificity' is vitally important in cancer therapy and particularly so when considering strategies that increase the biological effects of ionising radiation. If DDR inhibition were to sensitise normal tissues to the same degree as tumour cells, then no therapeutic gain would be made, since any increased tumour effect would be accompanied by an unacceptable increase in normal tissue toxicity.

Supporting the prospect of tumour-specific radiosensitisation, important differences between the DDR of tumours and normal tissues have been well documented. At the most fundamental level, the DDR presents a barrier to carcinogenesis during the early stages of tumour development [51]. Cellular populations in the process of carcinogenesis face selective pressures that promote survival of cells bearing mutations associated with altered DDR that increase their ability to tolerate oncogenic proliferative stress. At the population level, dysfunctional DDR can be advantageous, endowing a minority of tumour cells the capacity to generate and tolerate genomic instability and heterogeneity, leading to adaptability and a survival advantage in the hostile tumour microenvironment. Consistent with this, there is evidence to suggest that tumours may be profoundly deficient in some aspects of DDR, rendering them overly dependent on other DDR pathways to carry out necessary DNA repair. Examples of this behaviour are seen in the widespread loss of G1/S checkpoint integrity in solid tumours due to p53 mutation and resulting dependence upon G2/M checkpoint integrity. A further example is seen in the context of 'synthetic lethality' in HR-deficient tumours, which are sensitive to therapies such as PARP inhibitors that create DNA lesions requiring HR for repair. Given that genomic instability is now considered a 'hallmark' of cancer, it is likely that DDR abnormalities are common in cancer cells [52]. Indeed the main reason why radiotherapy is a successful cancer treatment is because tumour cells are less able than the surrounding normal tissues to deal with the DNA damage caused by ionising radiation. The intact DDR of normal tissues ensures that a therapeutic ratio exists between tumour and normal tissue, allowing radiation to eradicate tumour cells whilst normal tissues are able to survive or tolerate the resulting DNA damage. Therefore, pharmacological inhibition of DDR exploits an inherent vulnerability of many cancer cells and represents a valid and promising therapeutic strategy.

Recently, a variety of small molecule inhibitors have become commercially available that possess the ability to specifically and potently inhibit individual DDR proteins. Although many of these are not yet sufficiently advanced to be anything more than laboratory tools, others such as the PARP inhibitor class have been licensed as single agents and are entering phase I and II clinical trials in combination with radiotherapy. A discussion on the current landscape of DDR inhibition in the context of radiation therapy now follows.

PARP Inhibition

PARP inhibitors represent the most developed class of DDR modifiers, largely due to early successful trials as monotherapy in the 'synthetic lethality' setting [53]. There are now several PARP inhibitors entering clinical trials as radiosensitisers including AZD2281 (olaparib), AG014699 (rucaparib) and ABT888 (veliparib). Extensive preclinical investigation into their role as radiosensitising agents has been carried out and is summarised below.

In vitro work has demonstrated that PARP inhibitors (PARPi) provide modest radiosensitisation. Sensitiser enhancement ratios (SER), which are a measure of the fold increase in radiation dose necessary to produce a given level of survival observed in the absence of the sensitising drug, have been reported in the range of 1.1–1.7, depending on the PARP inhibitor and cell line tested.

Brock et al. [54] demonstrated this effect in fibroblast and murine sarcoma cell lines, with SERs (at 10 % survival) of 1.4–1.6 using the PARP inhibitor INO-1001. Interestingly they also showed an enhanced sensitisation effect when INO-1001 was combined with fractionated radiotherapy, suggesting that PARPi was able to block interfraction repair of sublethal damage. This effect was also reported in a study of glioblastoma cell lines [55].

Other authors have confirmed the radiosensitising effects of PARPi in vitro in a variety of different tumour cell lines; these are summarised in Table 1.1 and include head and neck squamous cancer; prostate cancer; glioblastoma; pancreatic, colon and cervix cancer; and lung carcinoma cell lines.

PARP inhibitors have been shown to decrease clonogenic survival and increase apoptosis and mitotic catastrophe in irradiated cells in vitro. The pro-apoptotic effects of PARPi vary between studies and are likely to be cell line dependent. Noel et al. demonstrated lack of radiosensitisation of asynchronously dividing human cell lines treated with PARPi, whilst HeLa cells synchronised in S phase were significantly sensitised to radiation by the addition of PARPi, suggesting that sensitisation was dependent upon DNA replication [61]. This was confirmed by Dungey et al. [55] who showed that radiosensitisation was enhanced by synchronisation in S phase and abrogated by aphidicolin (which creates an early S phase block). PARPi delayed repair of DNA damage and was associated with a replication-dependent increase in DNA DSBs as measured by gamma H2AX and Rad51 foci. Again radiosensitisation was increased with a fractionated schedule, indicating impaired repair of sublethal damage in PARPi-treated cultures. The authors proposed a mechanism whereby PARPi reduced the rate of SSB repair which, in replicating cells, increased the burden of DSBs due to generation of collapsed replication forks during S phase (see Fig. 1.7). They also proposed that the DNA lesions produced by collapsed replication forks in the presence of PARPi might be more complex and hence more difficult to repair. Persistent binding of chemically inhibited PARP to DNA (via steric hindrance) would prevent efficient recruitment of DNA repair proteins to the lesion, providing a potential explanation for this theory [62]. The observation that DNA replication is required in order for PARP inhibition to radiosensitise cells indicates that direct effects on DSB repair are unlikely.

Table 1.1 Summary of in vitro studies of radiosensitising effects of PARP inhibitors

Author	Parp inhibitor and radiation dose	Cell line	Assays	Outcome
Brock et al. [54]	INO-1001 10 µM, IR 0–8 Gy	CHO rodent fibroblast, c37 human fibroblast, SaNH murine sarcoma cell lines	Clonogenic survival and apoptosis	Decreased clonogenic survival in PARPi plus IR, effect enhanced by fractionation No increase in apoptosis
Albert et al. [56]	ABT888 (veliparib) 5 µM, IR 0–6 Gy	H460 lung carcinoma cell lines	Clonogenic survival, apoptosis, endothelial damage assay	Decreased clonogenic survival in PARPi plus IR vs. IR alone Increased apoptosis Inhibition of endothelial tubule formation
Dungey et al. [55]	AZD2881 (olaparib) 1 µM , IR 0–5 Gy	T98G and U87MG glioblastoma cell lines	Clonogenic survival, gamma H2AX foci	Decreased clonogenic survival in PARPi plus IR vs. IR alone, decreased DNA repair, DNA replication-dependent effect of PARPi, fractionation-sensitive effect
Loser et al. [57]	AZD2881 (olaparib) 500 nmol/l plus IR 0–8 Gy	Human and murine primary cells defective in Artemis, ATM, DNA ligase IV	Clonogenic survival, alkaline comet assay, gamma H2AX foci	PARPi radiosensitisation enhanced in ATM, Artemis and DNA ligase IV-deficient cells. Clonogenic survival decreased in rapidly dividing and DNA repair-deficient cells
Calabrese et al. [58]	AG14361 0.4 µM plus IR 8 Gy	LoVo and SW620 human colonic carcinoma cell lines	Clonogenic survival	PARPi plus IR decreased survival by inhibiting recovery from potentially lethal damage
Russo et al. [59]	E7016 3–5 µM plus IR 0–8 Gy	U251 glioblastoma, MiaPaCa pancreatic, DU145 prostatic carcinoma cell lines	Clonogenic survival, gamma H2AX foci, mitotic catastrophe, apoptosis	PARPi plus IR increased clonogenic cell kill and mitotic catastrophe, however no increase in apoptosis
Liu et al. [60]	ABT 888 (veliparib) 2.5 µM plus IR 5 Gy	H1299 lung cancer cells, DU145 and 22RV1 prostate carcinoma cell lines	Clonogenic survival, repair foci assay	PARPi plus IR reduced clonogenic survival, with effect seen in acute hypoxic cells and oxic cells

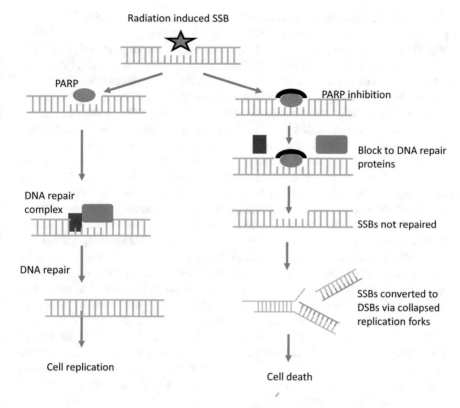

Fig. 1.7 Mechanism of radiosensitisation by PARP-1 inhibition. PARP inhibition does not affect binding of PARP-1 to DNA SSBs but prevents their efficient repair by inhibiting recruitment of key BER effectors and by blocking access of repair elements to damaged sites. This results in delayed SSB repair and increases the likelihood of replication fork collapse by which mechanism SSBs are converted into cytotoxic DSBs during S phase

Loser et al. investigated the radiosensitising effects of PARPi on cells that were deficient in various DDR pathways, an effect which has been termed 'synthetic sickness'. Pre-existing DDR pathway abnormalities were found to enhance the radiosensitising effects of PARPi when compared with effects in DDR competent cell lines. Whilst the underlying mechanism varied according to the specific DDR pathway abnormality, the addition of PARPi appeared to render DDR-deficient cells more vulnerable to radiation-induced DNA lesions that would otherwise have been repaired by alternative pathways [57].

Important work by Liu and colleagues [60] examined the effects of acute hypoxia on radiosensitisation by PARPi. Firstly, the clinical PARPi ABT-888 was shown to inhibit intracellular PARP activity in prostate and non-small cell lung carcinoma cell lines under conditions of hypoxia. Secondly, tumour cells under conditions of acute hypoxia were radiosensitised to the same degree as oxic cells. The authors concluded that ABT-888 remained an effective radiosensitiser under conditions of acute hypoxia, which is an important consideration in translating PARPi into clinical practice because most tumours are hypoxic to some degree [63, 64]. Chronic hypoxia induces downregulation of HR, which may allow targeting of chronically hypoxic cancer cells with a PARPi synthetic lethal strategy. Chan et al. have shown that PARPi-treated tumour xenografts with hypoxic subregions exhibited increased gamma H2AX signalling and reduced survival in an ex vivo clonogenic assay. However, the specific radiosensitising effects of PARPi in the context of chronic hypoxia were not investigated [65]. Nevertheless, the ability of PARPi to selectively target chronically hypoxic cancer cells is of significant clinical interest.

The radiosensitising effects of PARPi have been replicated by several authors in in vivo models. The results of these studies are summarised in Table 1.2. As an example, a recent paper by Tuli et al. demonstrated tumour growth inhibition and prolonged survival in an in vivo orthotopic model of pancreatic carcinoma [69].

Reviewing these data, there is an indication that the radiosensitising effects of PARPi are enhanced in in vivo models, with several studies showing radiosensitising effects that exceed those predicted by in vitro data. This is unlikely to be explained by radiotherapy fractionation effects alone, since several of the studies used large single fraction radiotherapy doses similar to those used in vitro. The enhanced effects observed in vivo may be at least partly explained by effects of PARPi on the tumour vasculature, which may in turn be attributed to the structural similarities of many PARPi to nicotinamide, which is a potent vasodilator. Vasodilatory effects of PARPi on tumour blood vessels might alleviate tumour hypoxia whilst simultaneously increasing drug delivery and enhancing radiosensitisation [58, 70]. As yet, the clinical relevance and therapeutic potential of these effects remain unproven.

The normal tissue toxicity implications of a PARPi radiosensitisation strategy have not been extensively investigated, partly because few animal models yield clinically meaningful radiation toxicity data. However, several mechanistic arguments predict at least a degree of tumour specificity, as described below. Likely toxicities will of course depend upon the tumour site irradiated. As single agents, PARP inhibitors have been shown to have highly favourable toxicity profiles [53], so toxicities outwith the irradiated field would be unexpected, unless concomitant chemotherapy was also incorporated into the treatment regimen.

Since PARP inhibition requires DNA replication to produce a radiosensitising effect, rapidly dividing tissues are likely to be radiosensitised by PARP inhibition. Hence, squamous cell carcinomas, glioblastoma and other highly mitotically active tumours may be most sensitised by PARPi. This also has implications for normal tissue toxicity, however, since tissues with high cellular turnover such as the skin, bone marrow and mucosal surfaces of the oesophagus, oropharynx and bowel might also be radiosensitised by PARPi, although only if these tissues were irradiated of course. Tissues such as the brain, spinal cord, heart and muscle, which are comprised mainly of infrequently dividing cells, are predicted not to be radiosensitised by PARPi, although it should be remembered that these tissues are heterogeneous and contain additional cell types such as vascular endothelial cells, which may have higher mitotic indices.

Table 1.2 Summary of in vivo studies of radiosensitising effects of PARP inhibitors

Author	PARP inhibitor and radiation dose	Cell line	Assay	Outcome
Khan et al. [66]	GPI-15427 10, 30, 100, 300 mg/kg po, IR 2 Gy for 2 days	JHU012 and JHU012 head and neck cancer xenografts	Tumour growth delay apoptosis	PARPi plus IR inhibited tumour regrowth vs. IR Increased apoptosis
Clarke et al. [67]	ABT 888 7.5 mg/kg po bd, Temozolomide 33 mg/kg/day, IR 20 Gy over 11 days	Glioblastoma intracranial xenografts (MGMT hypermethylated)	Animal survival, body weight	PARPi-TMZ-IR prolonged survival vs. IR alone, minimal weight loss
Donawho et al. [68]	ABT 888 25 mg/kg/day via osmotic pumps, IR 20 Gy over 10 days	HCT116 xenograft human colorectal carcinoma	Animal survival	PARPi plus IR increased mean survival time vs. IR alone
Albert et al. [56]	ABT 888 25 mg/kg ip for 5 days, IR 10 Gy over 5 days	H460 xenograft, human lung carcinoma	Tumour growth delay, Ki67 staining, apoptosis, blood vessel density	PARPi plus IR delayed tumour regrowth vs. IR alone Decreased tumour vasculature Decreased proliferation Increased apoptosis
Calabrese et al. [58]	AG143615 or 15 mg/kg/day ip, IR 10 Gy over 5 days	SW620 human colon carcinoma	Tumour growth delay	PARPi plus IR delayed tumour regrowth vs. IR alone
Russo et al. [59]	E7016 30 mg/kg po, IR 4 Gy single fraction	U251 glioblastoma xenograft	Tumour growth delay	PARPi-TMZ-IR delayed tumour regrowth vs. IR alone
Tuli et al. [69]	ABT 888 25 mg/kg, IR 5 Gy single fraction	Pancreatic carcinoma	Tumour growth delay and survival	PARPi plus IR delayed tumour regrowth and prolonged survival

Since vascular endothelial cells are present in every organ and tumour treated, they are worthy of specific consideration. The cell doubling time of endothelial cells in culture has been estimated from labelling studies to be in the region of 93 to 2300 days, which would classify the endothelium as an intermediate to late-responding tissue [71]. However, there is evidence to suggest that irradiation provides a proliferative stimulus that decreases cell doubling time and hence might increase the radiosensitising effects of PARPi on endothelial cell radiosensitivity [72]. To date, there is no direct evidence to support or refute such an effect either in animals or in patients.

It is also unknown whether the progenitor stem cells of slowly dividing tissues might be sensitised by PARPi strategies; this issue clearly has implications for late normal tissue toxicities. Intermediate tissues such as type I and II pneumocytes and the bladder epithelium would be expected to experience less radiosensitisation with PARPi than malignant tumours.

Considering potential mechanisms of tumour specificity, PARPi have been observed to accumulate in malignant tissue, an effect that might be related to increased levels of DNA damage (which would therefore bind more PARP) in malignant tissue. In theory, this phenomenon would increase the tumour-sensitising effects of PARPi [58] whilst limiting normal tissue toxicity [73] and might also have implications for scheduling of PARPi, particularly if cytotoxic chemotherapy agents form part of the therapeutic schedule and there is a risk of increased haematological toxicity in combinations with continuous PARPi dosing.

Taking the tumour selectivity argument a step further, there are theoretical grounds on which to predict that PARP inhibition could protect certain late-responding normal tissues from the adverse effects of radiation. In a variety of normal tissue models, damage-induced activation of PARP has been shown to deplete cells of NAD+, preventing them from activating energy-dependent apoptotic pathways and thereby promoting necrotic cell death and a consequent inflammatory cascade that exacerbates and disseminates tissue damage. If PARP activity is inhibited prior to the toxic insult, NAD+ levels are preserved, and cells are more likely to die via apoptosis, thus reducing overall levels of tissue damage. A broad and expanding literature describes the protective application of PARPi in animal models of myocardial reperfusion injury and acute lung injury that lend some support to this theory [74, 75]. Furthermore, it has been reported that PARP inhibition is protective in mouse models of irinotecan-induced gastrointestinal toxicity [76].

ATM Inhibition

The development of radiosensitisation strategies based on ATM inhibition is at a much earlier stage of development. Much of the in vitro work in this area has explored the use of ATM inhibition as a laboratory tool rather than preclinical investigation as a therapeutic radiosensitiser.

In recent studies, Golding et al. [77] evaluated ATM inhibition as a radiosensitiser for GBM. They demonstrated highly potent radiosensitisation of commercially available GBM cell lines using the ATM inhibitor KU-60019 and concluded that ATM inhibition had clinical potential as a highly effective radiosensitiser and inhibitor of DDR in this disease. In a subsequent paper, the team explored the combination of ATM inhibition with radiation and temozolomide on commercially available GBM cell lines [78]. SER_{37} values for radiation were calculated to be 1.8–2.1 depending on the dose of KU-60019 used, whilst the addition of temozolomide did not enhance the radiosensitising effects of ATM inhibition (nor did temozolomide radiosensitise in the absence of ATM inhibitor). In coculture models of glioma cells and human astrocytes, the combination of temozolomide and ATM inhibition reduced glioma cell growth by around 70%, but astrocytes did not exhibit in vitro radiosensitisation after exposure to KU-60019. Biddlestone-Thorpe et al. explored similar combinations in an orthotopic in vivo GBM model [79]. In vivo administration of KU-60019 required the use of intracranial osmotic pumps and convection-enhanced delivery, since the drug did not reach therapeutic concentrations in plasma following oral or intraperitoneal administration. In this context, KU-60019 delayed tumour growth and significantly prolonged survival when added to radiation treatment. The investigators also reported that p53 status had an important effect on the radiosensitising effects of ATM inhibition. U87 cells, which express wild-type p53, were infected with a mouse retrovirus expressing the p53-281G allele, generating p53-mutant U87 cells that were shown to be more susceptible to the radiosensitising effects of ATM inhibition in vitro than the parental cell populations. Similarly, mice bearing U87-281G xenografts experienced prolonged overall survival when treated with the combination of ATM inhibition and radiation in comparison to mice bearing U87 parental xenografts. Whilst the authors concluded that ATM inhibition may be of potential benefit in combination with radiotherapy for p53-mutant GBM, it should be recognised that aberrations in the p53 signalling pathway are observed in about 90% of GBM even though p53 mutations are seen in only 30–40% of cases [80].

These three papers represent the most in-depth preclinical studies of ATM inhibition to date. Other studies have demonstrated the potentiating effects of ATM inhibition on cisplatin-mediated radiosensitisation of non-small cell lung cancer cells and radiosensitisation of head and neck squamous carcinoma cell lines by ATM downregulation via RNA interference [81, 82]. Rainey et al. demonstrated that transient ATM inhibition for a period of 4 h was able to potently radiosensitise HeLa cells in vitro [83], whilst Choi et al. demonstrated distinct effects of ATM inhibition versus ATM loss, manifested by reduced sister chromatid exchange (a marker of homologous recombination) in ATM inhibited irradiated cells which was not apparent in irradiated ATM null cells [84].

Current dogma might suggest that inhibition of ATM in combination with radiotherapy would lead to overwhelming normal tissue toxicity, since ATM is one of the central DDR kinases. However, there is evidence to suggest that radiosensitivity following ATM inhibition may be tissue specific. A study by Schneider et al. demonstrated that astrocytes downregulate ATM expression but retain DNA repair competency via NHEJ [85]. In support of this, Gosink et al. demonstrated that astrocyte radiosensitivity was unaffected by ATM deficiency [86]. A further recent study by Moding et al. using a murine sarcoma model demonstrated that deletion of the ATM gene had much less of a radiosensitising effect on normal cardiac endothelia than on rapidly proliferating tumour endothelial cells [87]. These data suggest that ATM inhibition as a radiosensitising strategy may be clinically achievable; however, further study of the normal tissue effects of ATM inhibition is clearly required.

The low bioavailability of compounds used to inhibit ATM to date has been a barrier to both preclinical in vivo studies and clinical trials in combination with radiation. Recently however, a highly potent inhibitor of ATM that exhibits blood-brain barrier penetration has been described by Valerie et al. AZ32 in combination with a fractionated radiotherapy schedule significantly increased median survival in an orthotopic human glioma murine model [88].

ATR Inhibition

The effects of ATR inhibition on radiosensitivity have been the subject of several preclinical studies. Wang et al. investigated the effects of kinase-dead ATR expression on cellular radiosensitivity and demonstrated that loss of ATR kinase function radiosensitised cells through deficient S and G2 cell checkpoints and reduced HR [89]. Gilad et al. demonstrated a requirement for malignant cells to engage the ATR-Chk1 pathway in order to maintain genome stability following oncogenic expression of Ras, implying indirectly that suppression of ATR signalling may sensitise cancer cells to DNA-damaging agents such as radiation [90].

Until a recent study by Reaper et al. of the compound VE821, specific and potent inhibitors of ATR had not been available. VE-821 was shown to potentiate the lethal effects of cisplatin and ionising radiation, effects that were enhanced in cells with a deficiency in the ATM-p53 axis. The authors speculated that ATR inhibition generated DSBs via collapse of replication forks which would normally induce an ATM-dependent S phase checkpoint response. Cells deficient in ATM or p53 were unable to activate this response and exhibited increased sensitivity to ATR inhibition [91].

Prevo et al. investigated the radiosensitising effects of ATR inhibition in pancreatic carcinoma models using VE821, which was shown to ablate induction of Chk1 phosphorylation by radiation or gemcitabine. It also increased the sensitivity of established and primary pancreatic cancer cells to the combination of radiation and gemcitabine under both normoxic and hypoxic conditions and effectively inhibited radiation-induced G2/M arrest. ATR inhibition also appeared to increase DNA DSBs following treatment with radiation as assessed by persistent gamma H2AX and 53BP1 foci. In contrast, Rad51 foci formation was reduced 24 h after treatment with IR and VE821, suggesting inhibition of HR [92].

Fokas et al. subsequently used a more potent analogue, VE822, to study the effects of ATR inhibition on pancreatic cancer cell radiosensitivity in vivo. VE822 was found to inhibit Chk1 phosphorylation and sensitise pancreatic cancer cells to radiation, both alone and in combination with gemcitabine. In contrast, it had no effect on tube formation by human dermal microvascular endothelial cells after radiotherapy and did not affect clonogenic survival of fibroblasts, indicating favourable tumour specificity. As before, radiation-induced DSB repair foci (gamma H2AX and 53BP1) were increased by the combination of ATR and radiotherapy, whilst Rad51 foci were decreased, strengthening the concept that ATR inhibition is associated with an HR defect. In vivo, the combination of IR and ATR inhibition produced a significant increase in tumour growth delay in subcutaneous pancreatic tumour xenografts. This study also attempted to quantify the toxic effects of the IR plus ATR inhibitor combination on critical normal tissues by assessing apoptosis of jejunal cells and villus tip loss in mice treated with the combination. Neither of these parameters when compared with controls indicated additional toxicity with the addition of ATR inhibition [93].

In further studies on radiotherapy-resistant hypoxic tumour cells, Pires et al. demonstrated that inhibition of ATR with VE821 sensitised a wide variety of commercially available cancer cell lines to radiation with no evidence of a relationship with p53 mutation in these experiments. Severe hypoxia is known to cause replicative stress and consequent activation of ATM and ATR signalling; in this study, VE821 was demonstrated to abrogate hypoxia-mediated ATR signalling and to increase radiation-induced cell killing in physiologically relevant hypoxic conditions [94].

Finally, Sankunny et al. demonstrated that siRNA knockdown of ATR could radiosensitise oral squamous cell carcinoma with distal chromosome arm 11q loss (a marker of relative radioresistance and poor prognosis) [95], whilst Vavrova et al. have also demonstrated radiosensitisation of p53-deficient promyelocytic leukaemia cells by ATR inhibition [96].

Chk1 Inhibition

The radiosensitising effects of Chk1 have been investigated by several authors in various tumour models. Since Chk1 has important effects on G2/M checkpoint control and in the promotion of Rad51-mediated DNA DSB homologous recombination repair, Chk1 inhibitors are predicted to have potent radiosensitising effects. Many studies have addressed this question in p53-mutant models since these cells are expected to display increased dependency on G2/M checkpoint arrest. Koniaras et al. demonstrated that the G2/M checkpoint was independent of p53 and then showed that expression of a dominant negative Chk1 construct resulted in increased radiosensitivity [97]. Sorensen et al. further defined the role of Chk1 as an essential kinase for the maintenance of genomic integrity [98]. They demonstrated Chk1 inhibition with two different compounds (UCN01 and CEP3891) and noted an increase in phosphorylation of ATR targets, increased initiation of DNA replication and generation of DNA DSBs. Chen et al. investigated the role of Chk1 inhibition as a potential sensitiser to DNA-damaging agents [99] by comparing radiation responses of p53-mutated cancer cell lines following Chk1 inhibition to those of p53 wild-type cell lines and normal human fibroblasts. Chk1 inhibition was found to potentiate the effects of radiation in p53-mutant cells only.

Radiosensitising effects of additional Chk1 inhibitor compounds have subsequently been published in preclinical models of breast cancer and pancreatic cancer [100, 101].

Inhibition of NHEJ

Inhibition of NHEJ can be achieved using inhibitors of DNAPK, the apical kinase that plays a central role in this pathway. Since NHEJ is the predominant mechanism of DSB repair in normal mammalian cells, its inhibition might be predicted to cause non-specific radiosensitisation and severe normal tissue toxicity, an argument often used to suggest that NHEJ is not a promising therapeutic target. Nevertheless, it should be remembered firstly that malignant cells do not possess normal DDR and secondly that back up repair pathways such as MMEJ exist in normal cells. Inhibition of NHEJ thus remains an area of active interest as a radiosensitisation strategy.

DNAPK-deficient cell lines have been shown to be highly radiosensitive [102], but whilst several inhibitors of DNAPK are available, none as yet have been used in preclinical in vivo studies in combination with radiation. In cellular models, Veuger et al. demonstrated effective radiosensitisation in vitro using NU7026, which was shown to be a potent and specific DNAPK inhibitor in this study [102].

Rad51 Inhibition

Rad51 is a key element of the HR DSB repair pathway, and inhibition of this protein would be predicted to have significant effects on the repair of DSBs following irradiation. Investigating this hypothesis, Short et al. found that levels of Rad51 in human glioma cell lines were inversely related to their radiosensitivity and that knockdown of Rad51 led to increased sensitivity to both radiation and temozolomide (an alkylating cytotoxic agent). They and others have proposed that Rad51 inhibition represents a promising radiosensitisation strategy [103] but development of pharmacological inhibitors of Rad51 has lagged behind work on other DNA repair targets. Huang et al. recently described the development of a small molecule inhibitor of Rad51 which increased the chemosensitivity of in vitro cancer cells; however, the effects on radiosensitivity were not explored [104].

Combination DDR Inhibition

The ability to inhibit different targets within the DDR allows the prospect of inhibiting combinations of DDR proteins in order to manipulate radiation sensitivity. To date, only a few studies have adopted this approach. Vance et al. investigated radiosensitisation of pancreatic cancer cells exposed to combinations of Chk1 and PARP inhibitors [105]. This study demonstrated radiosensitisation of both p53 wild type and p53 mutants in isogenic cell lines by the combination treatment; however, radiosensitisation was greater in the p53-mutated cell lines. Single-agent sensitiser enhancement ratios for PARP and Chk1 were modest (1.5); however, the combination of agents produced sensitiser enhancement ratios of greater than 2. The combination of Chk1 and PARP inhibition caused G2/M dysfunction, inhibition of HR and persistent DDR in tumour cells but did not appear to radiosensitise normal intestinal epithelial cells in vitro. The authors speculated that the HR deficiency induced by Chk1 inhibition may sensitise to PARP inhibition via generation of a 'BRCAness' phenotype.

Hoglund et al. demonstrated that the combination of PARP inhibition and Chk2 functional loss elicits a synthetic lethal response in Myc-overexpressing lymphoma cells [106], whilst Booth et al. observed that combining PARP inhibition and Chk1 inhibition produced cytotoxic effects in mammary cells even in the absence of any exogenous DNA-damaging agent [107]. Furthermore, the actions of PARP and Chk1 inhibition were enhanced by ATM knockdown. Similarly Peasland et al. documented a synthetic lethal effect of combining the ATR inhibitor NU-6027 and PARP inhibition [108]. None of these studies evaluated the impact of adding ionising radiation.

Clearly the combination of different DDR inhibitors has the potential to enhance the effects of radiation, and given the redundancy encountered within DDR pathways, this may represent a particularly effective way of inducing potent radiosensitisation of resistant cancers. Nevertheless, the effects of combination DDR inhibition on normal tissue toxicity will require careful consideration.

DDR Kinase Inhibition and Cancer Stem Cell Theory

Cancer stem cell theory has gained prominence in a variety of solid tumour sites in the last decade. This theory states that only a subpopulation of tumour cells (cancer stem cells) possesses the ability to initiate tumour growth and that this subpopulation exhibits some of the features of normal tissue stem cells. Cancer stem cells have been shown by several authors to be resistant to conventional cancer treatments and in particular to be radiation resistant [109, 110]. These observations implicate the cancer stem cell population in tumour recurrence following treatment; hence, efforts to develop therapies that specifically target the cancer stem cell populations of solid tumours are urgently required.

Bao et al. demonstrated the radioresistance of glioblastoma cancer stem cells (GBM CSCs) and subsequently showed GBM CSCs to exhibit upregulated DNA damage responses [110]. Subsequent studies have demonstrated that GBM CSCs exhibit enhanced activation of the G2/M checkpoint and more efficient DNA DSB repair in G2 phase of the cell cycle following irradiation [109] compared to other GBM cell populations which did not exhibit the CSC phenotype. ATM inhibition was shown to be a potent radiosensitiser of GBM CSCs and was effective in abrogating both enhanced G2/M checkpoint activation and G2 DNA DSB repair advantage following radiation in the GBM CSC population. Ahmed et al. recently demonstrated that selective inhibition of parallel DNA damage response pathways optimised radiosensitisation of GBM CSCs. Individually, inhibition of ATR, PARP, Chk1 and ATM all radiosensitised GBM CSCs; however, only ATM inhibition or dual inhibition of ATR and PARP delivered increases in GBM CSC radiosensitivity that were significantly greater than those observed in tumour bulk (non-CSC) populations. These data demonstrate that multiple, parallel pathways contribute to GBM CSC radioresistance and that combined inhibition of cell cycle checkpoint and DNA repair targets provides the most effective means of overcoming radioresistance of GBM CSCs [111]. They also support the concept that upregulated DDR is integral to the radioresistance seen in GBM CSCs and that DDR inhibition is a promising radiosensitising strategy for this problematic cellular subpopulation.

Combining Radiotherapy and DDR Kinase Inhibition in the Clinic

Combining DDR kinase inhibition with radiotherapy in the clinic poses several challenges. Many DDR kinase inhibitors used for in vitro studies are potent and specific inhibitors of their targets but lack the bioavailability, tumour penetration or blood-brain barrier penetration necessary for them to be clinically useful compounds. In recent years, a number of clinically useful DDR kinase inhibitors have been developed, and these agents are starting to be combined with radiotherapy in early-phase clinical trials.

As discussed above, there is compelling evidence to suggest that a DDR inhibitor radiosensitiser strategy has the potential to provide tumour-specific radiosensitisation but that concomitant administration of cytotoxic systemic agents can complicate delivery of this strategy by increasing the risk of systemic toxicities. Many curative radiotherapy regimens now incorporate systemic chemotherapy agents, which have been demonstrated to provide small benefits in terms of tumour control, but which increase toxicity towards the ceiling of tolerance. DDR inhibition has been demonstrated to increase the haematological toxicity of chemotherapy drugs: early combination trials of PARP inhibitors with systemic cytotoxic agents reported severe haematological toxicity that limited the usefulness of the combination approach. However, improved scheduling of these agents with systemic treatments may provide a solution to this problem. Another solution would be to pioneer early-phase clinical trials in palliative (non-curative) radiotherapy treatments which do not include concurrent chemotherapy.

Clinical Trials of DDR Kinase Inhibition

Clinical trials of several DDR kinase inhibitor agents combined with radiation are either in progress or in advanced stages of development. Most are investigating the combination of PARP inhibitors with radiation, since these compounds are the most advanced in their clinical development. There are now several phase I clinical trials of PARP inhibitors in combination with radiotherapy in various tumour sites including breast cancer, non-small cell lung cancer, oesophageal cancer, brain metastases and glioblastoma. Many of the studies have adopted palliative (non-curative) radiotherapy regimens for locally advanced cancer in order that toxicity of combined PARP inhibitor and radiation therapy can be fully explored without compromising chances of cure. An example of one of these trials is the 'PARADIGM' study which is currently recruiting patients in the United Kingdom. This study will investigate the combination of olaparib with hypofractionated radiotherapy (40 Gy in 15 fractions) in glioblastoma patients who are unsuitable for concurrent chemoradiation. An initial phase I trial will identify a maximum tolerated dose of olaparib with radiotherapy before progressing to a randomised phase II trial which will investigate whether olaparib in combination with radiotherapy increases survival in this population, with a view to justifying a subsequent phase III trial.

The results of a phase I trial of the PARP inhibitor ABT888 (veliparib) in combination with palliative whole brain radiotherapy for brain metastases have been published recently [112]. This trial showed that the combination of whole brain radiotherapy and PARP inhibition was well tolerated; indeed a maximum tolerated dose of veliparib was not reached because predefined dose-limiting toxicities were not observed at any dose level. The toxicity of the combined regimen at the recommended phase 2 dose of veliparib was felt to be similar to that of whole brain radiation alone. Comparison to historical controls suggested an improvement in survival in patients receiving veliparib and radiotherapy; however, this was a phase 1 trial in a highly selected patient population, preventing any robust conclusions regarding efficacy. Nevertheless, the study provides promising evidence that PARP inhibition can be delivered in combination with whole brain radiotherapy with relatively modest toxicity.

The 'PATRIOT' study is the only 'non-PARP' DDR inhibitor/radiotherapy combination study currently under way. This phase I study is evaluating the ATR inhibitor AZD6738 both as monotherapy and in combination with radiation in solid tumours exhibiting abnormalities in the p53 pathway. The trial design incorporates three stages that enable investigation of optimal dose, optimal scheduling and overall safety of the combination of AZD6738 with palliative radiotherapy (20 or 30Gy). Recruitment to this trial has commenced, and results are eagerly awaited. Other inhibitors of the DDR are yet to be combined with radiation in a clinical setting, and to the authors' knowledge, no clinical trials of inhibitors of ATM or Chk1 in combination with radiotherapy are yet underway.

Biomarkers

Clinical application of DDR inhibitor radiosensitisation strategies will require the development of companion biomarkers that allow rational patient selection whilst ensuring optimal tumour radiosensitisation and minimal normal tissue toxicity. Next-generation sequencing technologies have enabled comprehensive sequencing of tumour genomes, facilitating detailed analysis of mutations, copy number variants and deletions in individual tumours. This information has the potential to enable selection of patients that will benefit from DDR inhibition and to identify the DDR inhibitor that will deliver optimal radiosensitisation. For example, a tumour deficient in the HR pathway may benefit from PARP inhibition, or cancers with high levels of replication stress may be optimally radiosensitised by ATR inhibition. Tumours lacking p53-mediated G1/S checkpoint may usefully be radiosensitised by Chk1 or ATM inhibition. In this way, radiosensitiser strategies could in the future be tailored to a patient's tumour allowing manipulation of the therapeutic ratio of radiation treatment to its maximum extent. Whilst the building blocks of this personalisation strategy are in place in the form of extensive, detailed understanding of the DDR pathways involved, clinically meaningful and deliverable molecular biomarkers have yet to be identified and will need to be validated in randomised clinical trials before they can be adopted in routine clinical practice.

Conclusion

Tumour radioresistance has been a fundamental problem facing radiation oncologists since ionising radiation was first used to treat cancer over one hundred years ago. Despite the knowledge that radiotherapy is essentially a DNA-damaging agent and that repair of radiation-induced DNA damage is a major determinant of tumour radioresistance, manipulation of the radiobiological response of tumours has not been a feasible prospect until the last few years. Recent advances in molecular biology have described the vast interconnected pathways responsible for maintaining the integrity of mammalian DNA, and it is clear that during the process of carcinogenesis fundamental alterations to the normal DNA damage response are necessary in order to generate the hallmark feature of genomic instability in cancer cells. Given the presence of altered DDR in many tumour cells, the targeting of specific DDR pathways by small molecule inhibitors provides the exciting prospect of tumour-specific radiosensitisation.

Recent research has centred upon inhibition of central DDR kinases such as ATM, ATR, DNAPKcs and Chk1. These agents deliver potent radiosensitisation in vitro, and there is some evidence to indicate tumour specificity in their actions. The effects of PARP inhibition on tumour radiation response have also been investigated by a number of authors, and this approach has been shown to be a promising way of radiosensitising normoxic and hypoxic tumour cells both in vitro and in vivo, in a potentially tumour-specific manner. Clinical development of DDR inhibitors is progressing, with PARP inhibitors entering phase I and II trials in combination with radiotherapy in a variety of tumour sites. Entry of other DDR inhibition strategies into clinical trials has been somewhat slower; however, ATR inhibitors are soon to enter phase I trials in combination with radiation.

The manipulation of DDR in radioresistant tumours will greatly enhance the biological effects of radiotherapy, allowing the treatment of cancers which have in the past proven difficult or impossible to cure using radiation. One of the challenges of developing DDR radiosensitiser strategies will be to identify which elements of DDR in a particular tumour can be safely targeted by inhibitors to produce tumour-specific radiosensitisation. Only a fuller understanding of the DDR mechanisms that determine radioresistance in tumours will achieve this aim, coupled with the development of clinically useful biomarkers. DDR inhibition has significant potential to enhance the beneficial biological effects of radiation on tumours and to open a new frontier in the treatment of malignant disease.

References

1. Shiloh Y, Ziv Y (2013) The ATM protein kinase: regulating the cellular response to genotoxic stress, and more. Nat Rev Mol Cell Biol 14(4):197–210
2. Taylor AM, Harnden DG, Arlett CF, Harcourt SA, Lehmann AR, Stevens S et al (1975) Ataxia telangiectasia: a human mutation with abnormal radiation sensitivity. Nature 258(5534):427–429
3. Bakkenist CJ, Kastan MB (2003) DNA damage activates ATM through intermolecular auto-phosphorylation and dimer dissociation. Nature 421(6922):499–506
4. You Z, Bailis JM, Johnson SA, Dilworth SM, Hunter T (2007) Rapid activation of ATM on DNA flanking double-strand breaks. Nat Cell Biol 9(11):1311–1318
5. Goodarzi AA, Noon AT, Deckbar D, Ziv Y, Shiloh Y, Lobrich M et al (2008) ATM signaling facilitates repair of DNA double-strand breaks associated with heterochromatin. Mol Cell 31(2):167–177
6. Riballo E, Kuhne M, Rief N, Doherty A, Smith GC, Recio MJ et al (2004) A pathway of double-strand break rejoining dependent upon ATM, Artemis, and proteins locating to gamma-H2AX foci. Mol Cell 16(5):715–724
7. Alvarez-Quilon A, Serrano-Benitez A, Lieberman JA, Quintero C, Sanchez-Gutierrez D, Escudero LM et al (2014) ATM specifically mediates repair of double-strand breaks with blocked DNA ends. Nat Commun 5:3347
8. Halazonetis TD, Gorgoulis VG, Bartek J (2008) An oncogene-induced DNA damage model for cancer development. Science 319(5868):1352–1355
9. Marechal A, Zou L. DNA damage sensing by the ATM and ATR kinases. Cold Spring Harb perspect Biol 2013;5(9). doi:10.1101/cshperspect.a012716
10. Brown EJ, Baltimore D (2000) ATR disruption leads to chromosomal fragmentation and early embryonic lethality. Genes Dev 14(4):397–402
11. Zeman MK, Cimprich KA (2014) Causes and consequences of replication stress. Nat Cell Biol 16(1):2–9
12. Liu H, Takeda S, Kumar R, Westergard TD, Brown EJ, Pandita TK et al (2010) Phosphorylation of MLL by ATR is required for execution of mammalian S-phase checkpoint. Nature 467(7313):343–346
13. Stiff T, O'Driscoll M, Rief N, Iwabuchi K, Lobrich M, Jeggo PA (2004) ATM and DNA-PK function redundantly to phosphorylate H2AX after exposure to ionizing radiation. Cancer Res 64(7):2390–2396
14. Lukas J, Lukas C, Bartek J (2004) Mammalian cell cycle checkpoints: signalling pathways and their organization in space and time. DNA Repair 3(8-9):997–1007
15. Deckbar D, Stiff T, Koch B, Reis C, Lobrich M, Jeggo PA (2010) The limitations of the G1-S checkpoint. Cancer Res 70(11):4412–4421
16. Mailand N, Falck J, Lukas C, Syljuasen RG, Welcker M, Bartek J et al (2000) Rapid destruction of human Cdc25A in response to DNA damage. Science 288(5470):1425–1429
17. Deckbar D, Birraux J, Krempler A, Tchouandong L, Beucher A, Walker S et al (2007) Chromosome breakage after G2 checkpoint release. J Cell Biol 176(6):749–755
18. Deckbar D, Jeggo PA, Lobrich M (2011) Understanding the limitations of radiation-induced cell cycle checkpoints. Crit Rev Biochem Mol Biol 46(4):271–283
19. Goodarzi AA, Jeggo PA (2012) Irradiation induced foci (IRIF) as a biomarker for radiosensitivity. Mutat Res 736(1–2):39–47
20. Frankenberg D, Frankenberg-Schwager M, Blocher D, Harbich R (1981) Evidence for DNA double-strand breaks as the critical lesions in yeast cells irradiated with sparsely or densely ionizing radiation under oxic or anoxic conditions. Radiat Res 88(3):524–532
21. Shibata A, Jeggo PA (2014) DNA double-strand break repair in a cellular context. Clin Oncol 26(5):243–249
22. Weterings E, Chen DJ (2008) The endless tale of non-homologous end-joining. Cell Res 18(1):114–124

23. Beucher A, Birraux J, Tchouandong L, Barton O, Shibata A, Conrad S et al (2009) ATM and Artemis promote homologous recombination of radiation-induced DNA double-strand breaks in G2. EMBO J 28(21):3413–3427

24. Shibata A, Conrad S, Birraux J, Geuting V, Barton O, Ismail A et al (2011) Factors determining DNA double-strand break repair pathway choice in G2 phase. EMBO J 30(6):1079–1092

25. Roth DB, Wilson JH (1986) Nonhomologous recombination in mammalian cells: role for short sequence homologies in the joining reaction. Mol Cell Biol 6(12):4295–4304

26. Wang H, Perrault AR, Takeda Y, Qin W, Wang H, Iliakis G (2003) Biochemical evidence for Ku-independent backup pathways of NHEJ. Nucleic Acids Res 31(18):5377–5388

27. McVey M, Lee SE (2008) MMEJ repair of double-strand breaks (director's cut): deleted sequences and alternative endings. Trends Genet 24(11):529–538

28. Bentley J, Diggle CP, Harnden P, Knowles MA, Kiltie AE (2004) DNA double strand break repair in human bladder cancer is error prone and involves microhomology-associated end-joining. Nucleic Acids Res 32(17):5249–5259

29. Jeggo PA, Geuting V, Lobrich M (2011) The role of homologous recombination in radiation-induced double-strand break repair. Radiother Oncol 101(1):7–12, Epub 2011/07/09

30. Helleday T, Lo J, van Gent DC, Engelward BP (2007) DNA double-strand break repair: from mechanistic understanding to cancer treatment. DNA Repair 6(7):923–935

31. San Filippo J, Sung P, Klein H (2008) Mechanism of eukaryotic homologous recombination. Annu Rev Biochem 77:229–257

32. Li X, Heyer WD (2008) Homologous recombination in DNA repair and DNA damage tolerance. Cell Res 18(1):99–113

33. Krejci L, Altmannova V, Spirek M, Zhao X (2012) Homologous recombination and its regulation. Nucleic Acids Res 40(13):5795–5818

34. Wold MS (1997) Replication protein A: a heterotrimeric, single-stranded DNA-binding protein required for eukaryotic DNA metabolism. Annu Rev Biochem 66:61–92

35. Eggler AL, Inman RB, Cox MM (2002) The Rad51-dependent pairing of long DNA substrates is stabilized by replication protein A. J Biol Chem 277(42):39280–39288

36. D'Amours D, Desnoyers S, D'Silva I, Poirier GG (1999) Poly(ADP-ribosyl)ation reactions in the regulation of nuclear functions. Biochem J 342(Pt 2):249–268

37. Burkle A, Virag L (2013) Poly(ADP-ribose): PARadigms and PARadoxes. Mol Aspects Med 34:1046–1065

38. Krishnakumar R, Kraus WL (2010) The PARP side of the nucleus: molecular actions, physiological outcomes, and clinical targets. Mol Cell 39(1):8–24

39. Khodyreva SN, Prasad R, Ilina ES, Sukhanova MV, Kutuzov MM, Liu Y et al (2010) Apurinic/apyrimidinic (AP) site recognition by the 5'-dRP/AP lyase in poly(ADP-ribose) polymerase-1 (PARP-1). Proc Natl Acad Sci U S A 107(51):22090–22095

40. Chasovskikh S, Dimtchev A, Smulson M, Dritschilo A (2005) DNA transitions induced by binding of PARP-1 to cruciform structures in supercoiled plasmids. Cytometry A 68(1):21–27

41. Lonskaya I, Potaman VN, Shlyakhtenko LS, Oussatcheva EA, Lyubchenko YL, Soldatenkov VA (2005) Regulation of poly(ADP-ribose) polymerase-1 by DNA structure-specific binding. J Biol Chem 280(17):17076–17083

42. Potaman VN, Shlyakhtenko LS, Oussatcheva EA, Lyubchenko YL, Soldatenkov VA (2005) Specific binding of poly(ADP-ribose) polymerase-1 to cruciform hairpins. J Mol Biol 348(3):609–615

43. Langelier MF, Ruhl DD, Planck JL, Kraus WL, Pascal JM (2010) The Zn3 domain of human poly(ADP-ribose) polymerase-1 (PARP-1) functions in both DNA-dependent poly(ADP-ribose) synthesis activity and chromatin compaction. J Biol Chem 285(24):18877–18887

44. Zahradka P, Ebisuzaki K (1982) A shuttle mechanism for DNA-protein interactions. The regulation of poly(ADP-ribose) polymerase. Eur J Biochem 127(3):579–585

45. Ferro AM, Olivera BM (1982) Poly(ADP-ribosylation) in vitro. Reaction parameters and enzyme mechanism. J Biol Chem 257(13):7808–7813

46. Lindahl T, Satoh MS, Poirier GG, Klungland A (1995) Post-translational modification of poly(ADP-ribose) polymerase induced by DNA strand breaks. Trends Biochem Sci 20 (10):405–411

47. Fisher AE, Hochegger H, Takeda S, Caldecott KW (2007) Poly(ADP-ribose) polymerase 1 accelerates single-strand break repair in concert with poly(ADP-ribose) glycohydrolase. Mol Cell Biol 27(15):5597–5605

48. Satoh MS, Lindahl T (1992) Role of poly(ADP-ribose) formation in DNA repair. Nature 356(6367):356–358

49. Strom CE, Johansson F, Uhlen M, Szigyarto CA, Erixon K, Helleday T (2011) Poly (ADP-ribose) polymerase (PARP) is not involved in base excision repair but PARP inhibition traps a single-strand intermediate. Nucleic Acids Res 39(8):3166–3175

50. El-Khamisy SF, Masutani M, Suzuki H, Caldecott KW (2003) A requirement for PARP-1 for the assembly or stability of XRCC1 nuclear foci at sites of oxidative DNA damage. Nucleic Acids Res 31(19):5526–5533

51. Bartkova J, Horejsi Z, Koed K, Kramer A, Tort F, Zieger K et al (2005) DNA damage response as a candidate anti-cancer barrier in early human tumorigenesis. Nature 434(7035):864–870

52. Hanahan D, Weinberg RA (2011) Hallmarks of cancer: the next generation. Cell 144(5): 646–674

53. Fong PC, Boss DS, Yap TA, Tutt A, Wu P, Mergui-Roelvink M et al (2009) Inhibition of poly(ADP-ribose) polymerase in tumors from BRCA mutation carriers. N Engl J Med 361(2):123–134

54. Brock WA, Milas L, Bergh S, Lo R, Szabo C, Mason KA (2004) Radiosensitization of human and rodent cell lines by INO-1001, a novel inhibitor of poly(ADP-ribose) polymerase. Cancer Lett 205(2):155–160

55. Dungey FA, Caldecott KW, Chalmers AJ (2009) Enhanced radiosensitization of human glioma cells by combining inhibition of poly(ADP-ribose) polymerase with inhibition of heat shock protein 90. Mol Cancer Ther 8(8):2243–2254

56. Albert JM, Cao C, Kim KW, Willey CD, Geng L, Xiao D, et al. Inhibition of poly(ADP-ribose) polymerase enhances cell death and improves tumor growth delay in irradiated lung cancer models. Clin Cancer Res. 2007;13(10):3033–42.

57. Loser DA, Shibata A, Shibata AK, Woodbine LJ, Jeggo PA, Chalmers AJ (2010) Sensitization to radiation and alkylating agents by inhibitors of poly(ADP-ribose) polymerase is enhanced in cells deficient in DNA double-strand break repair. Mol Cancer Ther 9(6):1775–1787

58. Calabrese CR, Almassy R, Barton S, Batey MA, Calvert AH, Canan-Koch S et al (2004) Anticancer chemosensitization and radiosensitization by the novel poly(ADP-ribose) polymerase-1 inhibitor AG14361. J Natl Cancer Inst 96(1):56–67

59. Russo, A. L.; Kwon, H. C.; Burgan, W. E.; Carter, D.; Beam, K.; Weizheng, X.; Zhang, J.; Slusher, B. S.; Chakravarti, A.; Tofilon, P. J.; Camphausen, K., In vitro and in vivo radiosensitization of glioblastoma cells by the poly (ADPribose) polymerase inhibitor E7016. Clin. Cancer. Res. 2009, 15(2), 607–12.

60. Liu SK, Coackley C, Krause M, Jalali F, Chan N, Bristow RG (2008) A novel poly(ADP-ribose) polymerase inhibitor, ABT-888, radiosensitizes malignant human cell lines under hypoxia. Radiother Oncol 88(2):258–268

61. Noel G, Godon C, Fernet M, Giocanti N, Megnin-Chanet F, Favaudon V (2006) Radiosensitization by the poly(ADP-ribose) polymerase inhibitor 4-amino-1,8-naphthalimide is specific of the S phase of the cell cycle and involves arrest of DNA synthesis. Mol Cancer Ther 5(3):564–574

62. Langelier MF, Planck JL, Roy S, Pascal JM (2012) Structural basis for DNA damage-dependent poly(ADP-ribosyl)ation by human PARP-1. Science 336(6082):728–732

63. Meng AX, Jalali F, Cuddihy A, Chan N, Bindra RS, Glazer PM et al (2005) Hypoxia down-regulates DNA double strand break repair gene expression in prostate cancer cells. Radiother Oncol 76(2):168–176

64. Bindra RS, Schaffer PJ, Meng A, Woo J, Maseide K, Roth ME et al (2004) Down-regulation of Rad51 and decreased homologous recombination in hypoxic cancer cells. Mol Cell Biol 24(19):8504–8518
65. Chan N, Pires IM, Bencokova Z, Coackley C, Luoto KR, Bhogal N et al (2010) Contextual synthetic lethality of cancer cell kill based on the tumor microenvironment. Cancer Res 70(20):8045–8054
66. Khan K, Araki K, Wang D, Li G, Li X, Zhang J, Xu W, Hoover RK, Lauter S, O'Malley B Jr, Lapidus RG, Li D. Head and neck cancer radiosensitization by the novel poly(ADP-ribose) polymerase inhibitor GPI-15427. Head Neck. 2010 Mar;32(3):381–91.
67. Clarke MJ, Mulligan EA, Grogan PT, Mladek AC, Carlson BL, Schroeder MA, Curtin NJ, Lou Z, Decker PA, Wu W, Plummer ER, Sarkaria JN. Effective sensitization of temozolomide by ABT-888 is lost with development of temozolomide resistance in glioblastoma xenograft lines. Mol Cancer Ther. 2009 Feb;8(2):407–14.
68. Donawho CK, Luo Y, Luo Y, Penning TD, Bauch JL, Bouska JJ, Bontcheva-Diaz VD, Cox BF, DeWeese TL, Dillehay LE, Ferguson DC, Ghoreishi-Haack NS, Grimm DR, Guan R, Han EK, Holley-Shanks RR, Hristov B, Idler KB, Jarvis K, Johnson EF, Kleinberg LR, Klinghofer V, Lasko LM, Liu X, Marsh KC, McGonigal TP, Meulbroek JA, Olson AM, Palma JP, Rodriguez LE, Shi Y, Stavropoulos JA, Tsurutani AC, Zhu GD, Rosenberg SH, Giranda VL, Frost DJ. ABT-888, an orally active poly(ADP-ribose) polymerase inhibitor that potentiates DNA-damaging agents in preclinical tumor models. Clin Cancer Res. 2007 May 1;13(9):2728–37.
69. Tuli R, Surmak AJ, Reyes J, Armour M, Hacker-Prietz A, Wong J et al (2014) Radiosensitization of pancreatic cancer cells in vitro and in vivo through poly (ADP-ribose) polymerase inhibition with ABT-888. Transl Oncol. doi:10.1016/j.tranon.2014.04.003
70. Ali M, Kamjoo M, Thomas HD, Kyle S, Pavlovska I, Babur M et al (2011) The clinically active PARP inhibitor AG014699 ameliorates cardiotoxicity but does not enhance the efficacy of doxorubicin, despite improving tumor perfusion and radiation response in mice. Mol Cancer Ther 10(12):2320–2329
71. Hobson B, Denekamp J (1984) Endothelial proliferation in tumours and normal tissues: continuous labelling studies. Br J Cancer 49(4):405–413
72. Haveman J, Rodermond H, van Bree C, Wondergem J, Franken NA (2007) Residual late radiation damage in mouse stromal tissue assessed by the tumor bed effect. J Radiat Res 48(2):107–112
73. Galia A, Calogero AE, Condorelli R, Fraggetta F, La Corte A, Ridolfo F et al (2012) PARP-1 protein expression in glioblastoma multiforme. Eur J Histochem 56(1), e9
74. Roesner JP, Mersmann J, Bergt S, Bohnenberg K, Barthuber C, Szabo C et al (2010) Therapeutic injection of PARP inhibitor INO-1001 preserves cardiac function in porcine myocardial ischemia and reperfusion without reducing infarct size. Shock 33(5):507–512
75. Hamahata A, Enkhbaatar P, Lange M, Yamaki T, Sakurai H, Shimoda K et al (2012) Administration of poly(ADP-ribose) polymerase inhibitor into bronchial artery attenuates pulmonary pathophysiology after smoke inhalation and burn in an ovine model. Burns 38(8):1210–1215
76. Tentori L, Leonetti C, Scarsella M, Muzi A, Mazzon E, Vergati M et al (2006) Inhibition of poly(ADP-ribose) polymerase prevents irinotecan-induced intestinal damage and enhances irinotecan/temozolomide efficacy against colon carcinoma. FASEB J 20(10):1709–1711
77. Golding SE, Rosenberg E, Valerie N, Hussaini I, Frigerio M, Cockcroft XF et al (2009) Improved ATM kinase inhibitor KU-60019 radiosensitizes glioma cells, compromises insulin, AKT and ERK prosurvival signaling, and inhibits migration and invasion. Mol Cancer Ther 8(10):2894–2902
78. Golding SE, Rosenberg E, Adams BR, Wignarajah S, Beckta JM, O'Connor MJ et al (2012) Dynamic inhibition of ATM kinase provides a strategy for glioblastoma multiforme radiosensitization and growth control. Cell Cycle 11(6):1167–1173
79. Biddlestone-Thorpe L, Sajjad M, Rosenberg E, Beckta JM, Valerie NC, Tokarz M et al (2013) ATM kinase inhibition preferentially sensitizes p53-mutant glioma to ionizing radiation. Clin Cancer Res 19(12):3189–3200

80. Cancer Genome Atlas Research N (2008) Comprehensive genomic characterization defines human glioblastoma genes and core pathways. Nature 455(7216):1061–1068
81. Toulany M, Mihatsch J, Holler M, Chaachouay H, Rodemann HP (2014) Cisplatin-mediated radiosensitization of non-small cell lung cancer cells is stimulated by ATM inhibition. Radiother Oncol 111(2):228–236
82. Zou J, Qiao X, Ye H, Yang Y, Zheng X, Zhao H et al (2008) Antisense inhibition of ATM gene enhances the radiosensitivity of head and neck squamous cell carcinoma in mice. J Exp Clin Cancer Res 27:56
83. Rainey MD, Charlton ME, Stanton RV, Kastan MB (2008) Transient inhibition of ATM kinase is sufficient to enhance cellular sensitivity to ionizing radiation. Cancer Res 68(18):7466–7474
84. Choi S, Gamper AM, White JS, Bakkenist CJ (2010) Inhibition of ATM kinase activity does not phenocopy ATM protein disruption: implications for the clinical utility of ATM kinase inhibitors. Cell Cycle 9(20):4052–4057
85. Schneider L, Fumagalli M (2012) d'Adda di Fagagna F. Terminally differentiated astrocytes lack DNA damage response signaling and are radioresistant but retain DNA repair proficiency. Cell Death Differ 19(4):582–591
86. Gosink EC, Chong MJ, McKinnon PJ (1999) Ataxia telangiectasia mutated deficiency affects astrocyte growth but not radiosensitivity. Cancer Res 59(20):5294–5298
87. Moding EJ, Lee CL, Castle KD, Oh P, Mao L, Zha S et al (2014) Atm deletion with dual recombinase technology preferentially radiosensitizes tumor endothelium. J Clin Invest 124(8):3325–3338
88. Blood-brain barrier penetrating ATM inhibitor (AZ32) radiosensitises intracranial gliomas in mice. Steve T. Durant, Jeremy Karlin, Kurt Pike, Nicola Colclough, N Mukhopadhyay, S F. Ahmad, J M. Bekta, M Tokarz, Catherine Bardelle, Gareth Hughes, Bhavika Patel, Andrew Thomason, Elaine Cadogan, Ian Barrett, Alan Lau, Martin Pass, Kristoffer Valerie DOI:10.1158/1538-7445.AM2016-3041 Published 15 July 2016
89. Wang H, Wang H, Powell SN, Iliakis G, Wang Y (2004) ATR affecting cell radiosensitivity is dependent on homologous recombination repair but independent of nonhomologous end joining. Cancer Res 64(19):7139–7143
90. Gilad O, Nabet BY, Ragland RL, Schoppy DW, Smith KD, Durham AC et al (2010) Combining ATR suppression with oncogenic Ras synergistically increases genomic instability, causing synthetic lethality or tumorigenesis in a dosage-dependent manner. Cancer Res 70(23):9693–9702
91. Reaper PM, Griffiths MR, Long JM, Charrier JD, Maccormick S, Charlton PA et al (2011) Selective killing of ATM- or p53-deficient cancer cells through inhibition of ATR. Nat Chem Biol 7(7):428–430
92. Prevo R, Fokas E, Reaper PM, Charlton PA, Pollard JR, McKenna WG et al (2012) The novel ATR inhibitor VE-821 increases sensitivity of pancreatic cancer cells to radiation and chemotherapy. Cancer Biol Ther 13(11):1072–1081
93. Fokas E, Prevo R, Pollard JR, Reaper PM, Charlton PA, Cornelissen B et al (2012) Targeting ATR in vivo using the novel inhibitor VE-822 results in selective sensitization of pancreatic tumors to radiation. Cell Death Dis 3, e441
94. Pires IM, Olcina MM, Anbalagan S, Pollard JR, Reaper PM, Charlton PA et al (2012) Targeting radiation-resistant hypoxic tumour cells through ATR inhibition. Br J Cancer 107(2):291–299
95. Sankunny M, Parikh RA, Lewis DW, Gooding WE, Saunders WS, Gollin SM (2014) Targeted inhibition of ATR or CHEK1 reverses radioresistance in oral squamous cell carcinoma cells with distal chromosome arm 11q loss. Genes Chromosomes Cancer 53(2):129–143
96. Vavrova J, Zarybnicka L, Lukasova E, Rezacova M, Novotna E, Sinkorova Z et al (2013) Inhibition of ATR kinase with the selective inhibitor VE-821 results in radiosensitization of cells of promyelocytic leukaemia (HL-60). Radiat Environ Biophys 52(4):471–479, Epub 2013/08/13

97. Koniaras K, Cuddihy AR, Christopoulos H, Hogg A, O'Connell MJ (2001) Inhibition of Chk1-dependent G2 DNA damage checkpoint radiosensitizes p53 mutant human cells. Oncogene 20(51):7453–7463

98. Sorensen CS, Hansen LT, Dziegielewski J, Syljuasen RG, Lundin C, Bartek J et al (2005) The cell-cycle checkpoint kinase Chk1 is required for mammalian homologous recombination repair. Nat Cell Biol 7(2):195–201

99. Chen Z, Xiao Z, Gu WZ, Xue J, Bui MH, Kovar P et al (2006) Selective Chk1 inhibitors differentially sensitize p53-deficient cancer cells to cancer therapeutics. Int J Cancer 119(12):2784–2794

100. Engelke CG, Parsels LA, Qian Y, Zhang Q, Karnak D, Robertson JR et al (2013) Sensitization of pancreatic cancer to chemoradiation by the Chk1 inhibitor MK8776. Clin Cancer Res 19(16):4412–4421

101. Ma Z, Yao G, Zhou B, Fan Y, Gao S, Feng X (2012) The Chk1 inhibitor AZD7762 sensitises p53 mutant breast cancer cells to radiation in vitro and in vivo. Mol Med Rep 6(4):897–903

102. Veuger SJ, Curtin NJ, Richardson CJ, Smith GC, Durkacz BW (2003) Radiosensitization and DNA repair inhibition by the combined use of novel inhibitors of DNA-dependent protein kinase and poly(ADP-ribose) polymerase-1. Cancer Res 63(18):6008–6015

103. Short SC, Giampieri S, Worku M, Alcaide-German M, Sioftanos G, Bourne S et al (2011) Rad51 inhibition is an effective means of targeting DNA repair in glioma models and CD133+ tumor-derived cells. Neuro Oncol 13(5):487–499

104. Huang F, Mazin AV (2014) A small molecule inhibitor of human RAD51 potentiates breast cancer cell killing by therapeutic agents in mouse xenografts. PLoS One 9(6), e100993

105. Vance S, Liu E, Zhao L, Parsels JD, Parsels LA, Brown JL et al (2011) Selective radiosensitization of p53 mutant pancreatic cancer cells by combined inhibition of Chk1 and PARP1. Cell Cycle 10(24):4321–4329

106. Hoglund A, Stromvall K, Li Y, Forshell LP, Nilsson JA (2011) Chk2 deficiency in Myc overexpressing lymphoma cells elicits a synergistic lethal response in combination with PARP inhibition. Cell Cycle 10(20):3598–3607

107. Booth L, Cruickshanks N, Ridder T, Dai Y, Grant S, Dent P (2013) PARP and CHK inhibitors interact to cause DNA damage and cell death in mammary carcinoma cells. Cancer Biol Ther 14(5):458–465

108. Peasland A, Wang LZ, Rowling E, Kyle S, Chen T, Hopkins A et al (2011) Identification and evaluation of a potent novel ATR inhibitor, NU6027, in breast and ovarian cancer cell lines. Br J Cancer 105(3):372–381

109. Carruthers R, Ahmed SU, Strathdee K, Gomez-Roman N, Amoah-Buahin E, Watts C et al (2015) Abrogation of radioresistance in glioblastoma stem-like cells by inhibition of ATM kinase. Mol Oncol 9(1):192–203

110. Bao S, Wu Q, McLendon RE, Hao Y, Shi Q, Hjelmeland AB et al (2006) Glioma stem cells promote radioresistance by preferential activation of the DNA damage response. Nature 444(7120):756–760

111. Ahmed SU, Carruthers R, Gilmour L, Yildirim S, Watts C, Chalmers AJ (2015) Selective Inhibition of Parallel DNA Damage Response Pathways Optimizes Radiosensitization of Glioblastoma Stem-like Cells. Cancer Res 75(20):4416–4428

112. Mehta MP, Wang D, Wang F, Kleinberg L, Brade A, Robins HI et al (2015) Veliparib in combination with whole brain radiation therapy in patients with brain metastases: results of a phase 1 study. J Neurooncol 122(2):409–417

Chapter 2
Receptor Tyrosine Kinases as Targets for Enhancing Tumor Radiosensitivity

Thomas J. Hayman and Joseph N. Contessa

Abstract The advent of the modern era of molecularly targeted therapies in oncology has generated considerable excitement in the field of oncology. While there have been successes with molecularly targeted agents as monotherapies, most solid tumors display only a transient and modest response to single-targeted agents. As such, there has been significant effort in combining molecularly targeted agents with radiotherapy. Receptor tyrosine kinases (RTKs) play central roles in oncogenesis, stress sensitivity, tumor maintenance/progression, and clinical prognosis. Secondary to these roles, receptor tyrosine kinases are attractive targets for cancer therapy and specifically in combination with radiation therapy to enhance tumor radiosensitivity. Significant preclinical and clinical investigations have been performed to understand their roles in regulating the cellular response to radiation. A number of RTKs with relevance to radiation oncology have been identified including EGFR, VEGFR, IGF-1R, c-MET, and HER2. This chapter will highlight the preclinical and clinical findings associated with the combination of radiotherapy and inhibitors of the aforementioned receptors.

Keywords Radiosensitization • Receptor tyrosine kinase • EGFR • VEGF • c-Met • FGFR • Her2 • Epidermal growth factor receptor • RTK

Introduction

Clinicians have long combined radiation therapy with systemically delivered agents to enhance the local effects of RT, improve tumor control, and enhance patient survival. This combined modality approach couples standard fractionated radiation treatment regimens with cytotoxic chemotherapies such as 5FU, mitomycin, cisplatin,

T.J. Hayman • J.N. Contessa (✉)
Department of Therapeutic Radiology, Yale University School of Medicine,
P.O Box 208040, New Haven, CT, USA
e-mail: Thomas.Hayman@yale.edu; Joseph.Contessa@yale.edu

© Springer International Publishing Switzerland 2017
P.J. Tofilon, K. Camphausen (eds.), *Increasing the Therapeutic Ratio of Radiotherapy*, Cancer Drug Discovery and Development, DOI 10.1007/978-3-319-40854-5_2

taxol, and gemcitabine. While these combinations have shown success for specific disease sites in the clinic, substantial limitations exist. Chief among these are the dose limitations and toxicity imposed by normal tissue responses to the nonspecific nature of cytotoxic chemotherapy.

The advent of the modern era of targeted therapies has been met with great excitement in the oncology community. By attacking aberrantly activated pathways only present in tumor cells, targeted therapies have the potential benefit of being able to minimize normal tissue toxicity while maximizing tumor effect. While there have been successes with the use of targeted agents as monotherapies (e.g., imatinib in the BCR-Abl-driven chronic myeloid leukemia) [1], most common solid tumors have shown only a modest and transient response to single-targeted agents [2]. As such, tremendous effort has been expended in studying the combinations of these molecularly targeted agents with standard chemotherapies and/or radiation.

One target-rich area of tumor biology that has received considerable interest is membrane receptor (or specifically receptor tyrosine kinase) signaling. These kinases have been shown to play an important role in oncogenesis, stress sensitivity, tumor maintenance/progression, and clinical prognosis [3]. Secondary to these roles, receptor tyrosine kinases (RTKs) are attractive targets for cancer therapy and specifically in combination with radiation therapy to tumor radiosensitivity. As such, considerable preclinical and clinical investigations have been performed to understand their roles in regulating the cellular response to radiation. A number of RTKs with relevance to radiation oncology have been identified including EGFR, VEGFR, IGF-1R, c-MET, and HER2 [2, 4, 5]. This chapter will highlight the substantial preclinical and clinical findings associated with the combination of radiotherapy and inhibitors of the aforementioned receptors.

EGFR

The erbB family of receptors has been the subject of extensive laboratory and clinical investigations. The erbB family consists of four distinct receptors: EGFR (erbB1), HER-2/NEU (erbB2), erbB3, and erbB4 [6]. EGFR or epidermal growth factor receptor is the most well studied of the family with regard to its role in modulating a tumor's response to radiation.

The EGFR is a 170-kDa transmembrane RTK that plays an important role in carcinogenesis, tumor progression, and response to therapy [6]. Structurally, EGFR is comprised of four extracellular domains, a hydrophobic transmembrane domain, a juxtamembrane sub-domain, an intracellular tyrosine kinase domain, and c-terminal phosphorylation sites [6]. The natural ligands of the EGFR include epidermal growth factor (EGF), transforming growth factor alpha (TGF-α), epiregulin, betacellulin, amphiregulin, and heparin-binding EGF-like growth factor (HB-EGF) [7]. The EGFR is present in a monomeric state, but ligand binding drives a conformational change of the extracellular domain that causes receptor homo- and heterodimerization with other ErbB family receptors [8]. This dimerization activates intracellular tyrosine kinase domain auto- and transphosphorylation and initiates downstream signal transduction [8]. The EGFR and other RTKs are also activated by ionizing radiation [9]. The mechanisms that underlie this phenomenon include (1) receptor clustering and dimerization [10, 11], (2) radiation-induced release of autocrine ligands [12], and (3) phosphatase inactivation [13].

Signal transduction downstream of the EGFR occurs through a number of critical pathways including RAS/RAF/MAPK, PI3K/AKT/mTOR, Jak/STAT, Src, and PLC-DAG/PKC [14–18]. While the goal of this chapter is not to describe in detail each of these pathways, it is important to highlight their respective roles in the radiation response and tumor biology in general. The PI3K/AKT/mTOR pathway has been shown to be directly involved in regulating cell survival after radiation both in vitro and in vivo [19–21]. Various investigations have demonstrated different mechanisms by which this pathway governs radiosensitivity: through regulation of metabolic demands through activation of the mechanistic target of rapamycin (mTOR) kinase, control of proliferative signaling via MAPK cascade stimulation, and activation of cell survival signaling through AKT [22]. Other work has also documented the roles of Jak/STAT and PKC pathways in influencing tumor cell radiosensitivity [23, 24]. Ultimately activation of these pathways modifies cellular responses and repair programs induced by DNA damage, and regulation of these critical oncogenic pathways by EGFR underscores its potential as a target for enhancing tumor radiosensitivity and improving patient outcomes.

EGFR has a well-documented role in cancer [6] that was initially implicated by increased expression levels in a wide range of cancers including ovarian, brain, breast, colorectal, non-small cell lung cancer (NSCLC), and head and neck squamous cell carcinomas (HNSCC) [25, 26]. Based upon this appreciation, several classes of EGFR inhibitors have been developed. These inhibitors belong broadly to two classes: monoclonal antibodies (mAb) that target the extracellular ligand-binding domain and small molecule inhibitors that target the intracellular kinase domain [2, 27]. mAbs to the EGFR recognize, inactivate, and remove the receptor from the cell surface, and several mAbs have been advanced to the clinic including cetuximab, panitumumab, and matuzumab [2, 27]. Cetuximab is FDA approved for the treatment of HNSCC in combination with radiation [2, 5, 27]. Small-molecule tyrosine kinase inhibitors (TKIs), which bind to the intracellular ATP-binding domain of the EGFR, prevent receptor phosphorylation and subsequent signal transduction [2, 27]. A number of these TKIs have been developed and tested in the laboratory and clinic. Gefitinib and erlotinib are two EGFR-specific TKIs developed as single agents for advanced NSCLC and that have demonstrated efficacy in clinical trials [28, 29].

The observation that prolonged exposure of head and neck cancer cells to EGF enhanced the effects of radiation by clonogenic survival began to spark interest in studying the effects of EGFR modulation and radiation [30, 31]. While these initial in vitro results seem counterintuitive, it is likely that prolonged EGF exposure resulted in EGFR internalization and degradation causing a decrease in EGFR signaling. Another early study by Balaban et al. showed that targeting of

EGFR via the anti-EGFR antibody LA22 resulted in an increase in radiation-induced apoptosis [32]. Additionally, several other groups demonstrated in pre-clinical models (in vitro and in vivo) that EGFR expression inversely correlated with radiation sensitivity [33–35]. This correlation was also observed in clinical samples, and in fact poor survival of HNSCC patients with high EGFR tumors was shown to be secondary to poorer local regional tumor control and not distant metastasis [36]. The in vitro observation that radiation activates EGFR receptor phosphorylation [9, 37] and several downstream signaling cascades such as Ras/MAPK and PI3K/AKT/mTOR [17, 38] provided a mechanistic rationale for targeting EGFR function concurrent with RT, and genetic models of EGFR blockade indeed provided evidence that radiosensitization could be achieved through EGFR inhibition [10, 39].

These initial preclinical results, as well as parallel work examining EGFR targeting as a monotherapy, led to the development of the mAb, C225 (now known as cetuximab). C225 was shown to enhance radiation effects in vitro in HNSCC cell lines despite also causing a G1 cell cycle arrest, a finding that supported the potential for clinical translation [40]. Preclinical and clinical research has also been performed on additional mAbs such as mAb806, which recognizes an activation-specific conformation of the receptor. This antibody has been shown to bind a cryptic EGFR epitope that is exposed in the presence of oncogenic mutations such as EGFRvIII or is coincident with overexpression and activation of wild-type EGFR [41]. The specificity of blocking activated EGFR signaling in tumor cells with this Mab represents an intriguing strategy to minimize normal tissue toxicity [41]. Phase I clinical trial testing with mAB806 (ABT806) has been completed in patients with advanced solid malignancies (NCT01255657) although results have not yet been reported [42].

Preclinical studies have also investigated combinations of radiation and mAbs or TKIs that target EGFR in NSCLC, breast adenocarcinoma, and glioblastoma [40, 43–45]. Effects on in vitro intrinsic radiosensitivity as determined by clonogenic survival assays have been modest but consistent in most instances [2]. In vivo results from the combination of radiation and EGFR inhibition have typically been more striking with concurrent treatment, resulting in greater than additive effects on tumor growth delay [2]. In vivo radiosensitization has been achieved with both single fractions of radiation as well as the more clinically relevant fractionated radiation schedules [7, 46]. For example, treatment of tumor xenografts with gefitinib [47, 48] in combination with radiation resulted in inhibition of tumor growth that was greater than either modality alone. The discrepancy between in vitro and in vivo results has been hypothesized to be related to several different mechanisms that would only be apparent in vivo including inhibition of angiogenesis and reduction in tumor cell invasion [2].

Secondary to the promising preclinical results in the aforementioned paragraphs, numerous clinical trials have been designed evaluating the efficacy of combining EGFR inhibitors with radiation [49]. Perhaps the most notable of these trials was a phase III multicentered randomized controlled trial with 424 patients with locoregionally advanced HNSCC [50]. The trial compared treatment with radiotherapy alone to radiotherapy plus cetuximab. The results were striking and showed an increase in overall survival (OS) from 29.3 months with radiotherapy alone to 49.0 months with the combination of radiotherapy and cetuximab (hazard ratio for death 0.73; $P = 0.03$). Local control rates were also significantly improved with the addition of cetuximab to radiotherapy (50 % vs. 41 % in the radiotherapy alone arm).

Building upon the Bonner et al. study, RTOG 0522 was designed to answer the question as to whether the addition of cetuximab to cisplatin-based standard chemoradiotherapy (CRT) improved outcomes [51]. This phase III clinical trial randomized patients to concurrent CRT (cisplatin + radiotherapy) alone or with cetuximab in patients with stage III/IV HNSCC. The results of the study showed no difference in OS or PFS with the addition of cetuximab to standard cisplatin-based CRT. However the critical unanswered question is whether cetuximab could replace cisplatin as a radiosensitizing agent for definitive CRT of locoregionally advanced HNSCC. RTOG 1016 was designed to answer this question in a subset of HPV-positive HNSCC [42] and randomizes patients with oropharyngeal cancer to CRT with cisplatin or cetuximab. This trial began recruiting in 2011 and outcomes are pending.

The combined results of the Bonner et al. trials, the preclinical data suggesting that EGFR is a target for radiosensitization, and data showing that the majority of NSCLCs overexpress EGFR led to the development of a 2×2 phase III trial in NSCLC evaluating the use of cetuximab and radiation dose escalation up to 74 Gy [52]. The results of this study, however, were disappointing and showed that addition of cetuximab to chemoradiotherapy in patients with locally advanced NSCLC did not affect patient survival. Why did cetuximab fail to radiosensitize NSCLC? The most likely explanation is that the radiosensitizing effect of EGFR inhibition was not additive with chemotherapy. Alternative explanations include the possibility that tumors from this primary site either contain parallel signaling mechanisms that compensate for EGFR inhibition or that EGFR is not a primary driver of cell survival.

The results of the RTOG 0617 and other negative clinical trials combining EGFR targeting with radiation/chemotherapies raise several important questions about how to advance this treatment strategy. The most important of these is how patients that respond to EGFR inhibition in combination with radiation can best be identified prior to treatment. This concept is currently undergoing extensive evaluations in both the laboratory and the clinic [2]. For example, it has been suggested that p16+ HNSCC are more sensitive to the combination of cetuximab and radiation [53]. In contrast, and somewhat surprisingly, EGFR expression has not shown to correlate to response to combination chemotherapy and cetuximab [54]. In fact responses to EGFR inhibition have been shown with a lack of EGFR staining by immunohistochemistry (IHC) [55], confirming that identification of mechanistic biomarkers will be valuable for directing future approaches for EGFR targeting and radiosensitization.

VEGF/VEGFR

Angiogenesis is a hallmark of tumor progression and metastasis, and the VEGF growth factor and its receptors play critical roles in the regulation of angiogenesis [56]. The VEGF family of proteins consists of VEGF A–E and placenta growth factor (PLGF) 1–2. VEGFA is the most abundant of the VEGF proteins and exerts its effects primarily by binding to VEGFR-1 and VEGFR-2 [56, 57]. Like the EGFR, both transmembrane RTKs are stimulated by ligands and undergo dimerization, autophosphorylation of its intracellular tyrosine residues, and initiation of downstream signaling [56]. These receptors exist primarily on vascular endothelial cells [56, 57]. VEGFR-1 is thought to be involved in vascular system development during angiogenesis, whereas VEGFR-2 is the primary mediator of the angiogenic, mitogenic, and vascular permeability-enhancing effects of VEGF. VEGFR-2 signals downstream via PI3K/AKT/mTOR and the RAS/MAPK pathways to enhance endothelial cell proliferation and survival [57].

VEGF is overexpressed in many solid tumors [57]. This increased expression has been shown to correlate with worse PFS and OS [56, 58]. As such anti-VEGF therapy has garnered significant interest as a cancer therapy, and development of bevacizumab, a humanized monoclonal antibody, is directed against VEGF that prevents its binding to VEGFR-1 and VEGFR-2 [59].

It was initially thought that antiangiogenic therapy would impair the effects of ionizing radiation by the induction of tumor hypoxia, as oxygen is thought to be critical to the formation of free radicals that cause DNA double-strand breaks and cell death [60]. However, early studies by Teicher et al. showed that this might not be true for all tumors as antiangiogenic therapy with the angiogenesis inhibitor TNP-470 and minocycline actually improved tumor oxygenation and the antitumor effects of radiotherapy [61]. Furthermore the interaction with EGFR signaling, which potentiates production of VEGF [62], suggests that enhanced angiogenesis is a mechanism for both tumor and vessel radioresistance [62]. Because of the increase in oxygenation with antiangiogenic therapies and data showing enhancement of VEGF levels by RT, it was postulated that strategies targeting angiogenesis might augment the radiation response.

In the first preclinical study of a targeted antiangiogenic therapy with radiation, it was shown that angiostatin, a natural product that inhibits angiogenesis, enhanced the effects of radiation on in vivo murine lung cancers as well as human glioblastoma, squamous cell carcinoma, and prostate carcinoma xenografts [63]. Gorski et al. showed that anti-VEGF antibodies in combination with radiation (20 and 40 Gy) in several tumor xenografts (lung carcinoma, squamous cell carcinoma, glioblastoma, and esophageal carcinoma) caused a greater than additive increase in tumor growth delay than either therapy alone [64]. DC101 an inhibitor of mouse VEGFR-2 has also been used in several preclinical studies to enhance the effects of radiation [65]. Kozin et al. showed that the use of DC101 before, during, and after fractionated radiation therapy decreased the dose of radiation required to control 50% of tumors locally in 54a (lung carcinoma) and U87 (glioma) xenografts by 1.7- and 1.3-fold, respectively [66].

Several potential mechanisms have been described with regard to anti-VEGF therapies and increased response to radiation. First, it has been suggested that anti-VEGF therapy increases the radiosensitivity of vascular endothelial cells [64]. Several studies have shown increased apoptosis of vascular endothelial cells with anti-VEGF therapy and radiation [65, 66]. The increased death of endothelial cells then can reduce vascular density and inhibit the formation of new blood vessels causing impaired nutrient delivery to the tumor [65]. Secondly, studies have shown that anti-VEGF agents can renormalize the vasculature causing an increase in tumor oxygenation and hence an increase in tumor radiosensitivity [67, 68].

Secondary to the promising preclinical findings mentioned above, clinical trials have been performed with anti-VEGF therapy both as monotherapy and in combination with radiation. Several phase I/II clinical trials have been published showing promising results in many tumor types (e.g., glioblastoma, rectal cancer, and HNSCC) [69]. These early clinical trials in patients with glioblastoma led to the development of two phase III clinical trials. The RTOG 0825 was a phase III double-blind randomized controlled trial comparing conventional concurrent chemoradiation and adjuvant temozolomide plus bevacizumab vs. conventional concurrent chemoradiation and adjuvant temozolomide in patients with newly diagnosed glioblastoma [70]. The data showed that there was no increase in OS with the addition of bevacizumab to standard therapy even though there was a trend toward increased PFS (HR, 0.79; 95 % CI, 0.66 to 0.94; $P = 0.007$). A similar study, AVAglio (Avastin in glioblastoma), was a phase III study that evaluated the efficacy of adding Avastin (bevacizumab) to standard chemoradiation and adjuvant temozolomide in patients with newly diagnosed glioblastoma [71]. After surgery or biopsy, patients were randomized to receive concurrent radiation and temozolomide plus either Avastin or placebo. After the completion of six cycles of maintenance temozolomide and Avastin or placebo, the patients continued on Avastin or placebo until disease progression or unacceptable side effects are presented. OS was nearly identical between the two arms. The improvement in PFS (10.6 months with Avastin vs. 6.2 months with placebo; HR 0.64; 95 % CI, 0.55–0.74; $P < 0.001$) observed in this study reflects the drug's clinical effectiveness for targeting angiogenesis without enhancing the radiosensitivity of glioblastoma tumor cells.

The disappointing results of these clinical trials in GBM suggest that the rationale for radiosensitization must be reevaluated. Chief among these concerns is the hypothesis that VEGFR inhibition does not increase hypoxia in human tumors as this effect could counteract the combination of antiangiogenic therapy with radiation. Additionally biomarkers and patient selection may also provide a way to identify patients most likely to benefit from anti-VEGF agents. We also know from preclinical results that treatment combinations with anti-VEGF agents and radiation are treatment dose dependent [72]. This emphasizes careful consideration and understanding of the clinical design of combinations of radiation and anti-VEGF agents. In addition, similar to anti-EGFR agents, patients being treated with anti-VEGF/VEGFR agents experience resistance to therapy [72]. In patients with glioblastoma who experienced clinical progression on cediranib (a potent TKI of VEGFRs), significant increases in plasma bFGF and stromal cell-derived growth factor (SDF1a) were noted [73]. This is in agreement with preclinical models where cross talk between many angiogenic factors including VEGF, PDGF, angiopoietins, ephrin, and Notch has been shown [56, 74]. Thus although inhibition of a single factor may not be sufficient to fully inhibit angiogenesis in all patients, study of rationale combinations of anti-VEGF therapy with other targeted agents in preclinical models may provide valuable insights for combining RT with targeting of angiogenesis.

c-Met

c-Met, also known as the hepatocyte growth factor (HGF) receptor, is a 170-KD transmembrane receptor tyrosine kinase that plays an important role in tumorigenesis and metastasis [75]. Like other RTKs, ligand binding activated receptor activity through dimerization and phosphorylation of intracellular tyrosine kinase domains [76]. Downstream signaling occurs through many of the previously mentioned oncogenic signaling pathways including PI3K/AKT/mTOR, RAS/MAPK, and JAK/STAT [77, 78].

HGF was originally identified as a cytokine that caused the dissociation of colonies of cells into single cells [79] and is a pro-migratory ligand that accumulates in the extracellular matrix and is linked to tumor cell invasion. HGF also promotes epithelial-mesenchymal transition (EMT) [79–82], which in turn causes further increases in tumor cell migration, invasion, and angiogenesis [77].

HGF/c-MET autocrine ligand signaling is aberrantly activated in a number of different cancers including breast, glioma, NSCLC, SCLC, and colon cancer [83–88]. Increased production of HGF by both cancer cells and the surrounding stroma as well as gene amplification and overexpression of c-Met has been described as mechanisms for activating this autocrine loop. Increased production/upregulation of the HGF/c-Met axis has also been shown to be a negative prognostic indicator [77, 89, 90]. For example, increased expression of HGF and c-Met in colon cancer is associated with worse disease stage [91], lymph node metastasis [91], and decreases in PFS and OS [86].

c-Met activation and signaling has been linked to resistance to both DNA-damaging chemotherapies and ionizing radiation [77]. One of the earliest studies to link HGF/c-Met and resistance to DNA-damaging therapies was done by Fan et al. [92]. This study showed that pretreating breast cancer cells with HGF decreased DNA fragmentation induced by DNA-damaging agents. In a further study, they showed this effect to be mediated by c-Met through the PI3K/AKT pathway [93]. In clinical studies increased c-Met expression has been shown to be an independent predictor of local failure in patients undergoing definitive radiation for SCC of the oropharynx [94].

Preclinical studies have explored the relationship between radiation and c-Met signaling. De Bacco et al. showed that irradiation induced c-Met expression in a variety of cell lines [95]. Furthermore they found that inhibition of c-Met activity with the small molecule tyrosine kinase inhibitors PHA665752 (or JNJ-38877605) sensitized glioma and breast cancer cells to irradiation in vitro and in tumor xeno-graft model systems [95]. Increased c-Met expression/activation after radiation has been reported in pancreatic cancer, glioblastoma, and neuroblastoma model systems [96–98], and Chu et al. reported that in glioblastoma cells, radiation-induced HGF secretion leads to activation of c-Met signaling in glioma cell lines [97].

Based upon the above observations several groups have begun to define the role of HGF/c-Met in mediating cell survival after exposure to ionizing radiation. Welsh et.al showed that inhibition of c-Met with siRNA and the small molecule inhibitor MP470 can radiosensitize glioma cells to radiation in vitro and in vivo [99]. In these studies, radiation-induced DNA damage repair via a decrease in Rad51 expression after irradiation was implicated as the mechanism for radiosen-sitization. In gastric carcinoma cells, inhibition of c-Met was shown to decrease phosphorylation of ATR and checkpoint kinase 1 (CHK1) [100]. Similar results demonstrating radiosensitization have been shown in other glioblastoma xenograft models as well as in vitro and in vivo models of prostate cancer, thyroid cancer, and NSCLC [101–105].

A number of different inhibitors of the HGF/c-Met signaling axis are available for clinical use [77, 106]. These include anti-HGF antibodies (ficlatuzumab, rilo-tumumab, and TAK-701), anti-Met antibodies (onartuzumab), and small molecule tyrosine kinase inhibitors (cabozantinib, foretinib, and tivantinib). Several of these molecules have been combined with other targeted agents including anti-EGFR inhibitors [77].

To date only one clinical trial of radiation and c-Met inhibition has been per-formed. This was a phase 1 safety trial of cabozantinib with temozolomide and radiation in newly diagnosed glioblastoma patients. The study closed in 2013 and the results have not been reported at the time of this publication [42]. Given the aforementioned preclinical and clinical data, it is logical to further explore the com-bination of radiation and c-Met inhibition with the goal of testing whether inhibition of Met signaling can enhance the effects of radiation therapy in malignant tumors.

Other RTKs

There are several other RTKs that have been studied with regard to their role in the radioresponse, however, to a lesser degree than the previously described receptors. One such studied RTK is the insulin-like growth factor-type 1 receptor (IGF-1R). The IGF family proteins are the primary ligand for IGF-1R [107]. Their binding acts similarly to the other RTKs discussed above [108]. IGF-1R signaling has been linked to malignant transformation, cellular proliferation, cell survival and differen-tiation [109], as well as increased local recurrence after RT [110].

With regard to regulation of the radiation response, several preclinical studies have been performed showing radiosensitization both in vitro and in vivo. Riesterer et al. showed that the use of A12, an anti-IGF-1R antibody, caused radiosensitiza-tion of HNSCC cell lines in vitro via the clonogenic survival assay as well as in vivo as measured by tumor growth delay [111]. Allen et al. published similar results with the combination of A12 and radiation in H226 lung cancer xenografts [112]. Recent data by Chitnis et al. reports IGF-1R inhibition by AZ12253801, a selective IGF-1R tyrosine kinase inhibitor that radiosensitizes tumor cell lines via an inhibition of both HR and NHEJ [113].

More recently several studies have begun to define the use of IGF-1R inhibitors in combination with radiation and EGFR blockade. The rationale for these studies lies in data showing cross talk between the EGFR and IGF-1R pathways at multiple levels [114, 115]. In fact, EGFR inhibition has been shown to cause increased response to IGF-1R ligands [114, 115]. Li et al. demonstrated that co-inhibition of EGFR and IGF-1R using specific small molecule tyrosine kinase inhibitors to both receptors caused synergistic radiosensitization in breast cancer cell in vitro and in tumor xenografts [116].

HER2 (or erbB2) is an RTK that has no known soluble ligand. However, it exerts its actions by formation of heterodimers with the other ErbB family members, notably EGFR. HER2 overexpression has been noted in approximately 30 % of breast cancers [117] and 20 % of gastroesophageal (GE) and gastric cancers [118]. Trastuzumab, a monoclonal antibody to the external domain of HER2, has been approved for clinical use in metastatic breast cancer and shows activity in preclinical models as well [119]. With regard to the role of HER2 in regulating radiosensitivity, much less is known, with only a few reports combining radiation with specific anti-HER2 therapies. One such study by Pietras et al. showed that trastuzumab treatment radiosensitized the breast cancer cell line MCF7 in vitro and in tumor xenografts only under conditions of HER2 overexpression [120]. Instead, most studies examining the role of Her2 in the radiation response have focused on the use of lapatinib a dual EGFR and Her2 inhibitor. Using lapatinib, several groups have shown an increase in radiosensitivity [121–123]. For example, Sambade et.al demonstrated that the effects of lapatinib plus radiation on tumor growth of HER2+/EGFR+ breast cancer xenografts were greater than additive of either therapy alone [121].

Although there is a paucity of preclinical data with regard to the combination of radiation and anti-HER2 therapies, there have been several clinical trials completed combining the two treatments. The Brown University Oncology Group performed a pilot study of trastuzumab in addition to chemoradiation in patients with HER2+ locally advanced esophageal adenocarcinoma [124]. Despite the patients' advanced burden of disease, a 3-year OS of 47 % was observed with no increase in adverse events. This study led to the development of RTOG 1010 in which patients with HER2+ locally advanced esophageal adenocarcinoma and GE junction tumors are randomized to chemoradiation plus concurrent and maintenance trastuzumab or chemoradiation [119]. This trial is still open to accrual [42]. In breast cancer, several large clinical trials including the NSABP B-31 and NCCTG N9831 trials have been completed [42]. These trials have compared the addition of trastuzumab to chemotherapy in node-positive or high-risk node-negative nonmetastatic, operable breast cancer patients [125]. Approximately 70 % of patients in both studies underwent adjuvant radiotherapy concurrently with trastuzumab. DFS ($P<0.001$; stratified HR, 0.52; 95 % CI, 0.45 to 0.60) and OS ($P<0.001$; stratified HR, 0.61; 95 % CI,

0.50–0.75) were significantly increased with the addition of trastuzumab. While this study was not directly comparing the effect of adding trastuzumab to adjuvant radiotherapy, some of the effects seen may have been due to this addition.

The fibroblast growth factor (FGF) pathway has also been studied with regard to its role in regulation of the cellular response to radiation. The FGFs mediate their biological effects through the FGF receptors (FGFRs). The four known FGFRs include FGFR-1, FGFR-2, FGFR-3, and FGFR-4 [125, 126]. Their activation is controlled by a unique combination of ligand (FGFs) binding as well as heparin sulfate glycosaminoglycan cofactors [127]. The FGF/FGFR signaling axis has a well-documented role in cancer [126]. Activating mutations, receptor overexpression, and alternative splicing have been shown to augment tumorigenesis in a variety of malignancies [126, 128–132]. Expression of FGFR-1 is a known predictor of poor overall survival and shorter time to progression in patients with glioblastoma [132, 133].

Several early reports began to define the role of the FGF/FGFR axis in regulating cellular survival after radiation [130, 133–135]. Fuks et al. showed that basal FGF (bFGF or FGF2) protected endothelial cell from radiation-induced apoptosis and that administration of bFGF to mice protected against the development of fatal radiation pneumonitis [134]. Other studies showed that expression of FGF2 in human tumor cell lines led to an increase in their relative radioresistance via the small GTPase RhoB [136]. A recent study by Ader et al. used an allosteric FGFR small molecule inhibitor, SSR128129E, to determine the effects of FGFR inhibition on glioma cell radiosensitivity [137]. They showed that inhibition of FGFR signaling enhanced in vitro radiosensitivity of two glioma cell lines via the clonogenic survival assay. Additionally the combination of radiation and SSR128129E significantly enhanced neurologic sign-free survival of mice bearing orthotopic glioma xenografts. Furthermore, Cazet et al. showed that disruption of glycosylation via inhibition of mannose phosphate isomerase inhibited FGFR signaling and enhanced radiosensitivity of glioma cell lines in vitro [133]. The preclinical results are promising and suggest further investigation into the role of FGF/FGFR signaling in regulating the cellular radioresponse both preclinically and clinically.

Conclusion

Significant progress has been made toward the understanding of receptor tyrosine kinase signaling in radiotherapy. The extensive body of literature reviewed above with regard to EGFR, VEGF/VEGFR, c-MET, IGF-1R, and HER2 illustrates this progress. These findings underscore the importance of the rational translation of preclinical data to the clinical setting. Perhaps the best example of this success is shown by the Bonner et al. showing substantial overall survival benefit with the addition of cetuximab to radiation therapy in HNSCC patients [50].

These successes in the preclinical and clinical settings are not without their limitation. First of all, resistance to these therapies is common [27, 119, 138]. As discussed above, the mechanisms of resistance are complicated and can possibly vary from tumor to tumor, and thus we are only beginning to understand the mechanisms of resistance. This understanding will allow us to pursue logical combinations of targeted agents in combinations with radiotherapy both preclinically and clinically. Secondly, it appears that with many of the agents that target RTKs, only a subset of tumors actually responds to a given therapy. This fact underscores the importance of being able to prospectively select patients for a given therapy. As illustrated above, this work has begun but has proved to be challenging and will require further investigation. Thirdly, in many of the clinical trials with agents targeting RTK pathways, there was a lack of true target engagement [2]. Being able to determine whether an agent is clearly inhibiting its target in the tumor and actually having an effect on downstream signaling is paramount to being able to judge success or failure in the clinic. While this may be challenging, it is of utmost importance to ensure proper interpretation of results.

Importantly an understanding of which molecular subtypes of tumors will respond to the combination of radiation and RTK inhibition will be of considerable significance. This has been an area of considerable interest with regard to inhibitors of RTKs as monotherapies [2, 27]. For instance, in lung carcinoma, it has been demonstrated that tumors that harbor KRAS mutations are resistant to EGFR inhibition [139]. Similarly PTEN deletion in glioblastoma patients causes resistance to EGFR-directed therapeutics. As both KRAS mutations and PTEN cause activation of signaling downstream of RTKs, it is rational to expect these mutations to confer resistance to inhibitors upstream molecules. A recent study by Bennett et al. extended these results to the combination of radiation and inhibition of RTK signaling via aclacinomycin (Acm) treatment [140]. They demonstrated that Acm was only effective as a radiosensitizer when used on cell lines that were EGFR dependent but not on cell lines that harbored KRAS mutations (EGFR independent) [141]. These results underscore the importance of choosing tumors with molecular characteristics that will be expected to respond to RTK-targeted therapies. As such future studies aimed at determining molecular signatures of responsive tumors will bear relevance to molecular radiation oncology.

While the mechanism of action of how these agents interact with radiation is beginning to be elucidated, much has yet to be learned. A mechanistic understanding of this interaction will allow for differing treatment schedules and rationale combinations with other therapies. Additionally, understanding the mechanisms of radiosensitization may allow us to exploit certain tumors based upon their specific genotypes or pathway alterations. As such continued investigation into all of the above RTKs should continue to provide a wealth of knowledge that will ultimately be able to benefit patients with many different types of tumors.

References

1. Druker BJ, Sawyers CL, Kantarjian H, Resta DJ, Reese SF, Ford JM, Capdeville R, Talpaz M (2001) Activity of a specific inhibitor of the BCR-ABL tyrosine kinase in the blast crisis of chronic myeloid leukemia and acute lymphoblastic leukemia with the Philadelphia chromosome. N Engl J Med 344(14):1038–1042. doi:10.1056/NEJM200104053441402

2. Nyati MK, Morgan MA, Feng FY, Lawrence TS (2006) Integration of EGFR inhibitors with radiochemotherapy. Nat Rev Cancer 6(11):876–885. doi:10.1038/nrc1953
3. Gschwind A, Fischer OM, Ullrich A (2004) The discovery of receptor tyrosine kinases: targets for cancer therapy. Nat Rev Cancer 4(5):361–370. doi:10.1038/nrc1360
4. Kim DW, Huamani J, Fu A, Hallahan DE (2006) Molecular strategies targeting the host component of cancer to enhance tumor response to radiation therapy. Int J Radiat Oncol Biol Phys 64(1):38–46. doi:10.1016/j.ijrobp.2005.02.008
5. Meyn RE, Munshi A, Haymach JV, Milas L, Ang KK (2009) Receptor signaling as a regulatory mechanism of DNA repair. Radiother Oncol 92(3):316–322. doi:10.1016/j.radonc.2009.06.031
6. Herbst RS (2004) Review of epidermal growth factor receptor biology. Int J Radiat Oncol Biol Phys 59(2 Suppl):21–26. doi:10.1016/j.ijrobp.2003.11.041
7. Zips D, Krause M, Yaromina A, Dorfler A, Eicheler W, Schutze C, Gurtner K, Baumann M (2008) Epidermal growth factor receptor inhibitors for radiotherapy: biological rationale and preclinical results. J Pharm Pharmacol 60(8):1019–1028. doi:10.1211/jpp.60.8.0008
8. Uberall I, Kolar Z, Trojanec R, Berkovcova J, Hajduch M (2008) The status and role of ErbB receptors in human cancer. Exp Mol Pathol 84(2):79–89. doi:10.1016/j.yexmp.2007.12.002
9. Schmidt-Ullrich RK, Valerie K, Fogleman PB, Walters J (1996) Radiation-induced autophosphorylation of epidermal growth factor receptor in human malignant mammary and squamous epithelial cells. Radiat Res 145(1):81–85
10. Contessa JN, Reardon DB, Todd D, Dent P, Mikkelsen RB, Valerie K, Bowers GD, Schmidt-Ullrich RK (1999) The inducible expression of dominant-negative epidermal growth factor receptor-CD533 results in radiosensitization of human mammary carcinoma cells. Clin Cancer Res 5(2):405–411
11. Li W, Li F, Huang Q, Frederick B, Bao S, Li CY (2008) Noninvasive imaging and quantification of epidermal growth factor receptor kinase activation in vivo. Cancer Res 68(13):4990–4997. doi:10.1158/0008-5472.CAN-07-5984
12. Dent P, Reardon DB, Park JS, Bowers G, Logsdon C, Valerie K, Schmidt-Ullrich R (1999) Radiation-induced release of transforming growth factor alpha activates the epidermal growth factor receptor and mitogen-activated protein kinase pathway in carcinoma cells, leading to increased proliferation and protection from radiation-induced cell death. Mol Biol Cell 10(8):2493–2506
13. Sturla LM, Amorino G, Alexander MS, Mikkelsen RB, Valerie K, Schmidt-Ullrichr RK (2005) Requirement of Tyr-992 and Tyr-1173 in phosphorylation of the epidermal growth factor receptor by ionizing radiation and modulation by SHP2. J Biol Chem 280(15):14597–14604. doi:10.1074/jbc.M413287200
14. Hennessy BT, Smith DL, Ram PT, Lu Y, Mills GB (2005) Exploiting the PI3K/AKT pathway for cancer drug discovery. Nat Rev Drug Discov 4(12):988–1004. doi:10.1038/nrd1902
15. Irwin ME, Bohin N, Boerner JL (2011) Src family kinases mediate epidermal growth factor receptor signaling from lipid rafts in breast cancer cells. Cancer Biol Ther 12(8):718–726. doi:10.4161/cbt.12.8.16907
16. Oliva JL, Griner EM, Kazanietz MG (2005) PKC isozymes and diacylglycerol-regulated proteins as effectors of growth factor receptors. Growth Factors 23(4):245–252. doi:10.1080/08977190500366043
17. Schmidt-Ullrich RK, Mikkelsen RB, Dent P, Todd DG, Valerie K, Kavanagh BD, Contessa JN, Rorrer WK, Chen PB (1997) Radiation-induced proliferation of the human A431 squamous carcinoma cells is dependent on EGFR tyrosine phosphorylation. Oncogene 15(10):1191–1197. doi:10.1038/sj.onc.1201275
18. Sebolt-Leopold JS, Herrera R (2004) Targeting the mitogen-activated protein kinase cascade to treat cancer. Nat Rev Cancer 4(12):937–947. doi:10.1038/nrc1503
19. Chen DJ, Nirodi CS (2007) The epidermal growth factor receptor: a role in repair of radiation-induced DNA damage. Clin Cancer Res 13(22 Pt 1):6555–6560. doi:10.1158/1078-0432.CCR-07-1610
20. Hayman TJ, Kramp T, Kahn J, Jamal M, Camphausen K, Tofilon PJ (2013) Competitive but not allosteric mTOR kinase inhibition enhances tumor cell radiosensitivity. Transl Oncol 6(3):355–362

21. Hayman TJ, Wahba A, Rath BH, Bae H, Kramp T, Shankavaram UT, Camphausen K, Tofilon PJ (2014) The ATP-competitive mTOR inhibitor INK128 enhances in vitro and in vivo radiosensitivity of pancreatic carcinoma cells. Clin Cancer Res 20(1):110–119. doi:10.1158/1078-0432.CCR-13-2136

22. Toulany M, Rodemann HP (2010) Membrane receptor signaling and control of DNA repair after exposure to ionizing radiation. Nuklearmed Nucl Med 49(Suppl 1):S26–S30

23. Bonner JA, Trummell HQ, Willey CD, Plants BA, Raisch KP (2009) Inhibition of STAT-3 results in radiosensitization of human squamous cell carcinoma. Radiother Oncol 92(3):339–344. doi:10.1016/j.radonc.2009.06.022

24. Willey CD, Xiao D, Tu T, Kim KW, Moretti L, Niermann KJ, Tawtawy MN, Quarles CC, Lu B (2010) Enzastaurin (LY317615), a protein kinase C beta selective inhibitor, enhances antiangiogenic effect of radiation. Int J Radiat Oncol Biol Phys 77(5):1518–1526. doi:10.1016/j.ijrobp.2009.06.044

25. Mendelsohn J (2001) The epidermal growth factor receptor as a target for cancer therapy. Endocr Relat Cancer 8(1):3–9

26. Ruddel J, Wennekes VE, Meissner W, Werner JA, Mandic R (2010) EGF-dependent induction of BCL-xL and p21CIP1/WAF1 is highly variable in HNSCC cells–implications for EGFR-targeted therapies. Anticancer Res 30(11):4579–4585

27. Cohen RB (2014) Current challenges and clinical investigations of epidermal growth factor receptor (EGFR)- and ErbB family-targeted agents in the treatment of head and neck squamous cell carcinoma (HNSCC). Cancer Treat Rev 40(4):567–577. doi:10.1016/j.ctrv.2013.10.002

28. Kris MG, Natale RB, Herbst RS, Lynch TJ Jr, Prager D, Belani CP, Schiller JH, Kelly K, Spiridonidis H, Sandler A, Albain KS, Cella D, Wolf MK, Averbuch SD, Ochs JJ, Kay AC (2003) Efficacy of gefitinib, an inhibitor of the epidermal growth factor receptor tyrosine kinase, in symptomatic patients with non-small cell lung cancer: a randomized trial. JAMA 290(16):2149–2158. doi:10.1001/jama.290.16.2149

29. Ellis PM, Coakley N, Feld R, Kuruvilla S, Ung YC (2015) Use of the epidermal growth factor receptor inhibitors gefitinib, erlotinib, afatinib, dacomitinib, and icotinib in the treatment of non-small-cell lung cancer: a systematic review. Curr Oncol 22(3):e183–e215. doi:10.3747/co.22.2566

30. Kwok TT, Sutherland RM (1989) Enhancement of sensitivity of human squamous carcinoma cells to radiation by epidermal growth factor. J Natl Cancer Inst 81(13):1020–1024

31. Bonner JA, Maihle NJ, Folven BR, Christianson TJ, Spain K (1994) The interaction of epidermal growth factor and radiation in human head and neck squamous cell carcinoma cell lines with vastly different radiosensitivities. Int J Radiat Oncol Biol Phys 29(2):243–247

32. Balaban N, Moni J, Shannon M, Dang L, Murphy E, Goldkorn T (1996) The effect of ionizing radiation on signal transduction: antibodies to EGF receptor sensitize A431 cells to radiation. Biochim Biophys Acta 1314(1-2):147–156

33. Sheridan MT, O'Dwyer T, Seymour CB, Mothersill CE (1997) Potential indicators of radiosensitivity in squamous cell carcinoma of the head and neck. Radiat Oncol Investig 5(4):180–186. doi:10.1002/(SICI)1520-6823(1997)5:4<180::AID-ROI3>3.0.CO;2-U

34. Milas L, Fan Z, Andratschke NH, Ang KK (2004) Epidermal growth factor receptor and tumor response to radiation: in vivo preclinical studies. Int J Radiat Oncol Biol Phys 58(3):966–971. doi:10.1016/j.ijrobp.2003.08.035

35. Akimoto T, Hunter NR, Buchmiller L, Mason K, Ang KK, Milas L (1999) Inverse relationship between epidermal growth factor receptor expression and radiocurability of murine carcinomas. Clin Cancer Res 5(10):2884–2890

36. Ang KK, Berkey BA, Tu X, Zhang HZ, Katz R, Hammond EH, Fu KK, Milas L (2002) Impact of epidermal growth factor receptor expression on survival and pattern of relapse in patients with advanced head and neck carcinoma. Cancer Res 62(24):7350–7356

37. Goldkorn T, Balaban N, Shannon M, Matsukuma K (1997) EGF receptor phosphorylation is affected by ionizing radiation. Biochim Biophys Acta 1358(3):289–299

38. Contessa JN, Hampton J, Lammering G, Mikkelsen RB, Dent P, Valerie K, Schmidt-Ullrich RK (2002) Ionizing radiation activates Erb-B receptor dependent Akt and p70 S6 kinase signaling in carcinoma cells. Oncogene 21(25):4032–4041. doi:10.1038/sj.onc.1205500

39. Lammering G, Hewit TH, Hawkins WT, Contessa JN, Reardon DB, Lin PS, Valerie K, Dent P, Mikkelsen RB, Schmidt-Ullrich RK (2001) Epidermal growth factor receptor as a genetic therapy target for carcinoma cell radiosensitization. J Natl Cancer Inst 93(12):921–929

40. Huang SM, Bock JM, Harari PM (1999) Epidermal growth factor receptor blockade with C225 modulates proliferation, apoptosis, and radiosensitivity in squamous cell carcinomas of the head and neck. Cancer Res 59(8):1935–1940

41. Gan HK, Burgess AW, Clayton AH, Scott AM (2012) Targeting of a conformationally exposed, tumor-specific epitope of EGFR as a strategy for cancer therapy. Cancer Res 72(12):2924–2930. doi:10.1158/0008-5472.CAN-11-3898

42. ClinicalTrials.gov [database on the Internet] (2000) National Library of Medicine (US). National Library of Medicine (US), Bethesda, MD. Available via National Library of Medicine (US). http://clinicaltrials.gov/. Accessed 1 Aug 2015

43. Hatanpaa KJ, Burma S, Zhao D, Habib AA (2010) Epidermal growth factor receptor in glioma: signal transduction, neuropathology, imaging, and radioresistance. Neoplasia 12(9):675–684

44. Raben D, Helfrich B, Bunn PA Jr (2004) Targeted therapies for non-small-cell lung cancer: biology, rationale, and preclinical results from a radiation oncology perspective. Int J Radiat Oncol Biol Phys 59(2 Suppl):27–38. doi:10.1016/j.ijrobp.2004.01.054

45. Rao GS, Murray S, Ethier SP (2000) Radiosensitization of human breast cancer cells by a novel ErbB family receptor tyrosine kinase inhibitor. Int J Radiat Oncol Biol Phys 48(5):1519–1528

46. Krause M, Schutze C, Petersen C, Pimentel N, Hessel F, Harstrick A, Baumann M (2005) Different classes of EGFR inhibitors may have different potential to improve local tumour control after fractionated irradiation: a study on C225 in FaDu hSCC. Radiother Oncol 74(2):109–115. doi:10.1016/j.radonc.2004.10.011

47. Solomon B, Hagekyriakou J, Trivett MK, Stacker SA, McArthur GA, Cullinane C (2003) EGFR blockade with ZD1839 ("Iressa") potentiates the antitumor effects of single and multiple fractions of ionizing radiation in human A431 squamous cell carcinoma. Epidermal growth factor receptor. Int J Radiat Oncol Biol Phys 55(3):713–723

48. Shintani S, Li C, Mihara M, Terakado N, Yano J, Nakashiro K, Hamakawa H (2003) Enhancement of tumor radioresponse by combined treatment with gefitinib (Iressa, ZD1839), an epidermal growth factor receptor tyrosine kinase inhibitor, is accompanied by inhibition of DNA damage repair and cell growth in oral cancer. Int J Cancer 107(6):1030–1037. doi:10.1002/ijc.11437

49. Cuneo KC, Nyati MK, Ray D, Lawrence TS (2015) EGFR targeted therapies and radiation: Optimizing efficacy by appropriate drug scheduling and patient selection. Pharmacol Ther. doi:10.1016/j.pharmthera.2015.07.002

50. Bonner JA, Harari PM, Giralt J, Azarnia N, Shin DM, Cohen RB, Jones CU, Sur R, Raben D, Jassem J, Ove R, Kies MS, Baselga J, Youssoufian H, Amellal N, Rowinsky EK, Ang KK (2006) Radiotherapy plus cetuximab for squamous-cell carcinoma of the head and neck. N Engl J Med 354(6):567–578. doi:10.1056/NEJMoa053422

51. Ang KK, Zhang Q, Rosenthal DI, Nguyen-Tan PF, Sherman EJ, Weber RS, Galvin JM, Bonner JA, Harris J, El-Naggar AK, Gillison ML, Jordan RC, Konski AA, Thorstad WL, Trotti A, Beitler JJ, Garden AS, Spanos WJ, Yom SS, Axelrod RS (2014) Randomized phase III trial of concurrent accelerated radiation plus cisplatin with or without cetuximab for stage III to IV head and neck carcinoma: RTOG 0522. J Clin Oncol 32(27):2940–2950. doi:10.1200/JCO.2013.53.5633

52. Bradley JD, Paulus R, Komaki R, Masters G, Blumenschein G, Schild S, Bogart J, Hu C, Forster K, Magliocco A, Kavadi V, Garces YI, Narayan S, Iyengar P, Robinson C, Wynn RB, Koprowski C, Meng J, Beitler J, Gaur R, Curran W Jr, Choy H (2015) Standard-dose versus high-dose conformal radiotherapy with concurrent and consolidation carboplatin plus paclitaxel with or without cetuximab for patients with stage IIIA or IIIB non-small-cell lung cancer (RTOG 0617): a randomised, two-by-two factorial phase 3 study. Lancet Oncol 16(2):187–199. doi:10.1016/S1470-2045(14)71207-0

53. Riaz N, Sherman EJ, Fury M, Lee N (2013) Should cetuximab replace Cisplatin for definitive chemoradiotherapy in locally advanced head and neck cancer? J Clin Oncol 31(2):287–288. doi:10.1200/JCO.2012.46.9049

54. Elie C, Geay JF, Morcos M, Le Tourneau A, Girre V, Broet P, Marmey B, Chauvenet L, Audouin J, Pujade-Lauraine E, Camilleri-Broet S (2004) Lack of relationship between EGFR-1 immunohistochemical expression and prognosis in a multicentre clinical trial of 93 patients with advanced primary ovarian epithelial cancer (GINECO group). Br J Cancer 91(3):470–475. doi:10.1038/sj.bjc.6601961

55. Chung KY, Shia J, Kemeny NE, Shah M, Schwartz GK, Tse A, Hamilton A, Pan D, Schrag D, Schwartz L, Klimstra DS, Fridman D, Kelsen DP, Saltz LB (2005) Cetuximab shows activity in colorectal cancer patients with tumors that do not express the epidermal growth factor receptor by immunohistochemistry. J Clin Oncol 23(9):1803–1810. doi:10.1200/JCO.2005.08.037

56. Ferrara N, Gerber HP, LeCouter J (2003) The biology of VEGF and its receptors. Nat Med 9(6):669–676. doi:10.1038/nm0603-669

57. Goel HL, Mercurio AM (2013) VEGF targets the tumour cell. Nat Rev Cancer 13(12):871–882. doi:10.1038/nrc3627

58. Kabbinavar F, Hurwitz HI, Fehrenbacher L, Meropol NJ, Novotny WF, Lieberman G, Griffing S, Bergsland E (2003) Phase II, randomized trial comparing bevacizumab plus fluorouracil (FU)/leucovorin (LV) with FU/LV alone in patients with metastatic colorectal cancer. J Clin Oncol 21(1):60–65

59. Ferrara N, Hillan KJ, Gerber HP, Novotny W (2004) Discovery and development of bevacizumab, an anti-VEGF antibody for treating cancer. Nat Rev Drug Discov 3(5):391–400. doi:10.1038/nrd1381

60. O'Reilly MS (2006) Radiation combined with antiangiogenic and antivascular agents. Semin Radiat Oncol 16(1):45–50. doi:10.1016/j.semradonc.2005.08.006

61. Teicher BA, Dupuis N, Kusomoto T, Robinson MF, Liu F, Menon K, Coleman CN (1994) Antiangiogenic agents can increase tumor oxygenation and response to radiation therapy. Radiat Oncol Investig 2(6):269–276

62. Wachsberger PR, Lawrence YR, Liu Y, Daroczi B, Xu X, Dicker AP (2012) Epidermal growth factor receptor expression modulates antitumor efficacy of vandetanib or cediranib combined with radiotherapy in human glioblastoma xenografts. Int J Radiat Oncol Biol Phys 82(1):483–491. doi:10.1016/j.ijrobp.2010.09.019

63. Mauceri HJ, Hanna NN, Beckett MA, Gorski DH, Staba MJ, Stellato KA, Bigelow K, Heimann R, Gately S, Dhanabal M, Soff GA, Sukhatme VP, Kufe DW, Weichselbaum RR (1998) Combined effects of angiostatin and ionizing radiation in antitumour therapy. Nature 394(6690):287–291. doi:10.1038/28412

64. Gorski DH, Beckett MA, Jaskowiak NT, Calvin DP, Mauceri HJ, Salloum RM, Seetharam S, Koons A, Hari DM, Kufe DW, Weichselbaum RR (1999) Blockage of the vascular endothelial growth factor stress response increases the antitumor effects of ionizing radiation. Cancer Res 59(14):3374–3378

65. Wachsberger P, Burd R, Dicker AP (2003) Tumor response to ionizing radiation combined with antiangiogenesis or vascular targeting agents: exploring mechanisms of interaction. Clin Cancer Res 9(6):1957–1971

66. Kozin SV, Boucher Y, Hicklin DJ, Bohlen P, Jain RK, Suit HD (2001) Vascular endothelial growth factor receptor-2-blocking antibody potentiates radiation-induced long-term control of human tumor xenografts. Cancer Res 61(1):39–44

67. Winkler F, Kozin SV, Tong RT, Chae SS, Booth MF, Garkavtsev I, Xu L, Hicklin DJ, Fukumura D, di Tomaso E, Munn LL, Jain RK (2004) Kinetics of vascular normalization by VEGFR2 blockade governs brain tumor response to radiation: role of oxygenation, angiopoietin-1, and matrix metalloproteinases. Cancer Cell 6(6):553–563. doi:10.1016/j.ccr.2004.10.011

68. Jain RK (2001) Normalizing tumor vasculature with anti-angiogenic therapy: a new paradigm for combination therapy. Nat Med 7(9):987–989. doi:10.1038/nm0901-987

69. Searle EJ, Illidge TM, Stratford IJ (2014) Emerging opportunities for the combination of molecularly targeted drugs with radiotherapy. Clin Oncol (R Coll Radiol) 26(5):266–276. doi:10.1016/j.clon.2014.02.006

70. Gilbert MR, Dignam JJ, Armstrong TS, Wefel JS, Blumenthal DT, Vogelbaum MA, Colman H, Chakravarti A, Pugh S, Won M, Jeraj R, Brown PD, Jaeckle KA, Schiff D, Stieber VW, Brachman DG, Werner-Wasik M, Tremont-Lukats IW, Sulman EP, Aldape KD, Curran WJ Jr, Mehta MP (2014) A randomized trial of bevacizumab for newly diagnosed glioblastoma. N Engl J Med 370(8):699–708. doi:10.1056/NEJMoa1308573

71. Chinot OL, Wick W, Mason W, Henriksson R, Saran F, Nishikawa R, Carpentier AF, Hoang-Xuan K, Kavan P, Cernea D, Brandes AA, Hilton M, Abrey L, Cloughesy T (2014) Bevacizumab plus radiotherapy-temozolomide for newly diagnosed glioblastoma. N Engl J Med 370(8):709–722. doi:10.1056/NEJMoa1308345

72. Jain RK, Duda DG, Clark JW, Loeffler JS (2006) Lessons from phase III clinical trials on anti-VEGF therapy for cancer. Nat Clin Pract Oncol 3(1):24–40. doi:10.1038/ncponc0403

73. Dietrich J, Wang D, Batchelor TT (2009) Cediranib: profile of a novel anti-angiogenic agent in patients with glioblastoma. Expert Opin Investig Drugs 18(10):1549–1557. doi:10.1517/13543780903183528

74. Holderfield MT, Hughes CC (2008) Crosstalk between vascular endothelial growth factor, notch, and transforming growth factor-beta in vascular morphogenesis. Circ Res 102(6):637–652. doi:10.1161/CIRCRESAHA.107.167171

75. Birchmeier C, Birchmeier W, Gherardi E, Vande Woude GF (2003) Met, metastasis, motility and more. Nat Rev Mol Cell Biol 4(12):915–925. doi:10.1038/nrm1261

76. Ponzetto C, Bardelli A, Zhen Z, Maina F, dalla Zonca P, Giordano S, Graziani A, Panayotou G, Comoglio PM (1994) A multifunctional docking site mediates signaling and transformation by the hepatocyte growth factor/scatter factor receptor family. Cell 77 (2):261–271

77. Bhardwaj V, Cascone T, Cortez MA, Amini A, Evans J, Komaki RU, Heymach JV, Welsh JW (2013) Modulation of c-Met signaling and cellular sensitivity to radiation: potential implications for therapy. Cancer 119(10):1768–1775. doi:10.1002/cncr.27965

78. Sipeki S, Bander E, Buday L, Farkas G, Bacsy E, Ways DK, Farago A (1999) Phosphatidylinositol 3-kinase contributes to Erk1/Erk2 MAP kinase activation associated with hepatocyte growth factor-induced cell scattering. Cell Signal 11(12):885–890

79. Stoker M, Gherardi E, Perryman M, Gray J (1987) Scatter factor is a fibroblast-derived modulator of epithelial cell mobility. Nature 327(6119):239–242. doi:10.1038/327239a0

80. Rosen EM, Knesel J, Goldberg ID, Jin L, Bhargava M, Joseph A, Zitnik R, Wines J, Kelley M, Rockwell S (1994) Scatter factor modulates the metastatic phenotype of the EMT6 mouse mammary tumor. Int J Cancer 57(5):706–714

81. Sonnenberg E, Meyer D, Weidner KM, Birchmeier C (1993) Scatter factor/hepatocyte growth factor and its receptor, the c-met tyrosine kinase, can mediate a signal exchange between mesenchyme and epithelia during mouse development. J Cell Biol 123(1):223–235

82. Santos OF, Barros EJ, Yang XM, Matsumoto K, Nakamura T, Park M, Nigam SK (1994) Involvement of hepatocyte growth factor in kidney development. Dev Biol 163(2):525–529. doi:10.1006/dbio.1994.1169

83. Raghav KP, Wang W, Liu S, Chavez-MacGregor M, Meng X, Hortobagyi GN, Mills GB, Meric-Bernstam F, Blumenschein GR Jr, Gonzalez-Angulo AM (2012) cMET and phospho-cMET protein levels in breast cancers and survival outcomes. Clin Cancer Res 18(8):2269–2277. doi:10.1158/1078-0432.CCR-11-2830

84. Moriyama T, Kataoka H, Koono M, Wakisaka S (1999) Expression of hepatocyte growth factor/scatter factor and its receptor c-Met in brain tumors: evidence for a role in progression of astrocytic tumors (Review). Int J Mol Med 3(5):531–536

85. Koochekpour S, Jeffers M, Rulong S, Taylor G, Klineberg E, Hudson EA, Resau JH, Vande Woude GF (1997) Met and hepatocyte growth factor/scatter factor expression in human gliomas. Cancer Res 57(23):5391–5398

86. Inno A, Di Salvatore M, Cenci T, Martini M, Orlandi A, Strippoli A, Ferrara AM, Bagala C, Cassano A, Larocca LM, Barone C (2011) Is there a role for IGF1R and c-MET pathways in resistance to cetuximab in metastatic colorectal cancer? Clin Colorectal Cancer 10(4):325–332. doi:10.1016/j.clcc.2011.03.028

87. Cheng TL, Chang MY, Huang SY, Sheu CC, Kao EL, Cheng YJ, Chong IW (2005) Overexpression of circulating c-met messenger RNA is significantly correlated with nodal stage and early recurrence in non-small cell lung cancer. Chest 128(3):1453–1460. doi: 10.1378/chest.128.3.1453

88. Maulik G, Kijima T, Ma PC, Ghosh SK, Lin J, Shapiro GI, Schaefer E, Tibaldi E, Johnson BE, Salgia R (2002) Modulation of the c-Met/hepatocyte growth factor pathway in small cell lung cancer. Clin Cancer Res 8(2):620–627

89. Masuya D, Huang C, Liu D, Nakashima T, Kameyama K, Haba R, Ueno M, Yokomise H (2004) The tumour-stromal interaction between intratumoral c-Met and stromal hepatocyte growth factor associated with tumour growth and prognosis in non-small-cell lung cancer patients. Br J Cancer 90(8):1555–1562. doi:10.1038/sj.bjc.6601718

90. Nakamura Y, Niki T, Goto A, Morikawa T, Miyazawa K, Nakajima J, Fukayama M (2007) c-Met activation in lung adenocarcinoma tissues: an immunohistochemical analysis. Cancer Sci 98(7):1006–1013. doi:10.1111/j.1349-7006.2007.00493.x

91. Liu Y, Li Q, Zhu L (2012) Expression of the hepatocyte growth factor and c-Met in colon cancer: correlation with clinicopathological features and overall survival. Tumori 98(1):105–112. doi:10.1700/1053.11508

92. Fan S, Wang JA, Yuan RQ, Rockwell S, Andres J, Zlatapolskiy A, Goldberg ID, Rosen EM (1998) Scatter factor protects epithelial and carcinoma cells against apoptosis induced by DNA-damaging agents. Oncogene 17(2):131–141. doi:10.1038/sj.onc.1201943

93. Fan S, Ma YX, Wang JA, Yuan RQ, Meng Q, Cao Y, Laterra JJ, Goldberg ID, Rosen EM (2000) The cytokine hepatocyte growth factor/scatter factor inhibits apoptosis and enhances DNA repair by a common mechanism involving signaling through phosphatidyl inositol 3' kinase. Oncogene 19(18):2212–2223. doi:10.1038/sj.onc.1203566

94. Aebersold DM, Kollar A, Beer KT, Laissue J, Greiner RH, Djonov V (2001) Involvement of the hepatocyte growth factor/scatter factor receptor c-met and of Bcl-xL in the resistance of oropharyngeal cancer to ionizing radiation. Int J Cancer 96(1):41–54

95. De Bacco F, Luraghi P, Medico E, Reato G, Girolami F, Perera T, Gabriele P, Comoglio PM, Boccaccio C (2011) Induction of MET by ionizing radiation and its role in radioresistance and invasive growth of cancer. J Natl Cancer Inst 103(8):645–661. doi:10.1093/jnci/djr093

96. Qian LW, Mizumoto K, Inadome N, Nagai E, Sato N, Matsumoto K, Nakamura T, Tanaka M (2003) Radiation stimulates HGF receptor/c-Met expression that leads to amplifying cellular response to HGF stimulation via upregulated receptor tyrosine phosphorylation and MAP kinase activity in pancreatic cancer cells. Int J Cancer 104(5):542–549. doi:10.1002/ijc.10997

97. Sheng-Hua C, Yan-Bin M, Zhi-An Z, Hong Z, Dong-Fu F, Zhi-Qiang L, Xian-Hou Y (2007) Radiation-enhanced hepatocyte growth factor secretion in malignant glioma cell lines. Surg Neurol 68(6):610–613. doi:10.1016/j.surneu.2006.12.050, discussion 613-614

98. Schweigerer L, Rave-Frank M, Schmidberger H, Hecht M (2005) Sublethal irradiation promotes invasiveness of neuroblastoma cells. Biochem Biophys Res Commun 330(3):982–988. doi:10.1016/j.bbrc.2005.03.068

99. Welsh JW, Mahadevan D, Ellsworth R, Cooke L, Bearss D, Stea B (2009) The c-Met receptor tyrosine kinase inhibitor MP470 radiosensitizes glioblastoma cells. Radiat Oncol 4:69. doi: 10.1186/1748-717X-4-69

100. Medova M, Aebersold DM, Blank-Liss W, Streit B, Medo M, Aebi S, Zimmer Y (2010) MET inhibition results in DNA breaks and synergistically sensitizes tumor cells to DNA-damaging agents potentially by breaching a damage-induced checkpoint arrest. Genes Cancer 1(10): 1053–1062. doi:10.1177/1947601910388030

101. Yu H, Li X, Sun S, Gao X, Zhou D (2012) c-Met inhibitor SU11274 enhances the response of the prostate cancer cell line DU145 to ionizing radiation. Biochem Biophys Res Commun 427(3):659–665. doi:10.1016/j.bbrc.2012.09.117

102. Li B, Torossian A, Sun Y, Du R, Dicker AP, Lu B (2012) Higher levels of c-Met expression and phosphorylation identify cell lines with increased sensitivity to AMG-458, a novel selec-

tive c-Met inhibitor with radiosensitizing effects. Int J Radiat Oncol Biol Phys 84(4):e525–e531. doi:10.1016/j.ijrobp.2012.06.025

103. Lin CI, Whang EE, Donner DB, Du J, Lorch J, He F, Jiang X, Price BD, Moore FD Jr, Ruan DT (2010) Autophagy induction with RAD001 enhances chemosensitivity and radiosensitivity through Met inhibition in papillary thyroid cancer. Mol Can Res 8(9):1217–1226. doi:10.1158/1541-7786.MCR-10-0162

104. Buchanan IM, Scott T, Tandle AT, Burgan WE, Burgess TL, Tofilon PJ, Camphausen K (2011) Radiosensitization of glioma cells by modulation of Met signalling with the hepatocyte growth factor neutralizing antibody, AMG102. J Cell Mol Med 15(9):1999–2006. doi:10.1111/j.1582-4934.2010.01122.x

105. Lal B, Xia S, Abounader R, Laterra J (2005) Targeting the c-Met pathway potentiates glioblastoma responses to gamma-radiation. Clin Cancer Res 11(12):4479–4486. doi:10.1158/1078-0432.CCR-05-0166

106. Peters S, Adjei AA (2012) MET: a promising anticancer therapeutic target. Nat Rev Clin Oncol 9(6):314–326. doi:10.1038/nrclinonc.2012.71

107. Liu JP, Baker J, Perkins AS, Robertson EJ, Efstratiadis A (1993) Mice carrying null mutations of the genes encoding insulin-like growth factor I (Igf-1) and type 1 IGF receptor (Igf1r). Cell 75(1):59–72

108. Jacobs CI (2008) A review of the role of insulin-like growth factor 2 in malignancy and its potential as a modifier of radiation sensitivity. Clin Oncol (R Coll Radiol) 20(5):345–352. doi:10.1016/j.clon.2008.02.004

109. Samani AA, Yakar S, LeRoith D, Brodt P (2007) The role of the IGF system in cancer growth and metastasis: overview and recent insights. Endocr Rev 28(1):20–47. doi:10.1210/er.2006-0001

110. Turner BC, Haffty BG, Narayanan L, Yuan J, Havre PA, Gumbs AA, Kaplan L, Burgaud JL, Carter D, Baserga R, Glazer PM (1997) Insulin-like growth factor-I receptor overexpression mediates cellular radioresistance and local breast cancer recurrence after lumpectomy and radiation. Cancer Res 57(15):3079–3083

111. Riesterer O, Yang Q, Raju U, Torres M, Molkentine D, Patel N, Valdecanas D, Milas L, Ang KK (2011) Combination of anti-IGF-1R antibody A12 and ionizing radiation in upper respiratory tract cancers. Int J Radiat Oncol Biol Phys 79(4):1179–1187. doi:10.1016/j.ijrobp.2010.10.003

112. Allen GW, Saba C, Armstrong EA, Huang SM, Benavente S, Ludwig DL, Hicklin DJ, Harari PM (2007) Insulin-like growth factor-I receptor signaling blockade combined with radiation. Cancer Res 67(3):1155–1162. doi:10.1158/0008-5472.CAN-06-2000

113. Chitnis MM, Lodhia KA, Aleksic T, Gao S, Protheroe AS, Macaulay VM (2014) IGF-1R inhibition enhances radiosensitivity and delays double-strand break repair by both non-homologous end-joining and homologous recombination. Oncogene 33(45):5262–5273. doi:10.1038/onc.2013.460

114. Jin Q, Esteva FJ (2008) Cross-talk between the ErbB/HER family and the type I insulin-like growth factor receptor signaling pathway in breast cancer. J Mammary Gland Biol Neoplasia 13(4):485–498. doi:10.1007/s10911-008-9107-3

115. Jones HE, Dutkowski CM, Barrow D, Harper ME, Wakeling AE, Nicholson RI (1997) New EGF-R selective tyrosine kinase inhibitor reveals variable growth responses in prostate carcinoma cell lines PC-3 and DU-145. Int J Cancer 71(6):1010–1018

116. Li P, Veldwijk MR, Zhang Q, Li ZB, Xu WC, Fu S (2013) Co-inhibition of epidermal growth factor receptor and insulin-like growth factor receptor 1 enhances radiosensitivity in human breast cancer cells. BMC Cancer 13:297. doi:10.1186/1471-2407-13-297

117. Slamon DJ, Clark GM, Wong SG, Levin WJ, Ullrich A, McGuire WL (1987) Human breast cancer: correlation of relapse and survival with amplification of the HER-2/neu oncogene. Science 235(4785):177–182

118. Janjigian YY, Werner D, Pauligk C, Steinmetz K, Kelsen DP, Jager E, Altmannsberger HM, Robinson E, Tafe LJ, Tang LH, Shah MA, Al-Batran SE (2012) Prognosis of metastatic gas-

tric and gastroesophageal junction cancer by HER2 status: a European and USA International collaborative analysis. Ann Oncol 23(10):2656–2662. doi:10.1093/annonc/mds104

119. Hong TS, Wo JY, Kwak EL (2013) Targeted therapies with chemoradiation in esophageal cancer: development and future directions. Semin Radiat Oncol 23(1):31–37. doi:10.1016/j.semradonc.2012.09.004

120. Pietras RJ, Poen JC, Gallardo D, Wongvipat PN, Lee HJ, Slamon DJ (1999) Monoclonal antibody to HER-2/neuroreceptor modulates repair of radiation-induced DNA damage and enhances radiosensitivity of human breast cancer cells overexpressing this oncogene. Cancer Res 59(6):1347–1355

121. Sambade MJ, Camp JT, Kimple RJ, Sartor CI, Shields JM (2009) Mechanism of lapatinib-mediated radiosensitization of breast cancer cells is primarily by inhibition of the Raf>MEK>ERK mitogen-activated protein kinase cascade and radiosensitization of lapatinib-resistant cells restored by direct inhibition of MEK. Radiother Oncol 93(3):639–644. doi:10.1016/j.radonc.2009.09.006

122. Kimple RJ, Vaseva AV, Cox AD, Baerman KM, Calvo BF, Tepper JE, Shields JM, Sartor CI (2010) Radiosensitization of epidermal growth factor receptor/HER2-positive pancreatic cancer is mediated by inhibition of Akt independent of ras mutational status. Clin Cancer Res 16(3):912–923. doi:10.1158/1078-0432.CCR-09-1324

123. Sambade MJ, Kimple RJ, Camp JT, Peters E, Livasy CA, Sartor CI, Shields JM (2010) Lapatinib in combination with radiation diminishes tumor regrowth in HER2+ and basal-like/EGFR+ breast tumor xenografts. Int J Radiat Oncol Biol Phys 77(2):575–581. doi:10.1016/j.ijrobp.2009.12.063

124. Safran H, Dipetrillo T, Akerman P, Ng T, Evans D, Steinhoff M, Benton D, Purviance J, Goldstein L, Tantravahi U, Kennedy T (2007) Phase I/II study of trastuzumab, paclitaxel, cisplatin and radiation for locally advanced, HER2 overexpressing, esophageal adenocarcinoma. Int J Radiat Oncol Biol Phys 67(2):405–409. doi:10.1016/j.ijrobp.2006.08.076

125. Perez EA, Romond EH, Suman VJ, Jeong JH, Davidson NE, Geyer CE Jr, Martino S, Mamounas EP, Kaufman PA, Wolmark N (2011) Four-year follow-up of trastuzumab plus adjuvant chemotherapy for operable human epidermal growth factor receptor 2-positive breast cancer: joint analysis of data from NCCTG N9831 and NSABP B-31. J Clin Oncol 29(25):3366–3373. doi:10.1200/JCO.2011.35.0868

126. Turner N, Grose R (2010) Fibroblast growth factor signalling: from development to cancer. Nat Rev Cancer 10(2):116–129. doi:10.1038/nrc2780

127. Eswarakumar VP, Lax I, Schlessinger J (2005) Cellular signaling by fibroblast growth factor receptors. Cytokine Growth Factor Rev 16(2):139–149. doi:10.1016/j.cytogfr.2005.01.001

128. Cappellen D, De Oliveira C, Ricol D, de Medina S, Bourdin J, Sastre-Garau X, Chopin D, Thiery JP, Radvanyi F (1999) Frequent activating mutations of FGFR3 in human bladder and cervix carcinomas. Nat Genet 23(1):18–20. doi:10.1038/12615

129. Dutt A, Salvesen HB, Chen TH, Ramos AH, Onofrio RC, Hatton C, Nicoletti R, Winckler W, Grewal R, Hanna M, Wyhs N, Ziaugra L, Richter DJ, Trovik J, Engelsen IB, Stefansson IM, Fennell T, Cibulskis K, Zody MC, Akslen LA, Gabriel S, Wong KK, Sellers WR, Meyerson M, Greulich H (2008) Drug-sensitive FGFR2 mutations in endometrial carcinoma. Proc Natl Acad Sci U S A 105(25):8713–8717. doi:10.1073/pnas.0803379105

130. Weiss J, Sos ML, Seidel D, Peifer M, Zander T, Heuckmann JM, Ullrich RT, Menon R, Maier S, Soltermann A, Moch H, Wagener P, Fischer F, Heynck S, Koker M, Schottle J, Leenders F, Gabler F, Dabow I, Querings S, Heukamp LC, Balke-Want H, Ansen S, Rauh D, Baessmann I, Altmuller J, Wainer Z, Conron M, Wright G, Russell P, Solomon B, Brambilla E, Brambilla C, Lorimier P, Sollberg S, Brustugun OT, Engel-Riedel W, Ludwig C, Petersen I, Sanger J, Clement J, Groen H, Timens W, Sietsma H, Thunnissen E, Smit E, Heideman D, Cappuzzo F, Ligorio C, Damiani S, Hallek M, Beroukhim R, Pao W, Klebl B, Baumann M, Buettner R, Ernestus K, Stoelben E, Wolf J, Nurnberg P, Perner S, Thomas RK (2010) Frequent and focal FGFR1 amplification associates with therapeutically tractable FGFR1 dependency in squamous cell lung cancer. Sci Transl Med 2(62):62ra93. doi:10.1126/scitranslmed.3001451

131. Colvin JS, Bohne BA, Harding GW, McEwen DG, Ornitz DM (1996) Skeletal overgrowth and deafness in mice lacking fibroblast growth factor receptor 3. Nat Genet 12(4):390–397. doi:10.1038/ng0496-390
132. Brooks AN, Kilgour E, Smith PD (2012) Molecular pathways: fibroblast growth factor signaling: a new therapeutic opportunity in cancer. Clin Cancer Res 18(7):1855–1862. doi: 10.1158/1078-0432.CCR-11-0699
133. Cazet A, Charest J, Bennett DC, Sambrooks CL, Contessa JN (2014) Mannose phosphate isomerase regulates fibroblast growth factor receptor family signaling and glioma radiosensitivity. PLoS One 9(10), e110345. doi:10.1371/journal.pone.0110345
134. Fuks Z, Persaud RS, Alfieri A, McLoughlin M, Ehleiter D, Schwartz JL, Seddon AP, Cordon-Cardo C, Haimovitz-Friedman A (1994) Basic fibroblast growth factor protects endothelial cells against radiation-induced programmed cell death in vitro and in vivo. Cancer Res 54(10):2582–2590
135. Gu Q, Wang D, Wang X, Peng R, Liu J, Jiang T, Wang Z, Wang S, Deng H (2004) Basic fibroblast growth factor inhibits radiation-induced apoptosis of HUVECs. I. The PI3K/AKT pathway and induction of phosphorylation of BAD. Radiat Res 161(6):692–702
136. Ader I, Toulas C, Dalenc F, Delmas C, Bonnet J, Cohen-Jonathan E, Favre G (2002) RhoB controls the 24 kDa FGF-2-induced radioresistance in HeLa cells by preventing post-mitotic cell death. Oncogene 21(39):5998–6006. doi:10.1038/sj.onc.1205746
137. Ader I, Delmas C, Skuli N, Bonnet J, Schaeffer P, Bono F, Cohen-Jonathan-Moyal E, Toulas C (2014) Preclinical evidence that SSR128129E--a novel small-molecule multi-fibroblast growth factor receptor blocker--radiosensitises human glioblastoma. Eur J Cancer 50(13):2351–2359. doi:10.1016/j.ejca.2014.05.012
138. Hsu HW, Wall NR, Hsueh CT, Kim S, Ferris RL, Chen CS, Mirshahidi S (2014) Combination antiangiogenic therapy and radiation in head and neck cancers. Oral Oncol 50(1):19–26. doi:10.1016/j.oraloncology.2013.10.003
139. Lopez-Chavez A, Carter CA, Giaccone G (2009) The role of KRAS mutations in resistance to EGFR inhibition in the treatment of cancer. Curr Opin Investig Drugs 10(12):1305–1314
140. Bennett DC, Charest J, Sebolt K, Lehrman M, Rehemtulla A, Contessa JN (2013) High-throughput screening identifies aclacinomycin as a radiosensitizer of EGFR-mutant non-small cell lung cancer. Transl Oncol 6(3):382–391
141. Mellinghoff IK, Wang MY, Vivanco I, Haas-Kogan DA, Zhu S, Dia EQ, Lu KV, Yoshimoto K, Huang JH, Chute DJ, Riggs BL, Horvath S, Liau LM, Cavenee WK, Rao PN, Beroukhim R, Peck TC, Lee JC, Sellers WR, Stokoe D, Prados M, Cloughesy TF, Sawyers CL, Mischel PS (2005) Molecular determinants of the response of glioblastomas to EGFR kinase inhibitors. N Engl J Med 353(19):2012–2024. doi:10.1056/NEJMoa051918

Chapter 3
Histone Deacetylase Inhibitors and Tumor Radiosensitization

Elizabeth I. Spehalski, Philip J. Tofilon, and Kevin Camphausen

Abstract Current strategies to increase the radiosensitivity of tumor cells have focused on the molecules and pathways that regulate response to radiation at the cellular level. One group of processes that is generating considerable interest is the modification of DNA histones, with a particular focus on the inhibition of histone acetylation. Histone acetylation is the process by which an acetyl group is covalently affixed to lysine residues within the N-terminus of histone proteins. Acetylation levels are determined by the opposing actions of two families of enzymes: histone acetyltransferases (HATs) and histone deacetylases (HDACs). HDACs function to regulate both chromatin structure and gene expression, two factors that are important in determining the response of tumors to radiation. In an attempt to alter the histone acetylation status of cells, considerable efforts at the development of inhibitors of HDAC activity have occurred. The result is the development of a large and structurally diverse number of compounds that are able to inhibit HDAC activity, leading to the hyperacetylation of histones. In preclinical studies, these compounds have been found to enhance the in vitro and in vivo radiosensitivity of a spectrum of human tumor lines. Although the mechanism of HDAC inhibitor-induced radiosensitization has not been fully elucidated, HDAC inhibitors have shown promise in clinical trials when used in combination with chemotherapy and radiation therapy.

Keywords Hyperacetylation • Histone deacetylase • HDAC inhibitors • Tumor radiosensitization

Introduction

Over half of all cancer patients receive radiation treatment during the course of their disease. The American Cancer Society has predicted there will be over 1.7 million cases of cancer diagnosed in the United States in 2016 (www.cancer.org),

E.I. Spehalski • P.J. Tofilon • K. Camphausen (✉)
Radiation Oncology Branch, National Cancer Institute, 10 Center Drive, MSC 1002, Building 10, B3B69B, Bethesda, MD 20892, USA
e-mail: camphauk@mail.nih.gov

© Springer International Publishing Switzerland 2017
P.J. Tofilon, K. Camphausen (eds.), *Increasing the Therapeutic Ratio of Radiotherapy*, Cancer Drug Discovery and Development, DOI 10.1007/978-3-319-40854-5_3

suggesting that a significant number of cancer patients would be positively impacted by the development of strategies that selectively enhance tumor radiosensitivity. Progress in radiation physics and computer technology in the last quarter of the twentieth century allowed for improvements in technological advances in radiation source quality, design, delivery, and study of altered fractionation [1]. In the 1950s, attempts to increase the radiosensitivity of tumors began to focus on combining radiation with standard cytotoxic chemotherapy, with an early focus on using drugs that target rapidly dividing cells [2]. Since that time, chemoradiation modalities have been extensively explored with conflicting levels of success. In some tumor histologies, combination therapy has been extremely effective, while in others it is less so, leading scientists to address the mechanism behind this discrepancy. Thus, current approaches for enhancing radiosensitivity emphasize targeting the molecules and processes that regulate cellular radioresponse, such as cell cycle checkpoints, DNA damage response, and altered death pathways. This approach has resulted in the discovery of a range of molecules have been shown to effect radiosensitivity in one or more experimental tumor models.

Epigenetic modifiers are thus an attractive class of molecularly targeted agents to examine as they can affect cell cycle control and DNA damage response. Epigenetics is the study of changes in gene expression that are caused by external factors such as posttranslational histone modifications, DNA methylation, and chromatin remodeling, rather than changes in the DNA sequence itself. Histones are nuclear proteins that serve two crucial functions in eukaryotic cell nuclei. First, histones are the chief protein component of chromatin, acting as spools around which DNA winds. This enables the compaction of the genome into units called nucleosomes and the organization of the genome into the cell nuclei. In addition to this structural function, histones also undergo posttranslational modifications, which serve to alter their interaction with the DNA and nuclear proteins. These modifications are the basis of the histone-code hypothesis, which posits that chromatin-DNA interactions and, importantly, gene expression are determined by specific combinations of these chemical modifications [3, 4].

The core histones, H2A, H2B, H3, and H4, include an N-terminal tail that protrudes from the histone core of the nucleosome and is covalently modified in multiple places. These modifications include methylation, phosphorylation, ubiquitylation, ADP-ribosylation, SUMOylation, and acetylation. Though this chapter will mainly focus on histone acetylation, it is well established that posttranslational histone modifications can be radically altered during neoplastic development and consequently may be a target for tumor radiosensitization [5]. For example, several tumor histologies show widespread changes in histone methylation patterns, including the methylation of histone H3 on lysine 27. The histone methyltransferase (HMT) responsible for this modification, EZH2, has been found to be overexpressed in both breast and prostate cancers [6]. An example of an important histone phosphorylation event in tumor biology is the phosphorylation of the histone variant H2AX on serine 139 to form γH2AX [7]. This modification is crucial for many mechanisms of the DNA damage response and is used as a marker of DNA damage in cancer cells. Since DNA double-strand breaks are the primary lesion caused by ionizing radiation, it may be possible to target γH2AX as a radiosensitizing agent [8] or to use γH2AX as a tool to monitor the efficacy of radiation and chemotherapeutics in tissues [9]. Additionally, HDACs are found to be overexpressed in numerous types of cancer [10], while the loss of genome-wide histone H4 acetylation has been attributed to the overexpression of histone deacetylases (HDACs), which results in the repression of many genes, including tumor suppressors.

Because of this, the inhibition of histone-modifying enzymes has generated considerable interest as a potential target for cancer therapy. A large number of compounds with diverse structures and pharmacokinetics are being developed and tested to inhibit histone modifiers for cancer therapy. For example, HDAC inhibitors have been reported to induce tumor cell differentiation, apoptosis, and growth arrest. Importantly, experimental and clinical results suggest that the cytotoxic effects of HDAC inhibitors are tumor selective [11–14].

This chapter will present evidence that inhibition of histone deacetylation is an important strategy for tumor cell radiosensitization, discuss possible mechanisms of HDAC inhibition, and address critical questions that remain to be elucidated in order to make possible the clinical application of HDAC inhibitors as radiosensitizing agents.

Histone Acetylation and Deacetylation

Histone acetylation is closely associated with transcriptional activation and involves the NH_3+ group of conserved lysines of the N-terminal tails. It is mediated by histone acetyltransferases (HATs), which transfer an acetyl group from acetyl coenzyme A to the specific lysine residue of the protein tail. A large number of acetylating proteins have been identified, and they are grouped into families that share homology within the catalytic histone acetyltransferase domain, but little or no other sequence homology. Additionally, besides their ability to acetylate histones, the HAT families share little similarity with each other and can mediate different biological functions.

Deacetylation of histones is likewise modified by a series of histone deacetylases (HDACs). HDACs catalyze the inverse reaction to HATs, removing the acetyl group from the acetyl-lysine residue. Numerous HDACs have been discovered in higher organisms, and they were categorized into three classes. Class I HDACs include HDACs 1, 2, 3, and 8. Class II HDACs are divided into classes IIa (HDAC 4, 5, 7, and 9) and IIb (HDACs 6 and 10) and have the ability to shuttle between the nucleus and the cytoplasm, likely because class IIb proteins have predominantly non-epigenetic functions such as regulation of protein folding and turnover [15, 16]. Class III HDACs (SIRT1-7), also known as sirtuins, share homology with yeast Sir2 and are evolutionarily unrelated to the other classes of HDACs. Mammals also express an additional zinc-dependent HDAC (HDAC 11) that is different than class I, II, and III proteins and is therefore regarded as a separate class (class IV). HDAC activity is summarized in Fig. 3.1.

Histone acetylation typically correlates with an increase in general transcription activity [17] while providing a platform for protein binding. Various transcription

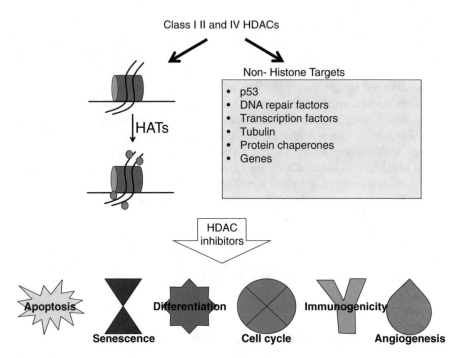

Fig. 3.1 Histone deacetylases are responsible for counteracting the reaction of HATs by removing the acetyl groups from acetyl-lysine residue. However, they also target non-histone proteins that control cellular processes such as cell cycle, DNA repair and gene expression. Thus, inhibitors of HDACs impact a wide range of cellular function

factors contain a bromodomain motif, which can recognize and bind to acetylated lysines on the histone tails [18, 19], serving to activate gene transcription by attracting further transcription complexes. On the contrary, histone deacetylation results in more closely condensed chromatin and the formation of more stable nucleosome interactions, leading to an overall inhibition of transcription [20–22]. Thus, HDACs function as enzymes, removing the acetyl group from a lysine of the histone tail. HDACs can also complex with transcriptional corepressors or protein-modifying enzymes to limit the accessibility of chromatin to transcription factors [23, 24] or to directly switch target transcription factors to their inactive form [25].

Given the effects of histone acetylation on chromatin dynamics, it is unsurprising that it has been implicated in the regulation of DNA repair, which is of utmost importance when considering targets for radiosensitization [26, 27]. The DNA damage response in human cells was first associated with histone acetylation when studies revealed that histones are very rapidly acetylated after ultraviolet radiation (UV) exposure [28]. This hyperacetylation of histones was accompanied by a more rapid repair of the DNA damage caused by the UV, leading to the hypothesis that the relaxing of chromatin initiated by acetylation allows the DNA repair machinery better access to the lesion [29]. The DNA damage caused by UV radiation is primarily thymine dimer formation, which is repaired differently from DNA double-strand breaks, the principal lesion caused by ionizing radiation (IR). As mentioned, one of the first chromatin events upon the formation of a DNA double-strand break in mammalian cells is the phosphorylation of H2AX to form γH2AX [7]. Acetylation of H2AX has also been observed to impact DNA repair after IR-induced DNA damage [30]. For example, the HAT TIP60 has been shown to acetylate H2AX on lysine 5 upon DNA damage [31]. TIP60 activity is regulated by SIRT1 which, when depleted, leads to hyperacetylation of H2AX lysine 5 and defective DNA damage response [32]. Deacetylation of histones has been shown to impact IR-induced DNA repair as well. Depletion of H3 lysine 56 acetylation has been shown to promote the nonhomologous end joining DNA repair pathway following IR [33].

Histone Acetylation and Metabolism

While alterations in global histone modification signatures are a hallmark of cancer, so is the metabolic reprogramming of tumor cells. Normal cells, under conditions of normal nutrient and oxygen levels, will generate energy (ATP) by utilizing the oxidation of pyruvate derived from glucose to carbon dioxide in the mitochondria via the tricarboxylic acid (TCA) cycle and the electron transport chain. In the absence of oxygen, cells are able to continue to produce energy via glycolysis and lactic acid fermentation in the cytosol. Cancer cells, as well as other populations of rapidly proliferating cells, preferentially employ glycolysis and lactic acid fermentation to produce ATP, even in the presence of sufficient levels of oxygen. This phenomenon is known as the Warburg effect, as it was first described by Otto Warburg in 1956 [34]. This process is far less efficient at generating ATP, but it may be advantageous for neoplastic cells to overutilize glycolysis, as it leads to increased biomass.

Interactions between metabolism and epigenetics are only beginning to be explored, but it is not surprising that the two are connected, as most histone-modifying enzymes require a substrate or cofactor that is a metabolic intermediate. Examples of this include the requirement for S-adenosyl methionine (SAM) during the transfer of methyl groups to histones by histone methyltransferases, the Jumanji-containing histone lysine demethylases dependence upon α-ketoglutarate, or the dependence of histone acetyl transferases on acetyl coenzyme A (acetyl-CoA) [35].

Given this relationship between histone acetylation and acetyl-CoA, a natural question to ask is if the levels of acetyl-CoA generated by glycolysis have an impact on chromatin structure and consequently transcription and DNA repair. Experiments have shown that feeding cell's elevated glucose concentrations will increase levels of glycolysis, leading to an increase in cytosolic acetyl-CoA [35], which has been directly linked to histone acetylation [36]. Inversely, depletion of ATP-citrate lyase results in a decrease in histone acetylation [36]. This data suggests that the cytosolic level of acetyl-

CoA produced during glycolysis is an important driver of histone acetylation. Furthermore, Liu and colleagues [37] explored the relationship between metabolism and DNA repair by inhibiting glycolysis using the inhibitor 2-deoxyglucose (2-DG) as well as siRNA against two rate-limiting enzymes in glycolysis (hexokinase I and pyruvate kinase) in a human lung carcinoma cell line. The inhibition of glycolysis in these cells produced a more compact chromatin structure in the nucleus. Since a more condensed chromatin assembly is often associated with histone deacetylation, they examined levels of protein acetylation in these cells and showed that acetylation of multiple lysine sites on histones H3, H4, H2A, and H2B were significantly decreased upon glycolysis inhibition, which was reversible with the addition of an HDAC inhibitor [37]. Furthermore, cells that were treated with inhibitors of glycolysis showed a decrease in DNA repair following treatment with a DNA-damaging agent, presumably because the condensed conformation of the chromatin prevented the DNA repair machinery from accessing the damage [37]. This is not the only study to examine the relationship between metabolism and DNA repair. Efimova and colleagues show that inhibition of glycolysis leads to the persistence of DNA double-strand breaks following DNA damage via ionizing irradiation as well as the acceleration of senescence [38]. Interestingly, this study was also able to show that the disruption of glutaminolysis impaired the DNA damage response of cells. Amplified glutamine uptake in cancer cells is, like glycolysis, thought to occur in order to increase the proliferating cell's demand for biomass. This study indicates that glutamine metabolism, too, may be important for genome repair.

This relationship between glycolytic metabolism and the modulation of histone acetylation has implications for the radiosensitization of cells. We have already established that the DNA damage response and DNA repair mechanisms are of utmost importance when considering the radioresponse of cells and that HATs are key regulators of the DNA damage response as well as transcription. Additional studies have shown that glycolysis inhibition can sensitize cancer cells to DNA-damaging chemotherapeutics and radiation [39, 40]. Taken together, it is clear that targeting HDACs for inhibition could both increase the efficacy of DNA-damaging chemotherapeutics as well as be used as a strategy to preferentially target cells that rely heavily upon glycolysis, such as tumor cells.

Inhibitors of Histone Deacetylation

Aberrant expression of HDACs has been repeatedly demonstrated in human tumors, and certain HDACs (1, 5, and 7) have been shown to act as molecular biomarkers for tumor tissue [41]. Additionally, the overexpression of individual HDACs in several types of cancer correlates with a significant decrease in both disease-free and overall survival in patients and was predictive of poor patient prognosis independent of variables such as tumor type and disease progression [42–45]. Given this, considerable focus has been put into the development of clinically applicable HDAC inhibitors.

While new inhibitors are being generated continually, the most commonly used HDAC inhibitors are divided into general classes based on their chemical structure: hydroxamates, carboxylic acids (also known as short-chain fatty or aliphatic acids), cyclic peptides, aminobenzamides, epoxyketones, and hybrid molecules [46]. The hydroxamic class of HDAC inhibitors includes suberoylanilide hydroxamic acid (SAHA), and trichostatin A (TSA). These compounds chelate zinc in the active site and contain a hydrophobic backbone that spans the active site of the hydrophobic pocket [47]. The carboxylic acids, which include sodium butyrate (NaB) and valproic acid (VPA), target the active site zinc and, due to their smaller size and lack of hydrophobic backbone, are significantly less potent than the hydroxamic acids [48]. The cyclic peptide class contains the drugs depsipeptide, apicidin, and romidepsin; all of which contain a cyclic ring. Aminobenzamides include MS-275 (entinostat), CI-994 (tacedinaline), and mocetinostat and function by attaching to the catalytic zinc ion as well [49]. Epoxyketones, which comprise trapoxins and 2-amino-8-oxo-9,10-epoxydecanoic acid, have an epoxyketone group that binds irreversibly to the catalytic site of the HDAC [50]. The final class, hybrid molecules, includes synthetic combinations of known compounds, specifically hydroxamic-acid-containing peptides having features of both hydroxamic acids and cyclic tetrapeptides [51]. Examples of this are tubacin and CUDC-101 [52].

The earliest inhibitors generated were not specific for a given HDAC but instead show slight preferences to either class I or II [53]. Despite this, current efforts to develop more advanced HDAC inhibitors trend toward isoform-selective deacetylase inhibitors [54]. Illustrations of this include tubacin, which was found to selectively inhibit HDAC6 deacetylation of α-tubulin [52], and PCI-34051, which was able to induce apoptosis in T-cell lymphomas by selectively binding HDAC8 [55]. Another focus of HDAC inhibitor development is the combination of inhibiting HDACs and other oncogenic proteins in the same molecule. These molecules allow the HDAC inhibition element to remain nonspecific, while targeting select oncogenic pathways like tyrosine kinases [56] or phosphatidylinositol 3-kinase (PI3K) [57]. The drug CUDC-101, which inhibits EGFR-2 and EGFR in addition to HDACs, has been shown to enhance the radiosensitivity of GBM cells in vitro [58]. Other hybrid expansions include pairing an HDAC inhibitor with a topoisomerase II inhibitor (fusing daunorubicin with SAHA) or with a nuclear receptor target via a vitamin D receptor agonist [59]. While these technologies provide a promising future for the treatment of cancers, it is important to note that compounds from the primary classes of HDAC inhibitors have been clinically evaluated for antitumor activity [60].

HDAC Inhibitors and Radiosensitization

In Vitro Radiosensitization

Inhibition of HDACs results in the hyperacetylation of histones, which loosens chromatin structure and has effects on the radiosensitivity of cells. Studies of HDAC inhibition combined with radiotherapy date back to the 1980s, when

J.T. Leith and colleagues demonstrated that the HDAC inhibitor sodium butyrate (NaB) increased the radiosensitivity of human colon carcinoma cell lines at relatively nontoxic concentrations [61]. At that time, NaB was considered a "differentiation-inducing agent," and its mechanism of action was yet to be elucidated. Radiation cell kill was attributed to "cell maturation," and the histone acetylation status of the tumor cells studied was not examined [62]. Because of its very short half-life and low achievable serum concentration, NaB has limited clinical applicability [63–65], but another HDAC inhibitor, trichostatin A (TSA), was also initially shown to produce a significant increase in the in vitro radiosensitivity of human colon carcinoma cell lines [66]. Like NaB, TSA showed excessive cytotoxicity, apparently due to actions involving the acetylation on nonhistone proteins, and is unstable under in vivo conditions [16, 67]. Thus, although the earliest studies done with agents that inhibit HDACs were promising in that they were able to enhance the level of radiation-induced cell death, the challenge remained to find drugs suitable for clinical use.

Advances in drug discovery have produced a number of HDAC inhibitors with more promising in vivo pharmacokinetic and toxicity profiles. One of the first clinically applicable HDAC inhibitors with respect to radiosensitizing potential is the benzamide entinostat (MS-275). MS-275 is a potent HDAC inhibitor, has been reported to have in vivo antitumor activity in a number of preclinical models [49], and was the first clinically relevant HDAC inhibitor to be evaluated as a radiosensitizing agent [68]. Utilizing a human prostate carcinoma line (DU145) and human glioma line (U251), the effect of MS-275 on histone acetylation status was determined by exposing the cells to the drug for 6–48 h. An increase in levels of acetylated histones could be detected after 6 h of drug treatment, reaching a maximum level between 24 and 48 h in both cell lines. As histone acetylation is a dynamic process with some species of histones having an acetylation half-life of minutes [69]. The investigators then determined the dependence of the elevated acetylation levels on the presence of MS-275. This was achieved by exposing the cultures to the HDAC inhibitor for 48 h to induce maximum acetylation levels, followed by removal of the drug. The result was that histone hyperacetylation was significantly reduced by 6 h following drug removal, with a reduction close to control levels by 16–24 h. The rapid decline in histone hyperacetylation following drug removal has a significant role in the radiosensitization mechanism of HDAC inhibitors.

The investigators then asked if MS-275-induced hyperacetylation was correlated with alterations in tumor cell radiosensitivity. To answer this question, DU145 and U251 cells were exposed to MS-275 for 48 h, irradiated, trypsinized, and plated sparsely as a single-cell suspension to determine colony formation efficiency and radiation cell survival. The result was a minor increase in DU145 cell radiosensitivity, with no effect on U251 cell radiosensitivity. Because the mechanism behind HDAC-induced radiosensitization was unknown, it was possible that the hyperacetylation needed to be maintained after irradiation to increase radiation-induced cell death. When radiation clonogenic studies were performed with MS-275 both pre-radiation treatment and post-radiation treatment, the result was a significant increase in the radiosensitivity of

DU145 and U251, with dose enhancement factors (DEFs) at a surviving fraction of 0.1 and 1.9 for DU145 and U251, respectively, compared to no increase in sensitivity when it was given only pre-radiation treatment. This work was significant because it was the first to demonstrate that there is a correlation between HDAC inhibitor-induced hyperacetylation and an increase in radiation sensitivity of tumor cells, as well as the first to show that the timing of the drug and radiation treatments were important.

These results led to parallel studies that examined other known HDAC inhibitors. One compound that had been studied extensively and quickly became of interest was valproic acid (VPA). Its clinical values were discovered in 1963, as an antiseizure drug [70], and it has since become a well-established treatment of epilepsy and other seizure disorders [71, 72]. In general, VPA is well tolerated by patients, has few serious side effects, and is highly effective, making it a standard therapy for chronic epilepsy [71]. It was not until 2001 that VPA's HDAC inhibitor activity was identified when Gottlicher and colleagues looked at VPA-treated hyperacetylation-hyperacetylation of histone species H3 and H4 in human teratocarcinoma and HeLa cells [73]. Treatment with concentrations of VPA as low as 0.25 mM caused a significant increase in acetylated histone H4. Shortly thereafter, Phiel et al. reported that VPA activates Wnt-dependent gene expression through a pathway that involves directly inhibiting HDAC1 [74]. The chemical structure of VPA is similar to NaB, an eight-carbon branched-chained fatty acid, but in place of the 30 min half-life of NaB, VPA exhibits a serum half-life of 9–18 h and can be administered orally [71]. Importantly, VPA's efficacy as an antiseizure medication proves that it can penetrate the blood-brain barrier and that it can be chronically administered with minimal toxicity. Combined, these factors generated considerable interest in VPA as a potential HDAC inhibitor for cancer patients.

Several studies have been done since, suggesting that VPA causes radiosensitization in vitro and in vivo. One study characterized the histone acetylation status of two human brain tumor lines, SF539 and U251, and showed that levels of acetylated H3 and H4 increased in a concentration-dependent manner after VPA treatment, reaching peak acetylation levels by 24 h [75]. Like MS-275, removal of VPA from cell culture media resulted in rapid loss of histone acetylation, indicating that histone hyperacetylation is dependent upon the continued presence of the HDAC inhibitor. In order to determine if VPA exposure, like MS-275, needed to be both pre- and post-irradiation in order to radiosensitize SF539 and U251 cells, experiments were carried out that mirrored the MS-275 study. The SF539 cells plated without post-irradiation VPA exhibited enhanced radiosensitivity with a DEF at a surviving fraction of 0.1 of 1.3, while the effect on U251 cells was negligible. However, the SF539 and U251 cultures that were plated with media containing VPA post-irradiation obtained DEFs of 1.6 and 1.5, respectively, demonstrating that exposure to VA, like MS-275, is required both before and after irradiation in order to increase tumor cell radiosensitivity. This effect of VPA on radiation sensitivity has been validated for other tumor types, including human erythroleukemic cells as well as esophageal squamous cell carcinomas [76, 77].

Numerous other HDAC inhibitors have shown radiosensitizing properties in various different tumor cell cultures, including SAHA in squamous cell carcinoma, prostate cancer cells, and pancreatic cancer cells as well as CI-994 and depsipeptide in glioblastoma [50, 78, 79]; phenylbutyrate in glioblastoma and hepatocellular carcinoma cells [80, 81]; tributyrin in melanoma cells [82]; PCI-24781 in cervical and colon carcinoma [83]; AR-42 in hepatocellular carcinoma cells [81]; and LBH589 in colon, breast, and lung cancer cells [84, 85].

In Vivo Radiosensitization

The in vitro data clearly demonstrates that HDAC inhibitors have the ability to enhance the radiosensitivity of a variety of tumor cell types by inhibiting HDAC function. Furthermore, these studies suggest that histone hyperacetylation may be used as a biomarker for radiosensitization. To further evaluate the antitumor potential of HDAC inhibitor and radiation combination therapy, in vivo xenograft model experiments have been performed.

The first xenograft experiments with MS-275 were performed by injection of MS-275 at 6 mg/kg every 12 h for up to three days. Mice were euthanized 6 h after 2, 4, or 6 injections in order to evaluate levels of acetylated histones in each tumor. Peak histone acetylation in DU145 xenografts was observed after 4 injections, with a rapid decrease in acetylation within 24 h of the last injection, consistent with the in vitro data [68]. A follow-up experiment was then designed in which radiation was delivered between the fourth and fifth of six MS-275 doses. Comparison of tumor growth rates revealed that MS-275 clearly enhanced radiation-induced tumor growth delay with a DEF of 2.8, signifying that MS-275 treatment increases the radiosensitivity of DU145 xenografts. In a similar study using U251 glioma xenografts, 150 mg/kg of VPA (a serum VPA concentration corresponding to that necessary to prevent seizures in humans) [72] was administered with a single dose of 4 Gy irradiation delivered 6 h after the third dose. Tumors showed a significant growth delay with a DEF of 2.6 for the combination treatments [75].

Other studies explored the actions of HDAC inhibitors FK228 and CBHA on human gastric and colorectal adenocarcinoma cells [86] and the effect of combination therapy of the HDAC inhibitor LBH589 on non-small cell lung cancers [87]. Collectively, these in vitro and in vivo analyses (summarized in Table 3.1) have afforded a rational basis for combining HDAC inhibitors with standard radiotherapy in both preclinical and clinical trials, a number of which are currently ongoing.

Tumor Versus Normal Cells

It is thought that tumor cells alone would be susceptible to the cytotoxic and cytostatic effects of HDAC inhibitors due to aberrant histone deacetylase activity in tumor cells as compared to normal cells. For the most part, experimental evidence has backed up this theory, as shown by cell culture studies [102, 104] and animal models administered with clinically relevant HDAC inhibitors at antitumor doses [105–107]. One such study shows that following NaB exposure, melanoma cell

Table 3.1 HDAC inhibitors in preclinical/clinical trials (partial list)

Agent	Class	In vitro studies	Select tumor lines studied	Shown radiation modifying effects	In vivo studies	Clinical trials	References
Vorinostat (SAHA)	Hydroxamic acid	Yes	Squamous cell carcinoma Prostate cancer Pancreatic cancer Leukemia	Yes	Yes	Yes	Almenara et al. [11], Folkvord et al. [88], Marks [89], Chinnaiyan et al. [78]
TSA	Hydroxamic acid	Yes	Colon carcinoma Melanoma	Yes	No	No	Kim et al. [90], Yoshida et al. [47]
NaB	Carboxylic acid	Yes	Melanoma	Yes	No	No	Remiszewski [48], Miller et al. [63], Perrine et al. [65]
VPA	Carboxylic acid	Yes	Erythroleukemia Esophageal squamous cell carcinoma Glioma	Yes	Yes	Yes	Camphausen et al. [75], Chavez-Blanco et al. [91], Chateauvieux et al. [92]
Depsipeptide (romidepsin, FK228)	Cyclic peptide	Yes	Gastric adenocarcinoma Colorectal adenocarcinoma	Yes	Yes	Yes	Miller et al. [102], Tan et al. (2010)
Apicidin	Cyclic peptide	Yes	Pancreatic carcinoma		No	No	Jose et al. [93], Bauden et al. [94]
Entinostat (MS-275)	Aminobenzamide	Yes	Glioma	Yes	Yes	Yes	Saito et al. [49], Camphausen et al. [68]

(continued)

Table 3.1 (continued)

Agent	Class	In vitro studies	Select tumor lines studied	Shown radiation modifying effects	In vivo studies	Clinical trials	References
Tacedinaline (CI-944)	Aminobenzamide	Yes	Colon carcinoma, AML, NSCLC	Yes	No	No	Beckers et al. [84]
Mocetinostat (MGCD103)	Aminobenzamide	Yes	Lung carcinoma, Colon carcinoma	No	Yes	Yes	Saito et al. [49], Fournel et al. (2008)
Trapoxin B	Epoxyketone	Yes	Colon carcinoma	No	Yes	No	Cerna et al. [50]
Tubacin	Hydroxamic acid	Yes	Burkitt lymphoma, ALL	No	No	No	Haggarty et al. [52]
PCI-34051	Hydroxamic acid	Yes	T-cell lymphoma	Yes	No	No	Adimoolam et al. [95], Balasubramanian et al. [55]
Phenylbutyrate	Carboxylic acid	Yes	Glioma, Hepatocellular carcinoma, Melanoma	Yes	Yes	Yes	Chung et al. [103], Lopez et al. [80], https://clinicaltrials.Gov
AR-42	Carboxylic acid	Yes	Hepatocellular carcinoma	Yes	Yes	Yes	Lu et al. [81]
Abexinostat (PCI-24781)	Cyclic peptide	Yes	Cervical carcinoma, Colon carcinoma, Neuroblastoma	Yes	Yes	Yes	Gressette et al. (2014), Banuelos et al. [83]
Panobinostat (LBH589)	Hydroxamic acid	Yes	Colon carcinoma, Breast carcinoma, Non-small cell lung carcinoma	Yes	Yes	Yes	Xiao et al. [96], Sholler et al. [97], Fouliard et al. [98]

CBHA	Hydroxamic acid	Yes	Gastric adenocarcinoma	Yes	Yes	No	Coffey et al. [51]
			Colorectal adenocarcinoma				
Belinostat (PXD-101)	Hydroxamic acid	Yes	Cervical carcinoma	No	Yes	Yes	Wagner et al. [99], Plumb et al. [100], Dejligbjerg et al. [101]
			Ovarian carcinoma				
			Colon carcinoma				

lines were significantly radiosensitized, while normal cells remain unaffected [82]. The same group then found that a tumor radiosensitizing treatment of SAHA delivered to normal fibroblasts also had no effect on radiosensitivity [50]. In accordance with these studies, Kim et al. found that while HDAC inhibitors amplified the in vitro sensitivity of tumor cells to DNA-damaging drugs, they had no effect on the drug sensitivity of normal breast or intestinal cells [108]. Finally, the HDAC inhibitor Garcinol was found to radiosensitize human cervical adeno-carcinoma line HeLa and large cell lung carcinoma line A549 to radiation, but not normal human fibroblasts [109].

In fact, HDAC inhibitors have been suggested as radioprotectors for normal tissue. Chung et al. were able to show that topical treatment with the histone deacetylases phenylbutyrate (PB), TSA, and VPA suppressed radiation-induced skin injury in a rat model and that later consequences of radiation such as skin fibrosis and tumorigenesis were avoided [103]. The same group explored the effects of the HDAC inhibitor PB on radiation-induced oral mucositis [110]. In this study, irradiated mucosa of hamsters treated with PB had significantly lower oxidative stress, TNF-α expression, and a reduction in oral tumor incidence than untreated, irradiated mucosa.

While there is a bulk of evidence suggesting that normal tissue is unaffected by HDAC inhibitors, a few studies have found that HDAC inhibitors have the capacity to reduce DNA repair capacity in normal cells. Stoilov et al. reported that normal lymphocytes treated with NaB exhibited a decrease in the repair of radiation-induced DNA double-strand breaks, as measured by premature chro-mosome condensation [111]. However, this study did not include a cell survival experiment, making it difficult to evaluate for a variation in lymphocyte radio-sensitivity as measured by cell death. Perrucker et al. examined the effects of four different HDAC inhibitors (NaB, VA, SAHA, and MS-275) on human fibro-blasts. They use both the persistence of γ-H2AX foci following treatment as well as clonogenic survival assays to show that HDAC inhibitors reduce the DNA double-strand break repair capacity of normal human fibroblasts [112]. Of note, this study shows that fibroblasts are radiosensitized differently depending on HDAC inhibitor used. Thus, HDAC inhibitors are a multifaceted class of mole-cules that have a complex effect on tissues, and in the absence of well-defined mechanistic insight, it remains necessary to continue to evaluate the effect of newer HDAC inhibitors on normal tissue, as well as to keep in mind the potential genotoxic effects when treating high-risk patient populations.

Clinical Application of HDAC Inhibitors and Radiotherapy

As a class of drugs, HDAC inhibitors enhance radiosensitivity in both in vitro and in vivo preclinical models of numerous tumor cell types derived from diverse histolo-gies including, but not limited to, colon carcinoma, glioma, melanoma, and pancre-atic adenocarcinoma. That said, there are various other factors that must be considered when matching the appropriate compound with the proper group of patients, including drug distribution, toxicity, and pharmacology. One example of this is that both VPA and CI-994 are able to cross the blood-brain barrier and thus would be a logical choice to use in combination with radiation in patients with brain tumors. Conversely, VPA would be an inappropriate choice for use in patients with pancreatic carcinomas, as one of the principal side effects of prolonged VPA exposure is pancreatitis. Thus, the agent selected to evaluate in each disease site should minimize the risk of toxicity while maximizing the chances of delivering therapeutic doses to the target tissues.

When performing preclinical studies, one goal is to model the future potential clinical studies. For example, the most profound HDAC inhibitor-induced radiosensitization measured preclinically was when the drugs were administered both pre- and post-radiation. This dosing protocol was used in a recent study that added twice daily VPA to the standard radiation therapy (RT) plus temozolomide (TMZ) treatment for patients with glioblastoma thus having a continuous pre- and post-RT exposure of drug. Thirty-seven patients diagnosed with glioblastoma were enrolled in the clinical study and given VPA twice daily for one week before the first day of RT and subsequently received twice daily VPA, with daily RT/TMZ [113]. This treatment protocol resulted in an overall survival of 29.6 months compared to 14.6 m for the standard treatment. Additionally, 70 % of patients were progression-free at 6 months, 86 % alive at 1 year, and 56 % alive more than 2 years after the initiation of therapy, a very favorable outcome. Moreover, there was little additional toxicity from this combination regimen. This survival benefit agrees with several retrospective studies that showed an improved survival rate in patients with GBM who were treated with either RT or combination RT/TMZ and had been given VPA for the management of seizures [114, 115].

Three additional studies have been reported with combination radiotherapy and HDAC inhibitor administration. The first was a Phase I study of the combination of vorinostat and RT for patients getting palliative RT to the pelvis. The second was a Phase I study of vorinostat plus RT in patients with brain metastases, and the third was a Phase I study of panobinostat plus RT in patients getting re-irradiation for recurrent high-grade gliomas. As all three reported trials were Phase I studies, no additional conclusions can be drawn about the efficacy of HDAC inhibitor administration plus RT. However, multiple additional studies are ongoing in various diseases including pediatric brain tumors, adult GBM, mycosis fungoides, as well as other sites.

Conclusion

The histone-code hypothesis theorizes that specific combinations of posttranslational chemical modifications to the histone determine chromatin-DNA interactions and gene expression of a cell, and this code can be drastically altered during neoplastic development and consequently may be a target for tumor radiosensitization. HDAC inhibitors, important regulators of this code, have been shown to be potent anticancer agents because of their ability to impact cell cycle, senescence, differentiation, and apoptosis via global control of gene expression. Preclinical data have demonstrated the efficacy of HDAC inhibitors as anticancer agents, especially in conjunction with other treatments such as radiation therapy. They are looked upon favorably in the clinic because they appear to have very little effect on normal tissues and generally low toxicity. The current number of active clinical trials that combine HDAC inhibitors and IR should help shed light into the mechanism of HDAC inhibitor-induced cell death, allowing for the full potential of these therapies to be utilized.

References

1. Lawrence TS, Haffty BG, Harris JR (2014) Milestones in the use of combined-modality radiation therapy and chemotherapy. J Clin Oncol 32(12):1173–1179
2. McGinn CJ, Shewach DS, Lawrence TS (1996) Radiosensitizing nucleosides. J Natl Cancer Inst 88(17):1193–1203
3. Jenuwein T, Allis CD (2001) Translating the histone code. Science 293(5532):1074–1080
4. Strahl BD, Allis CD (2000) The language of covalent histone modifications. Nature 403 (6765):41–45
5. Sharma S, Kelly TK, Jones PA (2010) Epigenetics in cancer. Carcinogenesis 31(1):27–36
6. Simon JA, Lange CA (2008) Roles of the EZH2 histone methyltransferase in cancer epigenetics. Mutat Res 647(1-2):21–29
7. Rogakou EP, Pilch DR, Orr AH, Ivanova VS, Bonner WM (1998) DNA double-stranded breaks induce histone H2AX phosphorylation on serine 139. J Biol Chem 273(10):5858–5868
8. Taneja N, Davis M, Choy JS, Beckett MA, Singh R, Kron SJ, Weichselbaum RR (2004) Histone H2AX phosphorylation as a predictor of radiosensitivity and target for radiotherapy. J Biol Chem 279(3):2273–2280
9. Bonner WM, Redon CE, Dickey JS, Nakamura AJ, Sedelnikova OA, Solier S, Pommier Y (2008) GammaH2AX and cancer. Nat Rev Cancer 8(12):957–967
10. Johnstone RW, Licht JD (2003) Histone deacetylase inhibitors in cancer therapy: Is transcription the primary target? Cancer Cell 4(1):13–18
11. Almenara J, Rosato R, Grant S (2002) Synergistic induction of mitochondrial damage and apoptosis in human leukemia cells by flavopiridol and the histone deacetylase inhibitor suberoylanilide hydroxamic acid (SAHA). Leukemia 16(7):1331–1343
12. Amin HM, Saeed S, Alkan S (2001) Histone deacetylase inhibitors induce caspase-dependent apoptosis and downregulation of daxx in acute promyelocytic leukaemia with t(15;17). Br J Haematol 115(2):287–297
13. Richon VM, Sandhoff TW, Rifkind RA, Marks PA (2000) Histone deacetylase inhibitor selectively induces p21WAF1 expression and gene-associated histone acetylation. Proc Natl Acad Sci U S A 97(18):10014–10019
14. Vrana JA, Decker RH, Johnson CR, Wang Z, Jarvis WD, Richon VM, Ehinger M, Fisher PB, Grant S (1999) Induction of apoptosis in U937 human leukemia cells by suberoylanilide hydroxamic acid (SAHA) proceeds through pathways that are regulated by Bcl-2/Bcl-XL, c-Jun, and p21CIP1, but independent of p53. Oncogene 18(50):7016–7025
15. Boyault C, Sadoul K, Pabion M, Khochbin S (2007) HDAC6, at the crossroads between cytoskeleton and cell signaling by acetylation and ubiquitination. Oncogene 26(37):5468–5476
16. Hubbert C, Guardiola A, Shao R, Kawaguchi Y, Ito A, Nixon A, Yoshida M, Wang XF, Yao TP (2002) HDAC6 is a microtubule-associated deacetylase. Nature 417(6887):455–458
17. Brown CE, Lechner T, Howe L, Workman JL (2000) The many HATs of transcription coactivators. Trends Biochem Sci 25(1):15–19

18. Cheung P, Allis CD, Sassone-Corsi P (2000) Signaling to chromatin through histone modifications. Cell 103(2):263–271
19. Winston F, Allis CD (1999) The bromodomain: a chromatin-targeting module? Nat Struct Biol 6(7):601–604
20. Glass CK, Rosenfeld MG (2000) The coregulator exchange in transcriptional functions of nuclear receptors. Genes Dev 14(2):121–141
21. Kouzarides T (1999) Histone acetylases and deacetylases in cell proliferation. Curr Opin Genet Dev 9(1):40–48
22. McKenna NJ, Lanz RB, O'Malley BW (1999) Nuclear receptor coregulators: cellular and molecular biology. Endocr Rev 20(3):321–344
23. Chen JD, Evans RM (1995) A transcriptional co-repressor that interacts with nuclear hormone receptors. Nature 377(6548):454–457
24. Chen JD, Umesono K, Evans RM (1996) SMRT isoforms mediate repression and anti-repression of nuclear receptor heterodimers. Proc Natl Acad Sci U S A 93(15):7567–7571
25. Verdin E, Dequiedt F, Kasler HG (2003) Class II histone deacetylases: versatile regulators. Trends Genet 19(5):286–293
26. Gong F, Miller KM (2013) Mammalian DNA repair: HATs and HDACs make their mark through histone acetylation. Mutat Res 750(1-2):23–30
27. Tamburini BA, Tyler JK (2005) Localized histone acetylation and deacetylation triggered by the homologous recombination pathway of double-strand DNA repair. Mol Cell Biol 25(12):4903–4913
28. Ramanathan B, Smerdon MJ (1986) Changes in nuclear protein acetylation in u.v.-damaged human cells. Carcinogenesis 7(7):1087–1094
29. Ramanathan B, Smerdon MJ (1989) Enhanced DNA repair synthesis in hyperacetylated nucleosomes. J Biol Chem 264(19):11026–11034
30. Miller KM, Jackson SP (2012) Histone marks: repairing DNA breaks within the context of chromatin. Biochem Soc Trans 40(2):370–376
31. Ikura T, Tashiro S, Kakino A, Shima H, Jacob N, Amunugama R, Yoder K, Izumi S, Kuraoka I, Tanaka K, Kimura H, Ikura M, Nishikubo S, Ito T, Muto A, Miyagawa K, Takeda S, Fishel R, Igarashi K, Kamiya K (2007) DNA damage-dependent acetylation and ubiquitination of H2AX enhances chromatin dynamics. Mol Cell Biol 27(20):7028–7040
32. Yamagata K, Kitabayashi I (2009) Sirt1 physically interacts with Tip60 and negatively regulates Tip60-mediated acetylation of H2AX. Biochem Biophys Res Commun 390(4):1355–1360
33. Miller KM, Tjeertes JV, Coates J, Legube G, Polo SE, Britton S, Jackson SP (2010) Human HDAC1 and HDAC2 function in the DNA-damage response to promote DNA nonhomologous end-joining. Nat Struct Mol Biol 17(9):1144–1151
34. Warburg O (1956) On the origin of cancer cells. Science 123(3191):309–314
35. Gut P, Verdin E (2013) The nexus of chromatin regulation and intermediary metabolism. Nature 502(7472):489–498
36. Wellen KE, Hatzivassiliou G, Sachdeva UM, Bui TV, Cross JR, Thompson CB (2009) ATP-citrate lyase links cellular metabolism to histone acetylation. Science 324(5930):1076–1080
37. Liu J, Wang H, Ma F, Xu D, Chang Y, Zhang J, Wang J, Zhao M, Lin C, Huang C, Qian H, Zhan Q (2015) MTA1 regulates higher-order chromatin structure and histone H1-chromatin interaction in-vivo. Mol Oncol 9(1):218–235
38. Efimova EV, Takahashi S, Shamsi NA, Wu D, Labay E, Ulanovskaya OA, Weichselbaum RR, Kozmin SA, Kron SJ (2016) Linking Cancer Metabolism to DNA Repair and Accelerated Senescence. Mol Cancer Res 14(2):173–184
39. Aghaee F, Pirayesh Islamian J, Baradaran B (2012) Enhanced radiosensitivity and chemosensitivity of breast cancer cells by 2-deoxy-d-glucose in combination therapy. J Breast Cancer 15(2):141–147
40. Suh DH, Kim MK, No JH, Chung HH, Song YS (2011) Metabolic approaches to overcoming chemoresistance in ovarian cancer. Ann N Y Acad Sci 1229:53–60

41. Ozdag H, Teschendorff AE, Ahmed AA, Hyland SJ, Blenkiron C, Bobrow L, Veerakumarasivam A, Burtt G, Subkhankulova T, Arends MJ, Collins VP, Bowtell D, Kouzarides T, Brenton JD, Caldas C (2006) Differential expression of selected histone modifier genes in human solid cancers. BMC Genomics 7:90

42. Krusche CA, Wulfing P, Kersting C, Vloet A, Bocker W, Kiesel L, Beier HM, Alfer J (2005) Histone deacetylase-1 and -3 protein expression in human breast cancer: a tissue microarray analysis. Breast Cancer Res Treat 90(1):15–23

43. Minamiya Y, Ono T, Saito H, Takahashi N, Ito M, Mitsui M, Motoyama S, Ogawa J (2011) Expression of histone deacetylase 1 correlates with a poor prognosis in patients with adenocarcinoma of the lung. Lung Cancer 74(2):300–304

44. Rikimaru T, Taketomi A, Yamashita Y, Shirabe K, Hamatsu T, Shimada M, Maehara Y (2007) Clinical significance of histone deacetylase 1 expression in patients with hepatocellular carcinoma. Oncology 72(1-2):69–74

45. Weichert W, Roske A, Gekeler V, Beckers T, Stephan C, Jung K, Fritzsche FR, Niesporek S, Denkert C, Dietel M, Kristiansen G (2008) Histone deacetylases 1, 2 and 3 are highly expressed in prostate cancer and HDAC2 expression is associated with shorter PSA relapse time after radical prostatectomy. Br J Cancer 98(3):604–610

46. West AC, Johnstone RW (2014) New and emerging HDAC inhibitors for cancer treatment. J Clin Invest 124(1):30–39

47. Yoshida M, Furumai R, Nishiyama M, Komatsu Y, Nishino N, Horinouchi S (2001) Histone deacetylase as a new target for cancer chemotherapy. Cancer Chemother Pharmacol 48(Suppl 1):S20–S26

48. Remiszewski SW (2002) Recent advances in the discovery of small molecule histone deacetylase inhibitors. Curr Opin Drug Discov Devel 5(4):487–499

49. Saito A, Yamashita T, Mariko Y, Nosaka Y, Tsuchiya K, Ando T, Suzuki T, Tsuruo T, Nakanishi O (1999) A synthetic inhibitor of histone deacetylase, MS-27-275, with marked in vivo antitumor activity against human tumors. Proc Natl Acad Sci U S A 96(8):4592–4597

50. Cerna D, Camphausen K, Tofilon PJ (2006) Histone deacetylation as a target for radiosensitization. Curr Topics Dev Biol 73:173–204

51. Coffey DC, Kutko MC, Glick RD, Butler LM, Heller G, Rifkind RA, Marks PA, Richon VM, La Quaglia MP (2001) The histone deacetylase inhibitor, CBHA, inhibits growth of human neuroblastoma xenografts in vivo, alone and synergistically with all-trans retinoic acid. Cancer Res 61(9):3591–3594

52. Haggarty SJ, Koeller KM, Wong JC, Grozinger CM, Schreiber SL (2003) Domain-selective small-molecule inhibitor of histone deacetylase 6 (HDAC6)-mediated tubulin deacetylation. Proc Natl Acad Sci U S A 100(8):4389–4394

53. Drummond DC, Noble CO, Kirpotin DB, Guo Z, Scott GK, Benz CC (2005) Clinical development of histone deacetylase inhibitors as anticancer agents. Annu Rev Pharmacol Toxicol 45:495–528

54. Marks PA (2010) Histone deacetylase inhibitors: a chemical genetics approach to understanding cellular functions. Biochim Biophys Acta 1799(10-12):717–725

55. Balasubramanian S, Ramos J, Luo W, Sirisawad M, Verner E, Buggy JJ (2008) A novel histone deacetylase 8 (HDAC8)-specific inhibitor PCI-34051 induces apoptosis in T-cell lymphomas. Leukemia 22(5):1026–1034

56. Mahboobi S, Dove S, Sellmer A, Winkler M, Eichhorn E, Pongratz H, Ciossek T, Baer T, Maier T, Beckers T (2009) Design of chimeric histone deacetylase- and tyrosine kinase-inhibitors: a series of imatinib hybrides as potent inhibitors of wild-type and mutant BCR-ABL, PDGF-Rbeta, and histone deacetylases. J Med Chem 52(8):2265–2279

57. Qian C, Lai CJ, Bao R, Wang DG, Wang J, Xu GX, Atoyan R, Qu H, Yin L, Samson M, Zifcak B, Ma AW, DellaRocca S, Borek M, Zhai HX, Cai X, Voi M (2012) Cancer network disruption by a single molecule inhibitor targeting both histone deacetylase activity and phosphatidylinositol 3-kinase signaling. Clin Cancer Res 18(15):4104–4113

58. Schlaff CD, Arscott WT, Gordon I, Camphausen KA, Tandle A (2015) Human EGFR-2, EGFR and HDAC triple- inhibitor CUDC-101 enhances radiosensitivity of GBM cells. Biomed Res J 2(1):105–119
59. Delcuve GP, Khan DH, Davie JR (2013) Targeting class I histone deacetylases in cancer therapy. Expert Opin Ther Targets 17(1):29–41
60. Mottamal M, Zheng S, Huang TL, Wang G (2015) Histone deacetylase inhibitors in clinical studies as templates for new anticancer agents. Molecules 20(3):3898–3941
61. Arundel CM, Glicksman AS, Leith JT (1985) Enhancement of radiation injury in human colon tumor cells by the maturational agent sodium butyrate (NaB). Radiat Res 104(3):443–448
62. Kruh J (1982) Effects of sodium butyrate, a new pharmacological agent, on cells in culture. Mol Cell Biochem 42(2):65–82
63. Miller AA, Kurschel E, Osieka R, Schmidt CG (1987) Clinical pharmacology of sodium butyrate in patients with acute leukemia. Eur J Cancer Clin Oncol 23(9):1283–1287
64. Novogrodsky A, Dvir A, Ravid A, Shkolnik T, Stenzel KH, Rubin AL, Zaizov R (1983) Effect of polar organic compounds on leukemic cells. Butyrate-induced partial remission of acute myelogenous leukemia in a child. Cancer 51(1):9–14
65. Perrine SP, Ginder GD, Faller DV, Dover GH, Ikuta T, Witkowska HE, Cai SP, Vichinsky EP, Olivieri NF (1993) A short-term trial of butyrate to stimulate fetal-globin-gene expression in the beta-globin disorders. N Engl J Med 328(2):81–86
66. Biade S, Stobbe CC, Boyd JT, Chapman JD (2001) Chemical agents that promote chromatin compaction radiosensitize tumour cells. Int J Radiat Biol 77(10):1033–1042
67. Blagosklonny MV, Robey R, Sackett DL, Du L, Traganos F, Darzynkiewicz Z, Fojo T, Bates SE (2002) Histone deacetylase inhibitors all induce p21 but differentially cause tubulin acetylation, mitotic arrest, and cytotoxicity. Mol Cancer Ther 1(11):937–941
68. Camphausen K, Scott T, Sproull M, Tofilon PJ (2004) Enhancement of xenograft tumor radiosensitivity by the histone deacetylase inhibitor MS-275 and correlation with histone hyperacetylation. Clin Cancer Res 10(18 Pt 1):6066–6071
69. Vidali G, Boffa LC, Mann RS, Allfrey VG (1978) Reversible effects of Na-butyrate on histone acetylation. Biochem Biophys Res Commun 82(1):223–227
70. Meunier H, Carraz G, Neunier Y, Eymard P, Aimard M (1963) Pharmacodynamic properties of N-dipropylacetic acid. Therapie 18:435–438
71. Perucca E (2002) Pharmacological and therapeutic properties of valproate: a summary after 35 years of clinical experience. CNS Drugs 16(10):695–714
72. Pinder RM, Brogden RN, Speight TM, Avery GS (1977) Sodium valproate: a review of its pharmacological properties and therapeutic efficacy in epilepsy. Drugs 13(2):81–123
73. Gottlicher M, Minucci S, Zhu P, Kramer OH, Schimpf A, Giavara S, Sleeman JP, Lo Coco F, Nervi C, Pelicci PG, Heinzel T (2001) Valproic acid defines a novel class of HDAC inhibitors inducing differentiation of transformed cells. EMBO J 20(24):6969–6978
74. Phiel CJ, Zhang F, Huang EY, Guenther MG, Lazar MA, Klein PS (2001) Histone deacetylase is a direct target of valproic acid, a potent anticonvulsant, mood stabilizer, and teratogen. J Biol Chem 276(39):36734–36741
75. Camphausen K, Cerna D, Scott T, Sproull M, Burgan WE, Cerra MA, Fine H, Tofilon PJ (2005) Enhancement of in vitro and in vivo tumor cell radiosensitivity by valproic acid. Int J Cancer 114(3):380–386
76. Karagiannis TC, Kn H, El-Osta A (2006) The epigenetic modifier, valproic acid, enhances radiation sensitivity. Epigenetics 1(3):131–137
77. Shoji M, Ninomiya I, Makino I, Kinoshita J, Nakamura K, Oyama K, Nakagawara H, Fujita H, Tajima H, Takamura H, Kitagawa H, Fushida S, Harada S, Fujimura T, Ohta T (2012) Valproic acid, a histone deacetylase inhibitor, enhances radiosensitivity in esophageal squamous cell carcinoma. Int J Oncol 40(6):2140–2146
78. Chinnaiyan P, Vallabhaneni G, Armstrong E, Huang S-M, Harari PM (2005) Modulation of radiation response by histone deacetylase inhibition. Int J Radiation Oncol Biol Phys 62(1):223–229

79. Zhang Y, Adachi M, Zhao X, Kawamura R, Imai K (2004) Histone deacetylase inhibitors FK228, N-(2-aminophenyl)-4-[N-(pyridin-3-yl-methoxycarbonyl)amino- methyl]benzamide and m-carboxycinnamic acid bis-hydroxamide augment radiation-induced cell death in gastrointestinal adenocarcinoma cells. Int J Cancer 110(2):301–308

80. Lopez CA, Feng FY, Herman JM, Nyati MK, Lawrence TS, Ljungman M (2007) Phenylbutyrate sensitizes human glioblastoma cells lacking wild-type P53 function to ionizing radiation. Int J Radiation Oncol Biol Phys 69(1):214–220

81. Lu YS, Chou CH, Tzen KY, Gao M, Cheng AL, Kulp SK, Cheng JC (2012) Radiosensitizing effect of a phenylbutyrate-derived histone deacetylase inhibitor in hepatocellular carcinoma. Int J Radiat Oncol Biol Phys 83(2):e181–e189

82. Munshi A, Kurland JF, Nishikawa T, Tanaka T, Hobbs ML, Tucker SL, Ismail S, Stevens C, Meyn RE (2005) Histone deacetylase inhibitors radiosensitize human melanoma cells by suppressing DNA repair activity. Clin Cancer Res 11(13):4912–4922

83. Banuelos CA, Banath JP, MacPhail SH, Zhao J, Reitsema T, Olive PL (2007) Radiosensitization by the histone deacetylase inhibitor PCI-24781. Clin Cancer Res 13(22 Pt 1):6816–6826

84. Beckers T, Burkhardt C, Wieland H, Gimmnich P, Ciossek T, Maier T, Sanders K (2007) Distinct pharmacological properties of second generation HDAC inhibitors with the benzamide or hydroxamate head group. Int J Cancer 121(5):1138–1148

85. Kim IA, No M, Lee JM, Shin JH, Oh JS, Choi EJ, Kim IH, Atadja P, Bernhard EJ (2009) Epigenetic modulation of radiation response in human cancer cells with activated EGFR or HER-2 signaling: potential role of histone deacetylase 6. Radiother Oncol 92(1):125–132

86. Zhang Y, Jung M, Dritschilo A, Jung M (2004) Enhancement of radiation sensitivity of human squamous carcinoma cells by histone deacetylase inhibitors. Radiat Res 161(6):667–674

87. Geng L, Cuneo KC, Fu A, Tu T, Atadja PW, Hallahan DE (2006) Histone deacetylase (HDAC) inhibitor LBH589 increases duration of gamma-H2AX foci and confines HDAC4 to the cytoplasm in irradiated non-small cell lung cancer. Cancer Res 66(23):11298–11304

88. Folkvord, S., A. H. Ree, T. Furre, T. Halvorsen and K. Flatmark (2009). "Radiosensitization by SAHA in Experimental Colorectal Carcinoma Models—In Vivo Effects and Relevance of Histone Acetylation Status." International Journal of Radiation Oncology*Biology*Physics 74(2):546–552

89. Marks, P. A. (2004). "The mechanism of the anti-tumor activity of the histone deacetylase inhibitor, suberoylanilide hydroxamic acid (SAHA)." Cell Cycle 3(5):534–535

90. Kim, J. H., J. H. Shin and I. H. Kim (2004). "Susceptibility and radiosensitization of human glioblastoma cells to trichostatin A, a histone deacetylase inhibitor." International Journal of Radiation Oncology*Biology*Physics 59(4):1174–1180

91. Chavez-Blanco, A., B. Segura-Pacheco, E. Perez-Cardenas, L. Taja-Chayeb, L. Cetina, M. Candelaria, D. Cantu, A. Gonzalez-Fierro, P. Garcia-Lopez, P. Zambrano, C. Perez-Plasencia, G. Cabrera, C. Trejo-Becerril, E. Angeles and A. Duenas-Gonzalez (2005). "Histone acetylation and histone deacetylase activity of magnesium valproate in tumor and peripheral blood of patients with cervical cancer. A phase I study." Mol Cancer 4(1):22

92. Chateauvieux, S., F. Morceau, M. Dicato and M. Diederich (2010). "Molecular and therapeutic potential and toxicity of valproic acid." J Biomed Biotechnol 2010

93. Jose, B., Y. Oniki, T. Kato, N. Nishino, Y. Sumida and M. Yoshida (2004). "Novel histone deacetylase inhibitors: cyclic tetrapeptide with trifluoromethyl and pentafluoroethyl ketones." Bioorg Med Chem Lett 14(21):5343–5346

94. Bauden, M., H. Tassidis and D. Ansari (2015). "In vitro cytotoxicity evaluation of HDAC inhibitor Apicidin in pancreatic carcinoma cells subsequent time and dose dependent treatment." Toxicol Lett 236(1):8–15

95. Adimoolam, S., M. Sirisawad, J. Chen, P. Thiemann, J. M. Ford and J. J. Buggy (2007). "HDAC inhibitor PCI-24781 decreases RAD51 expression and inhibits homologous recombination." Proc Natl Acad Sci U S A 104(49):19482–19487

96. Xiao, W., P. H. Graham, J. Hao, L. Chang, J. Ni, C. A. Power, Q. Dong, J. H. Kearsley and Y. Li (2013). "Combination therapy with the histone deacetylase inhibitor LBH589 and radiation is an effective regimen for prostate cancer cells." PLoS One 8(8):e74253

97. Sholler, G. S., E. A. Currier, A. Dutta, M. A. Slavik, S. A. Illenye, M. C. Mendonca, J. Dragon, S. S. Roberts and J. P. Bond (2013). "PCI-24781 (abexinostat), a novel histone deacetylase inhibitor, induces reactive oxygen speciesdependent apoptosis and is synergistic with bortezomib in neuroblastoma." J Cancer Ther Res 2:21

98. Fouliard, S., R. Robert, A. Jacquet-Bescond, Q. C. du Rieu, S. Balasubramanian, D. Loury, Y. Loriot, A. Hollebecque, I. Kloos, J. C. Soria, M. Chenel and S. Depil (2013). "Pharmacokinetic/pharmacodynamic modellingbased optimisation of administration schedule for the histone deacetylase inhibitor abexinostat (S78454/PCI-24781) in phase I." Eur J Cancer 49(13):2791–2797

99. Wagner, J. M., B. Hackanson, M. Lubbert and M. Jung (2010). "Histone deacetylase (HDAC) inhibitors in recent clinical trials for cancer therapy." Clin Epigenetics 1(3-4):117–136

100. Plumb, J. A., P. W. Finn, R. J. Williams, M. J. Bandara, M. R. Romero, C. J. Watkins, N. B. La Thangue and R. Brown (2003). "Pharmacodynamic response and inhibition of growth of human tumor xenografts by the novel histone deacetylase inhibitor PXD101." Mol Cancer Ther 2(8):721–728

101. Dejligbjerg, M., M. Grauslund, I. J. Christensen, J. Tjornelund, P. Buhl Jensen and M. Sehested (2008). "Identification of predictive biomarkers for the histone deacetylase inhibitor belinostat in a panel of human cancer cell lines." Cancer Biomark 4(2):101–109

102. Miller TA, Witter DJ, Belvedere S (2003) Histone deacetylase inhibitors. J Med Chem 46(24):5097–5116

103. Chung YL, Wang AJ, Yao LF (2004) Antitumor histone deacetylase inhibitors suppress cutaneous radiation syndrome: Implications for increasing therapeutic gain in cancer radiotherapy. Mol Cancer Ther 3(3):317–325

104. Cress WD, Seto E (2000) Histone deacetylases, transcriptional control, and cancer. J Cell Physiol 184(1):1–16

105. Atadja P, Gao L, Kwon P, Trogani N, Walker H, Hsu M, Yeleswarapu L, Chandramouli N, Perez L, Versace R, Wu A, Sambucetti L, Lassota P, Cohen D, Bair K, Wood A, Remiszewski S (2004) Selective growth inhibition of tumor cells by a novel histone deacetylase inhibitor, NVP-LAQ824. Cancer Res 64(2):689–695

106. Kelly WK, Richon VM, O'Connor O, Curley T, MacGregor-Curtelli B, Tong W, Klang M, Schwartz L, Richardson S, Rosa E, Drobnjak M, Cordon-Cordo C, Chiao JH, Rifkind R, Marks PA, Scher H (2003) Phase I clinical trial of histone deacetylase inhibitor: suberoylanilide hydroxamic acid administered intravenously. Clin Cancer Res 9(10 Pt 1):3578–3588

107. Patnaik A, Rowinsky EK, Villalona MA, Hammond LA, Britten CD, Siu LL, Goetz A, Felton SA, Burton S, Valone FH, Eckhardt SG (2002) A phase I study of pivaloyloxymethyl butyrate, a prodrug of the differentiating agent butyric acid, in patients with advanced solid malignancies. Clin Cancer Res 8(7):2142–2148

108. Kim MS, Blake M, Baek JH, Kohlhagen G, Pommier Y, Carrier F (2003) Inhibition of histone deacetylase increases cytotoxicity to anticancer drugs targeting DNA. Cancer Res 63(21):7291–7300

109. Oike T, Ogiwara H, Torikai K, Nakano T, Yokota J, Kohno T (2012) Garcinol, a histone acetyltransferase inhibitor, radiosensitizes cancer cells by inhibiting non-homologous end joining. Int J Radiat Oncol Biol Phys 84(3):815–821

110. Chung YL, Lee MY, Pui NN (2009) Epigenetic therapy using the histone deacetylase inhibitor for increasing therapeutic gain in oral cancer: prevention of radiation-induced oral mucositis and inhibition of chemical-induced oral carcinogenesis. Carcinogenesis 30(8):1387–1397

111. Stoilov L, Darroudi F, Meschini R, van der Schans G, Mullenders LH, Natarajan AT (2000) Inhibition of repair of X-ray-induced DNA double-strand breaks in human lymphocytes exposed to sodium butyrate. Int J Radiat Biol 76(11):1485–1491

112. Purrucker JC, Fricke A, Ong MF, Rube C, Rube CE, Mahlknecht U (2010) HDAC inhibition radiosensitizes human normal tissue cells and reduces DNA Double-Strand Break repair capacity. Oncol Rep 23(1):263–269

113. Krauze AV, Myrehaug SD, Chang MG, Holdford DJ, Smith S, Shih J, Tofilon PJ, Fine HA, Camphausen K (2015) A Phase 2 Study of Concurrent Radiation Therapy, Temozolomide, and the Histone Deacetylase Inhibitor Valproic Acid for Patients With Glioblastoma. Int J Radiat Oncol Biol Phys 92(5):986–992
114. Barker CA, Bishop AJ, Chang M, Beal K, Chan TA (2013) Valproic acid use during radiation therapy for glioblastoma associated with improved survival. Int J Radiat Oncol Biol Phys 86(3):504–509
115. Weller M, Gorlia T, Cairncross JG, van den Bent MJ, Mason W, Belanger K, Brandes AA, Bogdahn U, Macdonald DR, Forsyth P, Rossetti AO, Lacombe D, Mirimanoff RO, Vecht CJ, Stupp R (2011) Prolonged survival with valproic acid use in the EORTC/NCIC temozolomide trial for glioblastoma. Neurology 77(12):1156–1164

Chapter 4
Radioprotection as a Method to Enhance the Therapeutic Ratio of Radiotherapy

Su I. Chung, DeeDee K. Smart, Eun Joo Chung, and Deborah E. Citrin

Abstract Radiotherapy is a commonly used local and regional treatment for cancer. Although important advances in radiation treatment delivery have been made in recent years, normal tissue damage remains a major cause of toxicity from radiotherapy and chemoradiotherapy regimens. Efforts to reduce normal tissue injury have included technical improvements to minimize normal tissue exposure to high doses of irradiation. Extensive preclinical research and a growing field of clinical research are focusing on the development of agents to protect normal tissues from the deleterious effects of irradiation. In this review, we discuss the characteristics of these agents, the research required to translate these agents into clinical trials, and highlight some challenges and successes in these efforts.

Keywords Radiation protector • Radiation mitigator • Normal tissue toxicity

Background

Radiotherapy is a commonly used treatment modality for cancer, with more than half of all cancer patients receiving radiotherapy during the course of their malignancy [1, 2]. With a few exceptions, radiotherapy is used for the local and regional treatment of cancer. In many cases, radiation is combined with surgery or chemotherapy to improve the likelihood of long-term local and regional control of cancers. Advancements in radiation treatment delivery and medical imaging have revolutionized the field of radiation oncology, providing a greater certainty about the location of tumor in the body and allowing more precise delivery of complex dose

S.I. Chung • D.K. Smart • E.J. Chung • D.E. Citrin (✉)
Section of Translational Radiation Oncology, Radiation Oncology Branch, National Cancer Institute, Bethesda, MD 20892, USA
e-mail: citrind@mail.nih.gov

© Springer International Publishing Switzerland 2017
P.J. Tofilon, K. Camphausen (eds.), *Increasing the Therapeutic Ratio of Radiotherapy*, Cancer Drug Discovery and Development, DOI 10.1007/978-3-319-40854-5_4

distributions. Altered fractionation schemes have allowed improved tumor control [3]. Collectively, these advancements in technology have driven improvements in local control by allowing an escalation of dose to tumor while minimizing the volume of normal tissue exposed to high radiation doses.

Despite these improvements, normal tissue injury remains a common problem in modern treatments. Improving the ability of normal tissues to tolerate radiotherapy may further reduce toxicity of treatment, thus improving efficacy by minimizing treatment breaks and improving adherence to therapy. Further, the ability to spare normal tissues to even a moderate degree may allow further dose escalation to tumor at a similar or reduced rate of toxicity, thus potentially improving disease control.

The development of agents to protect normal tissues from irradiation to enhance the therapeutic index has long been a goal of radiobiologists. Herein, we will describe the mechanisms of injury in normal tissues after irradiation and highlight methods to prevent and treat this damage. We will focus on agents that have successfully been translated into the clinic and agents that are currently in development.

Methods to Improve the Therapeutic Index of Radiotherapy

Normal tissue damage from irradiation can result in both acute and late toxicities. Acute toxicities manifest within days or weeks after treatment, whereas late toxicities manifest months or years after radiation. Acute toxicities are often reversible, but may negatively impact treatment compliance or require treatment interruption. Examples of acute toxicities include dermatitis, mucositis, and cystitis. Late toxicities are often chronic, progressive, and, in many cases, irreversible. Examples of late toxicities are proctitis, fibrosis, myelitis, and brain necrosis. Both acute and late toxicities are radiation dose limiting.

The therapeutic index is a concept that can be applied to any treatment modality, including radiotherapy. For radiotherapy, the therapeutic index is the ratio between the radiation dose that results in tumor control and the dose that results in toxicity. A larger therapeutic index is favorable because it affords the selection of a higher dose of radiation that in turn results in a greater chance of cure with a minimal chance of toxicity. In practice, this ratio is often small, necessitating the clinician to tolerate a moderate chance of substantial toxicity from a radiation treatment.

A number of strategies may be employed to increase this ratio, including increasing the tolerance of normal tissue to a radiation treatment or enhancing the radiation response in a tumor. Strategies to improve normal tissue tolerance to radiotherapy include altered fractionation schedules, improvements in targeting and delivery, and the use of radiation modifiers. Altered fractionation schedules take advantage of differential responses between tumor and normal tissues to allow "escalation" of dose to tumor with similar normal tissue toxicity. Technological advancements allow improved accuracy and precision of radiation treatments, minimizing the amount of normal tissue exposed to high doses of irradiation.

Perhaps the greatest opportunity for improving the therapeutic ratio in radiotherapy in the future is the development of radiation protectors, radiation mitigators, and effective treatments for radiation injury in normal tissues. A basic understanding of these strategies is helpful to understanding their clinical implementation. Each of these strategies is briefly described below.

Radiation results in ionization events, which lead to free radical production. Often, these ionizations occur in water molecules, although direct damage to DNA and other cellular structures may occur (Fig. 4.1). It is thought that DNA double strand breaks are the lethal event that occurs after exposure to ionizing radiation. In cells that survive radiation exposure, signal transduction may be initiated, leading to the activation of multiple pathways important in cell survival and growth. At the tissue level, the loss of cells or the activation of these pathways may result in changes in tissue function or activation of additional processes like inflammation and wound healing. Intervening in these processes may result in modulation of normal tissue damage after irradiation. The three major categories of agents that can minimize normal tissue injury after irradiation fall into three classes: radioprotectors, radiation mitigators, and treatment.

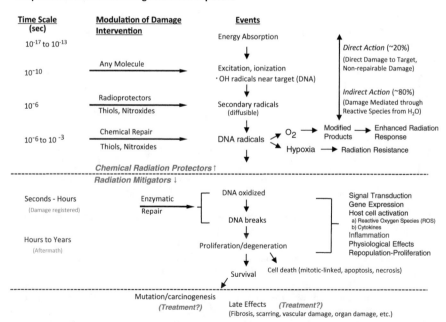

Fig. 4.1 Sequence of events following radiation exposure. The chart is divided into three parts by *dashed lines* suggesting events and reactions that might be modified by radiation protectors (*top*), radiation mitigators, and treatment (*bottom*). Reproduced from Citrin et al. [5]

Radioprotectors

A radioprotector is an agent that prevents the damage caused by radiation, generally, by scavenging the free radicals that cause DNA oxidation and DNA double strand breaks [4]. Because these agents prevent the damage from occurring, they must be given before or at the time of the radiation exposure. Free radicals have an extremely short half-life and, as a result, a limited range for diffusion. Thus, radioprotectors must have the ability to cross the nuclear membrane and accumulate near DNA. This accumulation allows scavenging of radicals that would otherwise lead to lethal DNA damage.

In order for a radioprotector to enhance the therapeutic ratio, the agent must selectively protect normal tissues from irradiation (Fig. 4.2). If the agent protects both normal and tumor tissues, there is no change in the ratio and hence, no benefit to the delivery of the agent [5]. The agent may selectively protect normal tissue

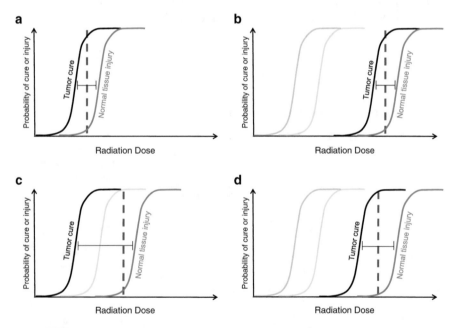

Fig. 4.2 Effects of radioprotectors on the therapeutic window. (**a**) The chosen treatment dose (*blue vertical line*) delivers a high chance of tumor cure (*black*) with a small chance of normal tissue injury (*red*). (**b**) A nonselective radioprotector indiscriminately protects tumor and normal tissue shifting both the tumor cure and normal tissue injury curve to the right. Consequently, the therapeutic window remains unchanged. Shifted curves are shown in *red and black*. The original curves are shown in *gray and pale red*. (**c**) A true selective radioprotector exclusively protects normal tissue and, thus, shifts only the normal tissue injury curve to the right. This affords a larger therapeutic window such that a higher dose can be given to achieve increased tumor cure with equal or less injury. A lower dose producing the same tumor probability can also be given with less tissue injury. (**d**) Some nonselective radioprotectors can protect the normal tissue to a greater extent shifting the normal tissue curve further to the right than the tumor cure curve and resulting in an increased therapeutic window

through a variety of mechanisms. For example, the radioprotector may be activated or taken up by normal tissue more effectively than tumor tissue, leading to a higher concentration of the agent in normal tissue. Conversely, the agent may be cleared or metabolized more rapidly by tumor tissue, also leading to a higher concentration of the agent in normal tissue.

Antioxidants are molecules that reduce cellular damage caused by free radicals. Some examples of antioxidants are ascorbic acid, polyphenols, and thiols. These low molecular weight antioxidants produce a more stable reactive species by donating a hydrogen atom to free radicals. Most radioprotectors are also antioxidants [5]. Of note, however, not every antioxidant has radioprotective effects [6, 7], as they are not all reactive toward the secondary species generated by radiation [7]. In addition to small molecule antioxidants, some antioxidants exist in the form of enzymes, such as superoxide dismutase, catalase, and glutathione peroxidase [5].

Amifostine

Amifostine is a thiol compound that scavenges free radicals, and it is the only FDA-approved radioprotector. Clinically, it has been administered to head and neck cancer patients receiving radiotherapy to prevent xerostomia (dry mouth) [8]. Amifostine is a prodrug that is only activated when dephosphorylated by alkaline phosphatase, a cell membrane protein [9]. It selectively protects normal tissue as it preferentially accumulates in normal tissue rather than tumor tissue [10]. It is thought that the hypovascularity and low pH of the tumor microenvironment limits the activation of amifostine. Furthermore, tumors have lower levels of alkaline phosphatase than normal tissues [11]. In addition to scavenging free radicals, amifostine metabolites induce hypoxia by increasing oxygen consumption [12, 13], which further protects tissues in which the metabolites concentrate.

Amifostine has been tested extensively in clinical trials in various cancer types for the prevention of both acute and late injury. At least 30 different studies have evaluated the use of amifostine in preventing oral mucositis, and the results from these studies have been conflicting. A systematic review of these studies found that data supporting the use of amifostine for oral mucositis was inconclusive [14]. In non-small lung cancer, several small studies showed that amifostine minimized esophagitis [15–17]. However, a study with a larger number of patients receiving chemoradiotherapy was unable to support a reduction in physician-assessed esophagitis; however, amifostine was reported to ameliorate patient-reported swallowing impairment and pain [18, 19]. Amifostine has been shown in some series to be effective against proctitis and dermatitis in patients with pelvic malignancies who underwent radiotherapy [20–22]. It has also been effective in reducing soft tissue [23] and lung fibrosis [23, 24] in patients receiving radiation.

Despite a large number of trials that have been conducted to evaluate amifostine, its usefulness is limited. Many of the studies were conducted with a small and heterogeneous patient population, and dosing schedules differed between studies. In addition, there are several limitations associated with the use of the drug. To be effective, amifostine must be given 15–30 min before radiation and is only approved for intravenous delivery, which may be logistically challenging. Systemic delivery of amifostine is also associated with several side effects, including nausea, vomiting, sleepiness, and low blood pressure. Finally there is much debate over the use of amifostine with radiotherapy and chemoradiotherapy not only because of its side effects but because there are concerns that it may reduce the effectiveness of radiation treatment.

Nitroxides

Nitroxides are recycling antioxidants that have been shown to prevent cytotoxicity induced by oxidative stress as well as by radiation. Nitroxides interconvert between the oxidized and reduced form. In their oxidized state, nitroxides are a stable free radical referred to as a nitroxide radical. These radicals undergo hydrogen reductions to generate hydroxylamine. Both nitroxide radicals and hydroxylamine have antioxidant functions [7, 25]; however only nitroxides exhibit radioprotective effects. In vitro studies using various cell types have shown that nitroxides can reduce DNA damage and cell death induced by radiation [26, 27]. More importantly, systematic administration of nitroxides to mice resulted in decrease lethality after total body irradiation exposures, further substantiating their therapeutic potential [28, 29].

One of the more clinically promising nitroxides is tempol (4-hydroxy-2,2,6,6-tetramethylpiperidine-1-oxyl). Tempol has been studied as a radioprotector in both topical and systemic applications. Topical application of tempol to the skin of guinea pigs exposed to single and fractionated doses of radiation was capable of ameliorating alopecia [30, 31]. Systemic administration of tempol was capable of reducing the lethality of total body irradiation exposures [28, 29]. Systemic administration of tempol has also been shown to protect salivary glands from radiation [32].

As mentioned previously, to enhance the therapeutic ratio, a radioprotector must selectively protect normal and not tumor tissue. The selectivity of tempol for normal tissues has been addressed in several preclinical studies. Systemic administration of tempol in tumor-bearing mice had no effect on tumor growth, and administration with radiation had no impact on the dose of radiation that results in cure in 50 % of tumors at 30 days after treatment [33]. However, systemic administration of tempol was capable of protecting salivary glands and the skin from irradiation [32].

The differential effect of tempol in normal and tumor tissue has been hypothesized to relate to faster reduction to the hydroxylamine metabolite in tumor compared to normal tissues [33]. This hypothesis was evaluated by temporally tracking nitroxide levels with magnetic resonance imaging (MRI). Tempol in its oxidized form acts as contrast agent and can be imaged by MRI. As tempol reduces into hydroxylamine, the contrast enhancement decreases because in its reduced form, it does not provide T_1 contrast. By following the intensity of contrast enhancement over time, it was deduced that tempol is reduced faster into its non-radioprotective

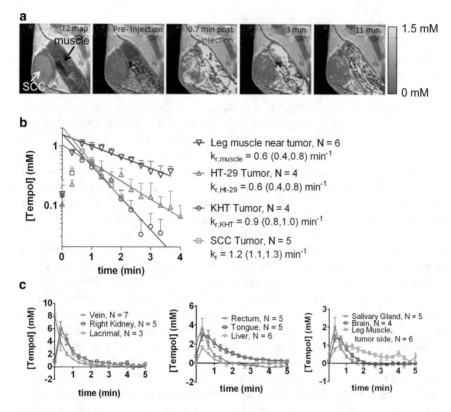

Fig. 4.3 Results from a redox imaging experiment of tumor and salivary glands. (**a**) Concentration maps overlaid on T2-weighted images corresponding to the hind leg region of a mouse. The tumor and the adjacent leg muscle are outlined in *red*. (**b**) The average tempol concentration inside the muscle and tumor was plotted as a function of time after injection. The concentration of tempol was determined in three different tumor models: SCCVII, KHT, and HT-29. For each time point after injection (20 s intervals), the average concentration was determined for each tissue. (**c**) Using the same technique as used in **a** and **b**, the concentration of tempol was determined in nine noncancerous tissue compartments. The *error bars* represent the standard error of the mean, and the lines connect the data points. Note the difference in tempol concentration in tumor compared to normal tissues as a function of time. Reproduced from Davis et al. [34]

form in the tumor compared to surrounding normal tissue (Fig. 4.3) [34]. The unique ability to image tempol may allow a determination of the optimal time of tempol delivery and may further allow the unique opportunity to test this relationship in each patient to be treated.

Clinical translation of tempol has met with initial success. In a phase I clinical trial, tempol was effective at reducing alopecia in patients who underwent whole-brain radiotherapy [35]. Pharmacokinetic studies found that tempol was only detectable in 50 % of plasma samples after topical application and that the levels were minimal in those in which it was detected, suggesting that tumor protection via systemic leak was not a major concern in patients treated with topical tempol.

Other Candidate Radioprotectors

Naturally occurring antioxidants have also been tested for their efficacy as radioprotectors. Antioxidants such as α-tocopherol (vitamin E) and β-carotene have been demonstrated to reduce various radiation-induced injuries including xerostomia [36] and mucositis [37, 38], and in combination with pentoxifylline, α-tocopherol has been shown to reduce lung fibrosis [39, 40]. The use of these nutritional antioxidants as radioprotectors has come under question due to concerns that these agents may also interfere with tumor control either through radioprotection or via enhancement in the rate of second malignancies. Combined α-tocopherol and β-carotene supplementation given during and after radiation was also shown to increase the local recurrence rate of head and neck tumors [37]. These findings highlight the need to consider the possibility of tumor radioprotection carefully.

One promising antioxidant that could be an effective radioprotector is superoxide dismutase (SOD). SOD is an endogenous enzyme that converts superoxide into oxygen and hydrogen peroxide. Transgene expression of SOD in animal models via gene therapy has been shown to protect against mucositis [41], esophagitis [42], and pneumonitis [43, 44]. Furthermore in animal models, SOD was demonstrated to selectively protect normal and not tumor tissue [45]. The major concern with this approach is the ability of SOD to access the primary target of radaition, DNA.

Melatonin is a hormone that has been shown in a number of studies to have radioprotective effects. It has the ability to directly scavenge free radicals and to increase the expression levels of antioxidant enzymes, including SOD, glutathione peroxidase, and catalase. It also has been reported to increase the efficiency of mitochondrial function, thereby reducing ROS levels generated by the electron transport chain [46]. In animal models, melatonin has been demonstrated to protect mice against lethal total body exposures [47, 48] and to protect a number of organs from radiation injury [49]. In vitro studies have demonstrated that melatonin sensitizes cancer cell lines to irradiation [50, 51].

Despite the fact that preclinical data supports that melatonin is a selective radioprotector, a phase II trial did not confirm activity in this regard. A Radiation Therapy Oncology Group (RTOG) trial randomized patients with brain metastases into two groups: morning versus nighttime high-dose melatonin. Melatonin was given to the patients during and following radiation. Results from this study were compared to historical controls who received only whole-brain radiotherapy. It was concluded that melatonin improved neither overall survival nor neurocognitive function after radiotherapy [52]. More recently, several in vitro studies have shown that melatonin at pharmacologic doses may actually have oxidant effects [53–55]. This finding has yet to be confirmed in vivo; nevertheless, it suggests caution and careful consideration of dosing is necessary when combining melatonin with radiotherapy.

Radiation Mitigators

Radiation mitigators reduce normal tissue damage after exposure to radiation through a variety of mechanisms. Unlike radioprotectors, which prevent damage from occurring, radiation mitigators minimize damage by acting upon physiologic processes that occur after radiation exposure but before the clinical manifestation of injury [4]. Radiation mitigators may be used to ameliorate both acute and late toxicities. Acute radiation toxicities, such as dermatitis and mucositis, are often caused by the death of rapidly dividing cells [56]. Damage to the rapidly proliferating stem cell compartment of organs, such as the skin and small intestine, eventually leads to loss of differentiated, specialized cells and results in the manifestation of tissue damage [57, 58]. Therefore, mitigators that effectively prevent acute injury often promote stem cell survival and proliferation.

Although the cellular response to radiation is almost immediate, the expression of late toxicities may be delayed for months to years after radiation exposure. Radiation activates a myriad of different signaling pathways that initiate pro-inflammatory, profibrotic, and vascular injury responses. These responses continue long after the initial radiation exposure and result in altered tissue homeostasis, fibrosis, vascular damage, atrophy, and necrosis [59]. Many radiation mitigators target key molecules or processes in the pathways that lead to late radiation injury. It is impossible to review every radiation mitigator identified in the space allowed. Thus, we have highlighted clinically approved or notable examples in the sections below.

Total Body Exposures

Normal tissue stem cells are responsible for regenerating tissues damaged by radiation and other processes. Stem cells are highly sensitive to radiation and are typically depleted in the radiation-damaged tissues [58, 60, 61]. Thus, a great deal of research has evaluated cytokines and growth factors that have the capacity to promote stem cell survival and proliferation. These approaches have been explored primarily as a method to reduce acute toxicity after localized and total body exposures.

Total body exposures can cause death through bone marrow failure and loss of intestinal integrity (gastrointestinal syndrome) [56]. At extreme doses death results from damage to the central nervous system and vascular collapse [56]. Intestinal damage is also a cause of major morbidity among transplant patients treated with total body irradiation. Many mitigant strategies for total body exposures are therefore geared toward preventing bone marrow failure and gastrointestinal syndrome by stimulating stem cell function. Intestinal injury is also a major dose-limiting factor during abdominal and pelvic radiation.

One example of this approach is the use of granulocyte colony-stimulating factor (G-CSF) as a radiation mitigant. In nonhuman primates, administration of G-CSF at 6 h after a total body exposure led to increased hematopoietic recovery [62]. In mice, administration of two separate doses of G-CSF at 24 h and 30 min before total body irradiation increased survival rates. Interestingly, there was no effect on survival when G-CSF was given 24 h after irradiation [63] suggesting that for the G-CSF to be effective, it must be given close to when radiation DNA damage occurs. This type of treatment may be useful in the setting of accidental total body exposures or in therapeutic exposures that require irradiation of extensive marrow compartments that are uninvolved by tumor. The use of G-CSF with therapeutic radiation must be approached with caution as G-CSF has been reported to drive epithelial to mesenchymal transition and tumor progression [64]. G-CSF is considered an effective treatment for accidental total body exposures and is part of the US Strategic National Stockpile [65].

Another agent in the stockpile, entolimod, is a toll-like receptor 5 (TLR5) agonist that has been shown to have mitigant efficacy in animal models of lethal total body exposures, dermatitis, and mucositis [66, 67], with no evidence of impaired tumor response [66, 67]. Entolimod, formerly known as CBLB502, is a *Salmonella* flagellin derivative that activates the NF-kB pathway by binding toll-like receptor 5 (TLR5). It is more potent but less immunogenic and toxic compared to purified flagellin [67]. At high radiation doses, delivery of entolimod in mice shortly before irradiation led to reduced gastrointestinal and hematological injury and subsequent improvement in survival. Enhanced survival was also observed with postirradiation delivery of entolimod but only at low radiation doses [67]. Efficacy of entolimod was further tested in nonhuman primates, and data showed that entolimod protected primates from hematopoietic and lymphoid organ damage and lethality incurred by radiation [67]. G-CSF and interleukin-6 (IL-6) are two potential biomarkers for entolimod efficacy in mitigating radiation-induced injury. In irradiated and nonirradiated animals, levels of these cytokines were stimulated by entolimod in a TLR5- and dose- dependent manner. Furthermore, inhibiting G-CSF and IL-6 with neutralizing antibodies blocked the radiation mitigating effects of entolimod suggesting that the two cytokines are major mediators of entolimod's mechanism of action [68]. The discovery of these two biomarkers may aid in determining the most optimal, efficacious dose to use in humans. Currently, entolimod is being evaluated in clinical trials for its capacity to mitigate radiation injury.

Palifermin is a truncated recombinant human keratinocyte growth factor (KGF). KGF is a mitogenic factor with diverse functions in proliferation, survival, differentiation, DNA repair, and reactive oxygen species detoxification [69]. Animal studies have shown that administration of palifermin can reduce xerostomia [70], mucositis [71], and gastrointestinal injury [72, 73] induced by radiation. Palifermin is FDA approved for prevention of severe mucositis in hematologic cancer patients who receive chemoradiotherapy prior to stem cell transplant [74]. Additionally, a phase II clinical trial for head and neck cancer found that delivery of palifermin to patients receiving concurrent chemotherapy and hyperfractionated radiotherapy minimized the incidence, severity, and duration of oral mucositis [75]. In the same study, it was concluded that palifermin had no effect on survival or progression-free survival [75], suggesting an absence of tumor-promoting effects. The selectivity of palifermin for normal tissue may depend on whether or not the fibroblast growth factor receptor 2b (FGFR2b), a cognate receptor for KGF, is expressed in tumor tissues. Preclinical studies have shown that KGF-FGFR2b signaling can promote tumor and metastatic phenotypes in breast, lung, and gastric cancer [76].

Because inflammation and vascular damage are two immediate radiation responses that can persist and cause late tissue damage, there has been much interest in mitigators that target inflammatory pathways. One such pathway is the thrombomodulin (THBD)-activated protein C (APC). THBD is a transmembrane glycoprotein that binds thrombin and activates thrombin activatable fibrinolysis inhibitor

(TAFI) [77]. In addition, it cleaves and activates the protein C zymogen, which in turn inactivates blood coagulation factors V and VIII via proteolysis [78]. The anti-coagulant APC also promotes fibrinolysis and induces anti-inflammatory and cyto-protective activities in endothelial, neuronal, and innate immune cells [78]. In clinical and preclinical studies, it has been shown that THBD is significantly reduced and never recovered in intestinal endothelial cells after radiation [79–81]. More interestingly, systematic delivery of soluble THBD and APC in mice exposed to total body irradiation resulted in protection from hematological injury and lethality [82]. Numerous candidate mitigants that expand hematopoiesis or gastrointestinal recovery after total body exposures have been studied, such as metformin, lyso-phosphatidic acid mimics, genistein, and GSK-3 inhibitors [83–89].

Dermatitis

Radiation dermatitis is an acute toxicity of radiotherapy that can cause pain, increase the risk of infection, and result in the need for treatment breaks. Radiation dermatitis typically begins as erythema and progresses with increasing skin dose to indura-tion, dry desquamation, moist desquamation, and finally to ulceration [56]. A number of agents have been tested as treatment for radiation dermatitis in small randomized trials. Several of these agents have been found to reduce the severity of radiation dermatitis to some degree [90–94]. Despite these findings, these agents are not in widespread clinical use at this time, and many patients are only treated with topical emollients for symptomatic relief. Mometasone furoate and betamethasone, topical steroids, have been shown in randomized trials to reduce the severity of radiation dermatitis [95, 96].

Fibrosis

Fibrosis is a common type of late tissue injury associated with radiation. TGF-β is the predominant signaling pathway that drives fibrosis [59], and accordingly, many radiation mitigators that target this pathway have been evaluated. Neutralizing anti-bodies against TGF-β have been shown to minimize fibrosis in animal models fol-lowing radiation [97]. Halofuginone, a small molecular inhibitor that targets TGF-β signaling, also had similar protective effects in mice and showed normal tissue selectivity as it had no effect on tumor radiosensitivity [98]. Downstream molecules of the TGF-β signaling pathway, such as Smad3, have also been demonstrated to be possible therapeutic targets [99, 100].

   It is noteworthy to mention that TGF-β has opposing, dual roles in cancer. In the early stages of cancer, it inhibits tumorigenesis but promotes metastasis as the disease progresses [101, 102]. Therefore, determining the appropriate dosing schedule for anti-TGF-β agents may be crucial in achieving therapeutic gain. Currently, there are no TGF-β-targeting agents in clinical trials specifically for mitigation of radiation-induced fibrosis, although there are several for fibrotic disease and scarring [103].

Statins are HMG-CoA reductase inhibitors that are traditionally used in clinic to lower cholesterol levels. Data from preclinical studies however suggest that statins may also be effective as a radiation mitigator for late and acute injury. In mice that received whole-lung irradiation, lovastatin was shown to reduce thrombopenia and mRNA levels of several pro-inflammatory and profibrotic genes including TNFα, IL-6, TGF-β, and connective tissue growth factor (CTGF) [104]. Lovastatin in a separate study was also shown to attenuate lung fibrosis and increase survival [105]. Moreover, other statins such as pravastatin were shown to attenuate CTGF expression and intestinal radiation fibrosis [106]. The mechanism by which statins regulate late tissue injury is unclear, but it has been hypothesized that it may involve the Rho pathways as inhibition of this pathway resulted in similar protective effects as seen with pravastatin [107, 108]. Statins are also known to inactivate Rho-GTPases further supporting the hypothesis [109]. Whether or not statins are safe to use during tumor radiotherapy remains to be determined. Several reports have shown that statins enhance the radiation cytotoxic effects in tumor tissue [110, 111], but further evaluation is needed.

Activation of the PDGF pathway has been implicated in the progression of radiation fibrosis. PDGFR inhibition via imatinib and other small molecule inhibitors has been shown to be effective in preclinical models of pulmonary and dermal fibrosis [112, 113]. One of the targets of imatinib, c-Abl, is known to be a downstream signaling intermediate of TGF-β in fibroblasts [114]. Furthermore, morphologic transformation and activation of gene expression in TGF-β-stimulated fibroblasts are dependent on the activation of c-Abl, suggesting that reduction in fibrosis with imatinib treatment may partially involve inhibition of TGF-β signaling.

Another group of agents thought to have efficacy in fibrosis and nephropathy are angiotensin-converting enzyme (ACE) inhibitors, agents that are widely used to treat hypertension and heart failure. These agents act by preventing the generation of Angiotensin II which is a vasoconstrictor [115]. More recently, animal studies have shown that ACE inhibitors can ameliorate radiation-induced normal tissue injury. For example, captopril, an ACE inhibitor, reduced pulmonary endothelial dysfunction in irradiated rats [116]. Captopril and other ACE inhibitors were also shown to minimize lung fibrosis caused by radiation [117, 118]. In addition to lung injury, ACE inhibitors have been reported to protect other organs such as the kidney [119] and skin [120, 121] from radiation injury. Importantly, ACE inhibitors have been shown to reduce radiation lethality from lung and kidney toxicity after total body exposures [119]. As for the effects of ACE inhibitors on tumors, a study of ramipril in mice bearing A549 xenografts had no effect on tumor response [121]. The mechanism by which captopril mitigates radiation injury is unclear. It has been hypothesized that it maybe through inhibition of angiotensin II production as angiotensin II is known to promote the expression of TGF-β, a known pro-fibrogenic factor [122, 123].

Small molecule inhibitors account for many of the agents thought to be effective as radiation mitigators. Another area of growing interest for radiation mitigation is cell-based therapies. Cell-based therapies can be used to inhibit inflammatory processes or to repopulate the damaged organ. The infusion of mesenchymal stem cells, an expandable, multipotent stem cell found in mesenchymal tissues, has been reported to mitigate radiation fibrosis in the lung and skin [124, 125]. These cells may be derived from a number of mesenchymal tissues such as bone marrow and adipose tissues. The use of these cells as a therapeutic option is of particular interest given that they can be harvested, expanded in vitro, and stored for future use. Further, these cells are considered immune privileged due to low expression of MHC-II, allowing the use of donor-derived mesenchymal stem cells as therapy. Importantly, the timing of delivery of these cells may be important in their efficacy. Evidence from skin fibrosis models suggests that the interaction of bone marrow stromal cells with activated macrophages results in macrophage repolarization, with elaboration of anti-inflammatory IL-10 [125]. Thus, it is possible that effective treatment with bone marrow stromal cells for mitigation requires a substantial accumulation of macrophages in the irradiated tissues, which is often not seen until several weeks after treatment. Stem cell-based therapies for radiation-induced organ dysfunction have also been studied for other types of radiation injury, such as liver injury and osteonecrosis [126–128].

Central Nervous System Injury

Patients with multiple brain tumors that cannot be surgically resected are commonly treated with whole-brain radiotherapy and/or stereotactic radiosurgery. Unfortunately, patients can experience cognitive impairments from tumor progression or radiation-induced demyelination, vascular damage, and white matter necrosis [129]. Although oxidative stress and inflammation have been implicated in promoting radiation-induced brain injury [130], more recent data suggests that brain tumors themselves may produce inflammatory changes in the CNS microenvironment that are independent of radiation [131]. Accordingly, agents that inhibit these cellular processes including ACE inhibitors, peroxisome proliferator-activated receptor-y (PPARy) agonists, and vascular endothelial growth factor (VEGF) inhibitors have been evaluated in animal models, and preclinical evidence suggests that it may be effective as radiation mitigators for brain injury [130, 132–137].

Clinical trials to mitigate radiation toxicity in the CNS have largely focused on technical approaches to reduce radiation dose to critical structures or off-label use of pharmacotherapies commonly used to treat dementia. RTOG 04 utilized intensity-modulated external beam radiation planning techniques to reduce the dose of radiation delivered to the hippocampus of patients requiring whole-brain radiation for treatment of brain metastases, with the hippocampal sparing technique producing improved performance on a neurocognitive evaluation at 4 months following treatment [138]. Acetylcholinesterase inhibitors, such as donepezil, have been evaluated for differences in neurocognition, mood, and quality of life outcomes in adult and in pediatric patients with some improvement compared to baseline at 24 weeks after radiation treatment [139, 140]. NMDA receptor antagonists such as memantine have produced some improvements in cognitive function over time and delayed neurocognitive decline 24 weeks after whole-brain radiotherapy [141].

Despite the current data demonstrating short-term benefits with some radiation mitigators in the CNS, there is a severe lack of understanding about the underlying biological processes which produce acute and long-term neurodegenerative changes. Most clinical strategies have relied on the assumption that the underlying biological process of neurocognitive decline seen in other conditions such as dementia also holds true for radiation-induced CNS damage. However, this assumption may be misplaced or may not reflect the entire spectrum of radiation-induced changes. The goal of current scientific investigations is to determine how the DNA damage response from radiotherapy to the CNS compartment translates to altered structural and biochemical changes so that more effective, targeted therapies may be developed to afford patients long-term, sustained benefits after radiation.

Treatment

Agents that are given after the development of radiation-induced symptoms are characterized as treatments. In general, preventing normal tissue injury with the use of radioprotectors and mitigators is preferable since some of these toxicities are irreversible and only limited treatments of variable efficacy exist. Treatments for radiation injury may be used for a short duration, or ongoing treatment may be required for prolonged periods to maintain clinical benefit. A comprehensive discussion of treatment of radiation injury is outside the scope of this section; however a few examples are highlighted below. In addition to the examples provided, a number of treatments have been studied for gastrointestinal toxicity, dermatologic toxicity, and mucositis with varying degrees of efficacy.

Fibrosis is a particularly challenging toxicity of radiotherapy, often considered to be irreversible. One treatment that has shown efficacy in this setting is pentoxifylline combined with vitamin E. A double blind, placebo-controlled trial of pentoxifylline and vitamin E in patients with radiation fibrosis of the skin and subcutaneous tissues after treatment for breast cancer found a marked regression in fibrotic surface area with treatment [142]. These findings were confirmed in a study of patients with radiation fibrosis at multiple sites, who were found to have improved range of motion and reduced pain with pentoxifylline treatment [143]. Importantly, long-term treatment with pentoxifylline and vitamin E appears to be necessary, with the possibility of rebound effects if treatment is discontinued too early [144]. Studies of pentoxifylline have also been completed for patients suffering from radiation injury in a number of organs with variable success [145–149].

Radiation pneumonitis may occur in up to 15 % of patients treated with thoracic radiotherapy [150]. Pneumonitis is characterized by fever, cough, and dyspnea with radiographic changes corresponding to the radiated field and may occur within the first 18 months after irradiation. Radiation pneumonitis is a diagnosis of exclusion, meaning that infection, tumor spread, and other causes of lung inflammation must be excluded. Radiation pneumonitis evolves into radiation fibrosis over time, although symptomatic pneumonitis is not a prerequisite for developing radiation fibrosis. Glucocorticoids remain the most effective treatment for radiation pneumonitis but are not considered an effective treatment for radiation fibrosis [151, 152]. Oxygen is also used as needed to limit hypoxia.

In patients receiving radiotherapy to the brain or head and neck, radiation brain necrosis may occur as a side effect. Traditionally, radiation necrosis has been managed with glucocorticoids, with surgical resection reserved for patients in whom radiation necrosis causes persistent symptoms. More recently, bevacizumab, a VEGF inhibitor, has been reported to substantially ameliorate radiation-induced brain necrosis [153–156]. In a randomized trial of bevacizumab versus placebo in 14 patients with biopsy or radiographically confirmed radiation necrosis, treatment with bevacizumab improved neurologic symptoms and signs in all patients [154]. All patients treated with placebo were allowed to cross over into the bevacizumab arm. No response was seen after treatment with the placebo; however, after bevacizumab treatment, only two patients developed a recurrence of radiation necrosis.

Challenges

A number of challenges exist in the effective preclinical and clinical development of the agents for use as radioprotectors and radiation mitigators. One major concern is the ability of animal models to predict the behavior of the human condition. Animals may have different pharmacokinetic responses to drugs, which may alter the appropriate timing and dosing of agents. Conventional radiotherapy often continues daily for up to 8 weeks, a condition challenging to replicate in animal models of injury in which one to ten fractions are typically delivered. Animals also tend to be of similar genetic background with no comorbidities that may affect drug metabolism, drug penetration, and susceptibility to radiation toxicity. And it cannot be forgotten that mice have fundamental biological differences from humans.

Another factor complicating the study of these agents is the use of chemotherapy concurrently with radiotherapy in a growing number of cancers. As a result, testing of these agents as radioprotectors or mitigators often requires assessment of effect in the context of combined radiation and chemotherapy, not just radiotherapy alone. This increases the level of complexity of preclinical studies, increases cost substantially, and complicates analysis of efficacy. To ensure that candidate radiation protectors or mitigators do not impair tumor control, additional studies should always be completed in tumor models before clinical translation if it is expected that they will be delivered in close proximity to radiotherapy.

Perhaps the greatest challenge for the development of effective radiation protectors and radiation mitigators is determining which patients would benefit most from treatment. Unless an agent has minimal cost and minimal toxicity, it would be unreasonable to treat every patient prophylactically unless the toxicity was so severe it would cause death or serious chronic injury in a substantial number of patients. In order to determine which patients would benefit the most from the use of these agents, it is necessary to develop effective means of predicting who will develop injury.

Finally, the clinical translation of agents used to prevent, mitigate, or treat radiation injury can be difficult because of the challenges involved in designing clinical trials capable of determining efficacy. Patients included in these trials will have different comorbidities and genetic background, which may variably affect the likelihood or predisposition to developing toxicity. Patients will have tumors of varying sizes or with characteristics that require treatment of different volumes or doses with radiotherapy. With newer techniques such as intensity-modulated radiation therapy, dose delivered to organs becomes increasingly complex to consider as a variable in these studies. Perhaps most importantly, the endpoint of these studies and grading scales used to assess efficacy must be carefully chosen to accurately reflect clinical benefit.

Despite these challenges, the development of radiation protectors, radiation mitigators, and treatment for radiation injury holds great promise for the growing number of patients that survive aggressive cancer therapy. Encouraging progress has been made in reducing normal tissue injury from radiotherapy, but clearly additional work is needed.

Acknowledgment This research was supported by the Intramural Research Program of the National Institutes of Health, National Cancer Institute.

Disclosures and Conflicts of Interests

The authors have no conflicts of interests or relationships to disclose.

References

1. Durante M, Loeffler JS (2010) Charged particles in radiation oncology. Nat Rev Clin Oncol 7(1):37–43
2. Moding EJ, Kastan MB, Kirsch DG (2013) Strategies for optimizing the response of cancer and normal tissues to radiation. Nat Rev Drug Discov 12(7):526–542
3. Fu KK, Pajak TF, Trotti A et al (2000) A Radiation Therapy Oncology Group (RTOG) phase III randomized study to compare hyperfractionation and two variants of accelerated fractionation to standard fractionation radiotherapy for head and neck squamous cell carcinomas: first report of RTOG 9003. Int J Radiat Oncol Biol Phys 48(1):7–16
4. Stone HB, Moulder JE, Coleman CN et al (2004) Models for evaluating agents intended for the prophylaxis, mitigation and treatment of radiation injuries. Report of an NCI Workshop, December 3-4, 2003. Radiat Res 162(6):711–728
5. Citrin D, Cotrim AP, Hyodo F et al (2010) Radioprotectors and mitigators of radiation-induced normal tissue injury. Oncologist 15(4):360–371
6. Camphausen K, Citrin D, Krishna MC et al (2005) Implications for tumor control during protection of normal tissues with antioxidants. J Clin Oncol 23(24):5455–5457
7. Xavier S, Yamada K, Samuni AM et al (2002) Differential protection by nitroxides and hydroxylamines to radiation-induced and metal ion-catalyzed oxidative damage. Biochim Biophys Acta 1573(2):109–120
8. Kouvaris JR, Kouloulias VE, Vlahos LJ (2007) Amifostine: the first selective-target and broad-spectrum radioprotector. Oncologist 12(6):738–747
9. Calabro-Jones PM, Fahey RC, Smoluk GD et al (1985) Alkaline phosphatase promotes radioprotection and accumulation of WR-1065 in V79-171 cells incubated in medium containing WR-2721. Int J Radiat Biol Relat Stud Phys Chem Med 47(1):23–27

10. Yuhas JM (1980) Active versus passive absorption kinetics as the basis for selective protection of normal tissues by S-2-(3-aminopropylamino)-ethylphosphorothioic acid. Cancer Res 40(5):1519–1524

11. Giatromanolaki A, Sivridis E, Maltezos E et al (2002) Down-regulation of intestinal-type alkaline phosphatase in the tumor vasculature and stroma provides a strong basis for explaining amifostine selectivity. Semin Oncol 29(6 Suppl 19):14–21

12. Purdie JW, Inhaber ER, Schneider H et al (1983) Interaction of cultured mammalian cells with WR-2721 and its thiol, WR-1065: implications for mechanisms of radioprotection. Int J Radiat Biol Relat Stud Phys Chem Med 43(5):517–527

13. Glover D, Negendank W, Delivoria-Papadopoulos M et al (1984) Alterations in oxygen transport following WR-2721. Int J Radiat Oncol Biol Phys 10(9):1565–1568

14. Nicolatou-Galitis O, Sarri T, Bowen J et al (2013) Systematic review of amifostine for the management of oral mucositis in cancer patients. Support Care Cancer 21(1):357–364

15. Werner-Wasik M, Axelrod RS, Friedland DP et al (2002) Phase II: trial of twice weekly amifostine in patients with non-small cell lung cancer treated with chemoradiotherapy. Semin Radiat Oncol 12(1 Suppl 1):34–39

16. Antonadou D (2002) Radiotherapy or chemotherapy followed by radiotherapy with or without amifostine in locally advanced lung cancer. Semin Radiat Oncol 12(1 Suppl 1):50–58

17. Komaki R, Lee JS, Milas L et al (2004) Effects of amifostine on acute toxicity from concurrent chemotherapy and radiotherapy for inoperable non-small-cell lung cancer: report of a randomized comparative trial. Int J Radiat Oncol Biol Phys 58(5):1369–1377

18. Movsas B, Scott C, Langer C et al (2005) Randomized trial of amifostine in locally advanced non-small-cell lung cancer patients receiving chemotherapy and hyperfractionated radiation: radiation therapy oncology group trial 98-01. J Clin Oncol 23(10):2145–2154

19. Sarna L, Swann S, Langer C et al (2008) Clinically meaningful differences in patient-reported outcomes with amifostine in combination with chemoradiation for locally advanced non-small-cell lung cancer: an analysis of RTOG 9801. Int J Radiat Oncol Biol Phys 72(5):1378–1384

20. Kouvaris J, Kouloulias V, Kokakis J et al (2002) The cytoprotective effect of amifostine in acute radiation dermatitis: a retrospective analysis. Eur J Dermatol 12(5):458–462

21. Singh AK, Menard C, Guion P et al (2006) Intrarectal amifostine suspension may protect against acute proctitis during radiation therapy for prostate cancer: a pilot study. Int J Radiat Oncol Biol Phys 65(4):1008–1013

22. Simone NL, Menard C, Soule BP et al (2008) Intrarectal amifostine during external beam radiation therapy for prostate cancer produces significant improvements in Quality of Life measured by EPIC score. Int J Radiat Oncol Biol Phys 70(1):90–95

23. Koukourakis MI, Panteliadou M, Abatzoglou IM et al (2013) Postmastectomy hypofractionated and accelerated radiation therapy with (and without) subcutaneous amifostine cytoprotection. Int J Radiat Oncol Biol Phys 85(1):e7–e13

24. Antonadou D, Coliarakis N, Synodinou M et al (2001) Randomized phase III trial of radiation treatment +/- amifostine in patients with advanced-stage lung cancer. Int J Radiat Oncol Biol Phys 51(4):915–922

25. Samuni A, Goldstein S, Russo A et al (2002) Kinetics and mechanism of hydroxyl radical and OH-adduct radical reactions with nitroxides and with their hydroxylamines. J Am Chem Soc 124(29):8719–8724

26. Soule BP, Hyodo F, Matsumoto K et al (2007) Therapeutic and clinical applications of nitroxide compounds. Antioxid Redox Signal 9(10):1731–1743

27. Soule BP, Hyodo F, Matsumoto K et al (2007) The chemistry and biology of nitroxide compounds. Free Radic Biol Med 42(11):1632–1650

28. Hahn SM, Tochner Z, Krishna CM et al (1992) Tempol, a stable free radical, is a novel murine radiation protector. Cancer Res 52(7):1750–1753

29. Hahn SM, Krishna CM, Samuni A et al (1994) Potential use of nitroxides in radiation oncology. Cancer Res 54 (7 Suppl):2006s–2010s

30. Cuscela D, Coffin D, Lupton GP et al (1996) Protection from radiation-induced alopecia with topical application of nitroxides: fractionated studies. Cancer J Sci Am 2(5):273–278
31. Goffman T, Cuscela D, Glass J et al (1992) Topical application of nitroxide protects radiation-induced alopecia in guinea pigs. Int J Radiat Oncol Biol Phys 22(4):803–806
32. Cotrim AP, Hyodo F, Matsumoto K et al (2007) Differential radiation protection of salivary glands versus tumor by Tempol with accompanying tissue assessment of Tempol by magnetic resonance imaging. Clin Cancer Res 13(16):4928–4933
33. Hahn SM, Sullivan FJ, DeLuca AM et al (1997) Evaluation of tempol radioprotection in a murine tumor model. Free Radic Biol Med 22(7):1211–1216
34. Davis RM, Mitchell JB, Krishna MC (2011) Nitroxides as cancer imaging agents. Anticancer Agents Med Chem 11(4):347–358
35. Metz JM, Smith D, Mick R et al (2004) A phase I study of topical Tempol for the prevention of alopecia induced by whole brain radiotherapy. Clin Cancer Res 10(19):6411–6417
36. Chitra S, Shyamala Devi CS (2008) Effects of radiation and alpha-tocopherol on saliva flow rate, amylase activity, total protein and electrolyte levels in oral cavity cancer. Indian J Dent Res 19(3):213–218
37. Bairati I, Meyer F, Gelinas M et al (2005) Randomized trial of antioxidant vitamins to prevent acute adverse effects of radiation therapy in head and neck cancer patients. J Clin Oncol 23(24):5805–5813
38. Ferreira PR, Fleck JF, Diehl A et al (2004) Protective effect of alpha-tocopherol in head and neck cancer radiation-induced mucositis: a double-blind randomized trial. Head Neck 26(4):313–321
39. Misirlioglu CH, Demirkasimoglu T, Kucukplakci B et al (2007) Pentoxifylline and alpha-tocopherol in prevention of radiation-induced lung toxicity in patients with lung cancer. Med Oncol 24(3):308–311
40. Jacobson G, Bhatia S, Smith BJ et al (2013) Randomized trial of pentoxifylline and vitamin E vs standard follow-up after breast irradiation to prevent breast fibrosis, evaluated by tissue compliance meter. Int J Radiat Oncol Biol Phys 85(3):604–608
41. Guo H, Seixas-Silva JA Jr, Epperly MW et al (2003) Prevention of radiation-induced oral cavity mucositis by plasmid/liposome delivery of the human manganese superoxide dismutase (SOD2) transgene. Radiat Res 159(3):361–370
42. Stickle RL, Epperly MW, Klein E et al (1999) Prevention of irradiation-induced esophagitis by plasmid/liposome delivery of the human manganese superoxide dismutase transgene. Radiat Oncol Investig 7(4):204–217
43. Epperly MW, Bray JA, Krager S et al (1999) Intratracheal injection of adenovirus containing the human MnSOD transgene protects athymic nude mice from irradiation-induced organizing alveolitis. Int J Radiat Oncol Biol Phys 43(1):169–181
44. Epperly MW, Travis EL, Sikora C et al (1999) Manganese [correction of Magnesium] superoxide dismutase (MnSOD) plasmid/liposome pulmonary radioprotective gene therapy: modulation of irradiation-induced mRNA for IL-I, TNF-alpha, and TGF-beta correlates with delay of organizing alveolitis/fibrosis. Biol Blood Marrow Transplant 5(4):204–214
45. Epperly MW, Defilippi S, Sikora C et al (2000) Intratracheal injection of manganese superoxide dismutase (MnSOD) plasmid/liposomes protects normal lung but not orthotopic tumors from irradiation. Gene Ther 7(12):1011–1018
46. Acuna-Castroviejo D, Martin M, Macias M et al (2001) Melatonin, mitochondria, and cellular bioenergetics. J Pineal Res 30(2):65–74
47. Vijayalaxmi MML, Reiter RJ et al (1999) Melatonin and protection from whole-body irradiation: survival studies in mice. Mutat Res 425(1):21–27
48. Blickenstaff RT, Brandstadter SM, Reddy S et al (1994) Potential radioprotective agents. 1. Homologs of melatonin. J Pharm Sci 83(2):216–218
49. Mihandoost E, Shirazi A, Mahdavi SR et al (2014) Can melatonin help us in radiation oncology treatments? Biomed Res Int 2014:578137
50. Jang SS, Kim WD, Park WY (2009) Melatonin exerts differential actions on X-ray radiation-induced apoptosis in normal mice splenocytes and Jurkat leukemia cells. J Pineal Res 47(2):147–155

51. Alonso-Gonzalez C, Gonzalez A, Martinez-Campa C et al (2015) Melatonin sensitizes human breast cancer cells to ionizing radiation by downregulating proteins involved in double-strand DNA break repair. J Pineal Res 58(2):189–197

52. Berk L, Berkey B, Rich T et al (2007) Randomized phase II trial of high-dose melatonin and radiation therapy for RPA class 2 patients with brain metastases (RTOG 0119). Int J Radiat Oncol Biol Phys 68(3):852–857

53. Zhang HM, Zhang Y (2014) Melatonin: a well-documented antioxidant with conditional pro-oxidant actions. J Pineal Res 57(2):131–146

54. Medina-Navarro R, Duran-Reyes G, Hicks JJ (1999) Pro-oxidating properties of melatonin in the in vitro interaction with the singlet oxygen. Endocr Res 25(3-4):263–280

55. Wolfler A, Caluba HC, Abuja PM et al (2001) Prooxidant activity of melatonin promotes fas-induced cell death in human leukemic Jurkat cells. FEBS Lett 502(3):127–131

56. Hall EJ, Giaccia AJ (2006) Radiobiology for the Radiologist. Lippincott Williams & Wilkins, Philadelphia

57. Blanpain C, Fuchs E (2006) Epidermal stem cells of the skin. Annu Rev Cell Dev Biol 22: 339–373

58. Metcalfe C, Kljavin NM, Ybarra R et al (2014) Lgr5+ stem cells are indispensable for radiation-induced intestinal regeneration. Cell Stem Cell 14(2):149–159

59. Bentzen SM (2006) Preventing or reducing late side effects of radiation therapy: radiobiology meets molecular pathology. Nat Rev Cancer 6(9):702–713

60. Iglesias-Bartolome R, Patel V, Cotrim A et al (2012) mTOR inhibition prevents epithelial stem cell senescence and protects from radiation-induced mucositis. Cell Stem Cell 11(3): 401–414

61. Mizumatsu S, Monje ML, Morhardt DR et al (2003) Extreme sensitivity of adult neurogenesis to low doses of X-irradiation. Cancer Res 63(14):4021–4027

62. Bertho JM, Frick J, Prat M et al (2005) Comparison of autologous cell therapy and granulocyte-colony stimulating factor (G-CSF) injection vs. G-CSF injection alone for the treatment of acute radiation syndrome in a non-human primate model. Int J Radiat Oncol Biol Phys 63(3):911–920

63. Uckun FM, Souza L, Waddick KG et al (1990) In vivo radioprotective effects of recombinant human granulocyte colony-stimulating factor in lethally irradiated mice. Blood 75(3):638–645

64. Cui YH, Suh Y, Lee HJ et al (2015) Radiation promotes invasiveness of non-small-cell lung cancer cells through granulocyte-colony stimulating factor. Oncogene 34:5372–5382

65. Singh VK, Romaine PL, Seed TM (2015) Medical countermeasures for radiation exposure and related injuries: characterization of medicines, FDA-approval status and inclusion into the strategic national stockpile. Health Phys 108(6):607–630

66. Burdelya LG, Gleiberman AS, Toshkov I et al (2012) Toll-like receptor 5 agonist protects mice from dermatitis and oral mucositis caused by local radiation: implications for head-and-neck cancer radiotherapy. Int J Radiat Oncol Biol Phys 83(1):228–234

67. Burdelya LG, Krivokrysenko VI, Tallant TC et al (2008) An agonist of toll-like receptor 5 has radioprotective activity in mouse and primate models. Science 320(5873):226–230

68. Krivokrysenko VI, Shakhov AN, Singh VK et al (2012) Identification of granulocyte colony-stimulating factor and interleukin-6 as candidate biomarkers of CBLB502 efficacy as a medical radiation countermeasure. J Pharmacol Exp Ther 343(2):497–508

69. Finch PW, Rubin JS (2004) Keratinocyte growth factor/fibroblast growth factor 7, a homeostatic factor with therapeutic potential for epithelial protection and repair. Adv Cancer Res 91:69–136

70. Lombaert IM, Brunsting JF, Wierenga PK et al (2008) Keratinocyte growth factor prevents radiation damage to salivary glands by expansion of the stem/progenitor pool. Stem Cells 26(10):2595–2601

71. Farrell CL, Rex KL, Kaufman SA et al (1999) Effects of keratinocyte growth factor in the squamous epithelium of the upper aerodigestive tract of normal and irradiated mice. Int J Radiat Biol 75(5):609–620

72. Farrell CL, Bready JV, Rex KL et al (1998) Keratinocyte growth factor protects mice from chemotherapy and radiation-induced gastrointestinal injury and mortality. Cancer Res 58(5): 933–939
73. Cai Y, Wang W, Liang H et al (2013) Keratinocyte growth factor pretreatment prevents radiation-induced intestinal damage in a mouse model. Scand J Gastroenterol 48(4): 419–426
74. Spielberger R, Stiff P, Bensinger W et al (2004) Palifermin for oral mucositis after intensive therapy for hematologic cancers. N Engl J Med 351(25):2590–2598
75. Brizel DM, Murphy BA, Rosenthal DI et al (2008) Phase II study of palifermin and concurrent chemoradiation in head and neck squamous cell carcinoma. J Clin Oncol 26(15): 2489–2496
76. Finch PW, Mark Cross LJ, McAuley DF et al (2013) Palifermin for the protection and regeneration of epithelial tissues following injury: new findings in basic research and pre-clinical models. J Cell Mol Med 17(9):1065–1087
77. Bouma BN, Marx PF, Mosnier LO et al (2001) Thrombin-activatable fibrinolysis inhibitor (TAFI, plasma procarboxypeptidase B, procarboxypeptidase R, procarboxypeptidase U). Thromb Res 101(5):329–354
78. Mosnier LO, Zlokovic BV, Griffin JH (2007) The cytoprotective protein C pathway. Blood 109(8):3161–3172
79. Wang J, Zheng H, Ou X et al (2002) Deficiency of microvascular thrombomodulin and up-regulation of protease-activated receptor-1 in irradiated rat intestine: possible link between endothelial dysfunction and chronic radiation fibrosis. Am J Pathol 160(6):2063–2072
80. Richter KK, Fink LM, Hughes BM et al (1998) Differential effect of radiation on endothelial cell function in rectal cancer and normal rectum. Am J Surg 176(6):642–647
81. Richter KK, Fink LM, Hughes BM et al (1997) Is the loss of endothelial thrombomodulin involved in the mechanism of chronicity in late radiation enteropathy? Radiother Oncol 44(1):65–71
82. Geiger H, Pawar SA, Kerschen EJ et al (2012) Pharmacological targeting of the thrombomodulin-activated protein C pathway mitigates radiation toxicity. Nat Med 18(7): 1123–1129
83. Xu G, Wu H, Zhang J et al (2015) Metformin ameliorates ionizing irradiation-induced long-term hematopoietic stem cell injury in mice. Free Radic Biol Med 87:15–25
84. Deng W, Kimura Y, Gududuru V et al (2015) Mitigation of the hematopoietic and gastrointestinal acute radiation syndrome by octadecenyl thiophosphate, a small molecule mimic of lysophosphatidic acid. Radiat Res 183(4):465–475
85. Patil R, Szabo E, Fells JI et al (2015) Combined mitigation of the gastrointestinal and hematopoietic acute radiation syndromes by an LPA2 receptor-specific nonlipid agonist. Chem Biol 22(2):206–216
86. Lee CL, Lento WE, Castle KD et al (2014) Inhibiting glycogen synthase kinase-3 mitigates the hematopoietic acute radiation syndrome in mice. Radiat Res 181(5):445–451
87. Landauer M, Kohler PA, Kortek Y et al (2009) Long-term care benefits and services in Europe. Gerontology 55(5):481–490
88. Zhou Y, Mi MT (2005) Genistein stimulates hematopoiesis and increases survival in irradiated mice. J Radiat Res 46(4):425–433
89. Davis TA, Clarke TK, Mog SR et al (2007) Subcutaneous administration of genistein prior to lethal irradiation supports multilineage, hematopoietic progenitor cell recovery and survival. Int J Radiat Biol 83(3):141–151
90. Chan RJ, Mann J, Tripcony L et al (2014) Natural oil-based emulsion containing allantoin versus aqueous cream for managing radiation-induced skin reactions in patients with cancer: a phase 3, double-blind, randomized, controlled trial. Int J Radiat Oncol Biol Phys 90(4): 756–764
91. Stefanelli A, Forte L, Medoro S et al (2014) Topical use of phytotherapic cream (Capilen(R) cream) to prevent radiodermatitis in breast cancer: a prospective historically controlled clinical study. G Ital Dermatol Venereol 149(1):107–113

92. Herst PM, Bennett NC, Sutherland AE et al (2014) Prophylactic use of Mepitel Film prevents radiation-induced moist desquamation in an intra-patient randomised controlled clinical trial of 78 breast cancer patients. Radiother Oncol 110(1):137–143

93. Kong M, Hong SE (2013) Topical use of recombinant human epidermal growth factor (EGF)-based cream to prevent radiation dermatitis in breast cancer patients: a single-blind randomized preliminary study. Asian Pac J Cancer Prev 14(8):4859–4864

94. Ryan JL, Heckler CE, Ling M et al (2013) Curcumin for radiation dermatitis: a randomized, double-blind, placebo-controlled clinical trial of thirty breast cancer patients. Radiat Res 180(1):34–43

95. Hindley A, Zain Z, Wood L et al (2014) Mometasone furoate cream reduces acute radiation dermatitis in patients receiving breast radiation therapy: results of a randomized trial. Int J Radiat Oncol Biol Phys 90(4):748–755

96. Ulff E, Maroti M, Serup J et al (2013) A potent steroid cream is superior to emollients in reducing acute radiation dermatitis in breast cancer patients treated with adjuvant radiotherapy. A randomised study of betamethasone versus two moisturizing creams. Radiother Oncol 108(2):287–292

97. Anscher MS, Thrasher B, Rabbani Z et al (2006) Antitransforming growth factor-beta antibody 1D11 ameliorates normal tissue damage caused by high-dose radiation. Int J Radiat Oncol Biol Phys 65(3):876–881

98. Xavier S, Piek E, Fujii M et al (2004) Amelioration of radiation-induced fibrosis: inhibition of transforming growth factor-beta signaling by halofuginone. J Biol Chem 279(15): 15167–15176

99. Flanders KC, Sullivan CD, Fujii M et al (2002) Mice lacking Smad3 are protected against cutaneous injury induced by ionizing radiation. Am J Pathol 160(3):1057–1068

100. Roberts AB, Piek E, Bottinger EP et al (2001) Is Smad3 a major player in signal transduction pathways leading to fibrogenesis? Chest 120(1 Suppl):43S–47S

101. Massague J (2008) TGFbeta in Cancer. Cell 134(2):215–230

102. Massague J, Heino J, Laiho M (1991) Mechanisms in TGF-beta action. Ciba Found Symp 157:51–59, discussion 59-65

103. Akhurst RJ, Hata A (2012) Targeting the TGFbeta signalling pathway in disease. Nat Rev Drug Discov 11(10):790–811

104. Ostrau C, Hulsenbeck J, Herzog M et al (2009) Lovastatin attenuates ionizing radiation-induced normal tissue damage in vivo. Radiother Oncol 92(3):492–499

105. Williams JP, Hernady E, Johnston CJ et al (2004) Effect of administration of lovastatin on the development of late pulmonary effects after whole-lung irradiation in a murine model. Radiat Res 161(5):560–567

106. Haydont V, Gilliot O, Rivera S et al (2007) Successful mitigation of delayed intestinal radiation injury using pravastatin is not associated with acute injury improvement or tumor protection. Int J Radiat Oncol Biol Phys 68(5):1471–1482

107. Haydont V, Bourgier C, Vozenin-Brotons MC (2007) Rho/ROCK pathway as a molecular target for modulation of intestinal radiation-induced toxicity. Br J Radiol 80(1):S32–S40

108. Bourgier C, Haydont V, Milliat F et al (2005) Inhibition of Rho kinase modulates radiation induced fibrogenic phenotype in intestinal smooth muscle cells through alteration of the cytoskeleton and connective tissue growth factor expression. Gut 54(3):336–343

109. Liao JK, Laufs U (2005) Pleiotropic effects of statins. Annu Rev Pharmacol Toxicol 45: 89–118

110. Miller AC, Kariko K, Myers CE et al (1993) Increased radioresistance of EJras-transformed human osteosarcoma cells and its modulation by lovastatin, an inhibitor of p21ras isoprenylation. Int J Cancer 53(2):302–307

111. Fritz G, Brachetti C, Kaina B (2003) Lovastatin causes sensitization of HeLa cells to ionizing radiation-induced apoptosis by the abrogation of G2 blockage. Int J Radiat Biol 79(8): 601–610

112. Horton JA, Chung EJ, Hudak KE et al (2013) Inhibition of radiation-induced skin fibrosis with imatinib. Int J Radiat Biol 89(3):162–170

113. Abdollahi A, Li M, Ping G et al (2005) Inhibition of platelet-derived growth factor signaling attenuates pulmonary fibrosis. J Exp Med 201(6):925–935

114. Daniels CE, Wilkes MC, Edens M et al (2004) Imatinib mesylate inhibits the profibrogenic activity of TGF-beta and prevents bleomycin-mediated lung fibrosis. J Clin Invest 114(9): 1308–1316

115. Brown NJ, Vaughan DE (1998) Angiotensin-converting enzyme inhibitors. Circulation 97(14):1411–1420

116. Ward WF, Kim YT, Molteni A et al (1988) Radiation-induced pulmonary endothelial dysfunction in rats: modification by an inhibitor of angiotensin converting enzyme. Int J Radiat Oncol Biol Phys 15(1):135–140

117. Molteni A, Moulder JE, Cohen EF et al (2000) Control of radiation-induced pneumopathy and lung fibrosis by angiotensin-converting enzyme inhibitors and an angiotensin II type 1 receptor blocker. Int J Radiat Biol 76(4):523–532

118. Kma L, Gao F, Fish BL et al (2012) Angiotensin converting enzyme inhibitors mitigate collagen synthesis induced by a single dose of radiation to the whole thorax. J Radiat Res 53(1): 10–17

119. Medhora M, Gao F, Wu Q et al (2014) Model development and use of ACE inhibitors for preclinical mitigation of radiation-induced injury to multiple organs. Radiat Res 182(5): 545–555

120. Matsuura-Hachiya Y, Arai KY, Ozeki R et al (2013) Angiotensin-converting enzyme inhibitor (enalapril maleate) accelerates recovery of mouse skin from UVB-induced wrinkles. Biochem Biophys Res Commun 442(1-2):38–43

121. Kohl RR, Kolozsvary A, Brown SL et al (2007) Differential radiation effect in tumor and normal tissue after treatment with ramipril, an angiotensin-converting enzyme inhibitor. Radiat Res 168(4):440–445

122. Wolf G, Mueller E, Stahl RA et al (1993) Angiotensin II-induced hypertrophy of cultured murine proximal tubular cells is mediated by endogenous transforming growth factor-beta. J Clin Invest 92(3):1366–1372

123. Hahn AW, Resink TJ, Bernhardt J et al (1991) Stimulation of autocrine platelet--derived growth factor AA-homodimer and transforming growth factor beta in vascular smooth muscle cells. Biochem Biophys Res Commun 178(3):1451–1458

124. Jiang X, Jiang X, Qu C et al (2015) Intravenous delivery of adipose-derived mesenchymal stromal cells attenuates acute radiation-induced lung injury in rats. Cytotherapy 17(5): 560–570

125. Horton JA, Hudak KE, Chung EJ et al (2013) Mesenchymal stem cells inhibit cutaneous radiation-induced fibrosis by suppressing chronic inflammation. Stem Cells 31(10):2231–2241

126. Chen Y, Li Y, Wang X et al (2015) Amelioration of hyperbilirubinemia in gunn rats after transplantation of human induced pluripotent stem cell-derived hepatocytes. Stem Cell Reports 5(1):22–30

127. Landis CS, Zhou H, Liu L et al (2015) Liver regeneration and energetic changes in rats following hepatic radiation therapy and hepatocyte transplantation by (3)(1)P MRSI. Liver Int 35(4):1145–1151

128. Jin IG, Kim JH, Wu HG et al (2015) Effect of bone marrow-derived stem cells and bone morphogenetic protein-2 on treatment of osteoradionecrosis in a rat model., J Craniomaxillofac Surg

129. Greene-Schloesser D, Robbins ME, Peiffer AM et al (2012) Radiation-induced brain injury: a review. Front Oncol 2:73

130. Steeg PS, Camphausen KA, Smith QR (2011) Brain metastases as preventive and therapeutic targets. Nat Rev Cancer 11(5):352–363

131. Smart D, Garcia Glaessner A, Palmieri D et al (2015) Analysis of radiation therapy in a model of triple-negative breast cancer brain metastasis. J Clin Exp Metastasis 32:717–727

132. Ryu S, Kolozsvary A, Jenrow KA et al (2007) Mitigation of radiation-induced optic neuropathy in rats by ACE inhibitor ramipril: importance of ramipril dose and treatment time. J Neurooncol 82(2):119–124

133. Lee TC, Greene-Schloesser D, Payne V et al (2012) Chronic administration of the angiotensin-converting enzyme inhibitor, ramipril, prevents fractionated whole-brain irradiation-induced perirhinal cortex-dependent cognitive impairment. Radiat Res 178(1):46–56

134. Jenrow KA, Brown SL, Liu J et al (2010) Ramipril mitigates radiation-induced impairment of neurogenesis in the rat dentate gyrus. Radiat Oncol 5:6

135. Greene-Schloesser D, Payne V, Peiffer AM et al (2014) The peroxisomal proliferator-activated receptor (PPAR) alpha agonist, fenofibrate, prevents fractionated whole-brain irradiation-induced cognitive impairment. Radiat Res 181(1):33–44

136. Zhao W, Payne V, Tommasi E et al (2007) Administration of the peroxisomal proliferator-activated receptor gamma agonist pioglitazone during fractionated brain irradiation prevents radiation-induced cognitive impairment. Int J Radiat Oncol Biol Phys 67(1):6–9

137. Jiang X, Engelbach JA, Yuan L et al (2014) Anti-VEGF antibodies mitigate the development of radiation necrosis in mouse brain. Clin Cancer Res 20(10):2695–2702

138. Gondi V, Pugh SL, Tome WA et al (2014) Preservation of memory with conformal avoidance of the hippocampal neural stem-cell compartment during whole-brain radiotherapy for brain metastases (RTOG 0933): a phase II multi-institutional trial. J Clin Oncol 32(34): 3810–3816

139. Shaw EG, Rosdhal R, D'Agostino RB Jr et al (2006) Phase II study of donepezil in irradiated brain tumor patients: effect on cognitive function, mood, and quality of life. J Clin Oncol 24(9):1415–1420

140. Castellino SM, Tooze JA, Flowers L et al (2012) Toxicity and efficacy of the acetylcholinesterase (AChe) inhibitor donepezil in childhood brain tumor survivors: a pilot study. Pediatr Blood Cancer 59(3):540–547

141. Brown PD, Pugh S, Laack NN et al (2013) Memantine for the prevention of cognitive dysfunction in patients receiving whole-brain radiotherapy: a randomized, double-blind, placebo-controlled trial. Neuro Oncol 15(10):1429–1437

142. Delanian S, Porcher R, Balla-Mekias S et al (2003) Randomized, placebo-controlled trial of combined pentoxifylline and tocopherol for regression of superficial radiation-induced fibrosis. J Clin Oncol 21(13):2545–2550

143. Okunieff P, Augustine E, Hicks JE et al (2004) Pentoxifylline in the treatment of radiation-induced fibrosis. J Clin Oncol 22(11):2207–2213

144. Delanian S, Porcher R, Rudant J et al (2005) Kinetics of response to long-term treatment combining pentoxifylline and tocopherol in patients with superficial radiation-induced fibrosis. J Clin Oncol 23(34):8570–8579

145. Gothard L, Cornes P, Brooker S et al (2005) Phase II study of vitamin E and pentoxifylline in patients with late side effects of pelvic radiotherapy. Radiother Oncol 75(3):334–341

146. Gothard L, Cornes P, Earl J et al (2004) Double-blind placebo-controlled randomised trial of vitamin E and pentoxifylline in patients with chronic arm lymphoedema and fibrosis after surgery and radiotherapy for breast cancer. Radiother Oncol 73(2):133–139

147. Magnusson M, Hoglund P, Johansson K et al (2009) Pentoxifylline and vitamin E treatment for prevention of radiation-induced side-effects in women with breast cancer: a phase two, double-blind, placebo-controlled randomised clinical trial (Ptx-5). Eur J Cancer 45(14): 2488–2495

148. Delanian S, Chatel C, Porcher R et al (2011) Complete restoration of refractory mandibular osteoradionecrosis by prolonged treatment with a pentoxifylline-tocopherol-clodronate combination (PENTOCLO): a phase II trial. Int J Radiat Oncol Biol Phys 80(3):832–839

149. Venkitaraman R, Price A, Coffey J et al (2008) Pentoxifylline to treat radiation proctitis: a small and inconclusive randomised trial. Clin Oncol (R Coll Radiol) 20(4):288–292

150. Yazbeck VY, Villaruz L, Haley M et al (2013) Management of normal tissue toxicity associated with chemoradiation (primary skin, esophagus, and lung). Cancer J 19(3):231–237

151. Abratt RP, Morgan GW, Silvestri G et al (2004) Pulmonary complications of radiation therapy. Clin Chest Med 25(1):167–177

152. Monson JM, Stark P, Reilly JJ et al (1998) Clinical radiation pneumonitis and radiographic changes after thoracic radiation therapy for lung carcinoma. Cancer 82(5):842–850

153. Gonzalez J, Kumar AJ, Conrad CA et al (2007) Effect of bevacizumab on radiation necrosis of the brain. Int J Radiat Oncol Biol Phys 67(2):323–326
154. Levin VA, Bidaut L, Hou P et al (2011) Randomized double-blind placebo-controlled trial of bevacizumab therapy for radiation necrosis of the central nervous system. Int J Radiat Oncol Biol Phys 79(5):1487–1495
155. Wang Y, Pan L, Sheng X et al (2012) Reversal of cerebral radiation necrosis with bevacizumab treatment in 17 Chinese patients. Eur J Med Res 17:25
156. Tye K, Engelhard HH, Slavin KV et al (2014) An analysis of radiation necrosis of the central nervous system treated with bevacizumab. J Neurooncol 117(2):321–327

Chapter 5
Application of Functional Molecular Imaging in Radiation Oncology

Sarwat Naz, Murali C. Krishna, and James B. Mitchell

Abstract Molecular imaging of tumors is rapidly gaining momentum as a tool with the capacity to improve cancer treatment. It has the potential to provide more precise diagnosis of cancer, improve radiation treatment planning, and monitor response to treatment as the treatment progresses. Noninvasive imaging platforms reporting on molecular, biochemical, metabolic, and physiological parameters coupled with existing high-resolution anatomical modalities hold the promise of providing clinicians with information regarding the *biology* of the tumor in the context of its anatomical location. The basic principles of established and emerging molecular imaging techniques as applied to radiation oncology are reviewed highlighting advantages and limitations. The application of molecular imaging monitoring normal tissue responses as well as tumor may provide a means to determine more precisely a therapeutic ratio of different experimental radiation or chemoradiation approaches.

Keywords Radiation oncology • Metabolic imaging • Functional imaging • Tumor heterogeneity • Molecular biomarker • Hypoxia • Glucose metabolism • PET/CT • ^{13}C hyperpolarization • Cell proliferation

Introduction

Radiation therapy is an effective non-invasive cancer therapy approach that can be administered to patients repetitively over a few to several weeks. Each year approximately 60 % of cancer patients, in the United States are given radiation therapy for definitive treatment, for palliation of symptoms, or as an adjunct to surgery or chemotherapy. A continuing challenge in the field of radiation oncology is to improve the therapeutic ratio, which is the balance of biological effectiveness of treatment and severity of treatment-related side effects on normal tissue. A major objective in

S. Naz • M.C. Krishna • J.B. Mitchell (✉)
Radiation Biology Branch, Center for Cancer Research, National Cancer Institute, National Institutes of Health, Bethesda, MD 20892, USA
e-mail: sarwat.naz@nih.gov; cherukum@mail.nih.gov; jbm@helix.nih.gov

© Springer International Publishing Switzerland 2017
P.J. Tofilon, K. Camphausen (eds.), *Increasing the Therapeutic Ratio of Radiotherapy*, Cancer Drug Discovery and Development, DOI 10.1007/978-3-319-40854-5_5

radiation oncology is to accurately delineate tumor volume and thereby, when possible, minimize radiation exposure to normal tissues. In the past decade, substantial technological progress in radiation oncology has achieved remarkable success in radiation dose delivery with high geometric precision. This has been possible with the introduction of stereotactic radiotherapy, radiosurgery, intensity-modulated radiotherapy (IMRT), and three-dimensional planning of brachytherapy. Computer-optimized intensity-modulated radiation therapy (IMRT) allows achieving high radiation doses to the primary tumor while limiting the dose to radiation-sensitive normal tissues adjacent to the tumor. Despite the advancement in accurate delivery of high-dose radiotherapy, overall survival rates of some specific tumors have not significantly improved. There are several reasons behind this including intrinsic and acquired resistance of tumors mediated through genetic and phenotypic tumor heterogeneity and influence of the tumor microenvironment. Several clinical trials conducted using targeted therapies have demonstrated the existence of genetic and phenotypic tumor heterogeneity [1]. As a result, patients with similar tumor types exhibit differential responses to the same therapy. Genetic heterogeneity in a tumor can arise from the clonal expansion of aggressive and therapy-resistant cancer cells combined with spatial heterogeneity arising from variety of stresses imposed by the tumor microenvironment. These changes within a tumor can lead to regional differences in stromal composition [2], oxygen consumption and hypoxia [3, 4], glucose metabolism [4], and varied gene expression [5]. Consequently, subregions within a given tumor exhibit spatially distinct patterns of blood flow [6, 7], vessel permeability [8], cellular proliferation [9], cell death [10] and other related features. Spatial heterogeneity is observed between different tumors within individual patients (*intertumor heterogeneity*) and within each lesion in an individual (*intratumor heterogeneity*) patient. To overcome these barriers, additional approaches are warranted to quantitatively estimate the exact tumor volume and the extent of phenotypic tumor heterogeneity for effective delivery of ionizing radiation.

One approach to quantitatively extract information pertaining to tumor heterogeneity is the development and introduction of molecular imaging methods. Functional molecular imaging is a noninvasive approach providing visual and quantitative information about a disease process. In addition, it can be combined with diagnostic imaging modalities to provide spatial orientation that may provide molecular, biochemical, or physiological information unique to the tumor or region within the tumor. It is anticipated that such information will be of paramount importance in diagnosis, staging, and selection of tailored treatments and assessment of treatment response. Likewise, alterations in these functional endpoints may also prove useful in monitoring and predicting toxicities in treated normal tissues. Not only can these imaging modalities help to define a more precise "gross tumor volume" (GTV) but also can aid in establishing a "biological target volume" (BTV). The biological target volume represents a subregion within a given tumor with specific characteristics such as hypoxia [11]. Given the accuracy of modern radiation delivery instrumentations, such tumor volumes that are resistant to radiation could be given extra dose of radiation, thus enabling the concept of "dose painting" or "dose sculpturing" to be founded on firm biological and physiological rationale [12].

Combining functional molecular imaging with standard or experimental treatment approaches holds the promise to help clinicians rapidly assess the effectiveness of an existing or new therapy in individual patients and help abandon ineffective treatments at an early stage.

The emergence of functional molecular imaging modalities coupled with the availability of an expanding array of molecular probes is beginning to augment the role of molecular medicine in the treatment of cancer [13]. In this chapter, we briefly outline the basic principles of the different imaging modalities and discuss functional molecular imaging techniques to study functional characteristics of tumor mainly tumor glucose metabolism and hypoxia, application of molecular imaging in chemo-/radiotherapy planning, dose painting, and monitoring treatment response. We aim to discuss the limitations and challenges associated with individual imaging methods in preclinical and clinical setup. Lastly, we give an overall perspective on the future direction of this immensely growing field and its impact on image-guided radiotherapy.

Principles of Established and Emerging Advanced Molecular Imaging Technology

Medical imaging began with radiography after the discovery of X-rays in 1895 by Wilhelm Roentgen, a German professor of physics. X-rays were put to diagnostic use very early, before the dangers of ionizing radiation were discovered. Since then, imaging human diseases has advanced unprecedentedly. Various molecular imaging techniques exist at preclinical and clinical stages including magnetic resonance imaging (MRI), X-ray computed tomography (CT), positron emission topography (PET), ultrasound, and optical approaches. In this chapter, we describe specifically two widely used approaches, namely, MRI and PET, to image malignancies.

CT Imaging

X-ray computed tomography (CT) is a technique for visualizing interior features within solid objects. CT images can be generated by rotating a low-energy X-ray source and detector around the subject to acquire a series of projections. These projections are then used to construct a three-dimensional image. Contrast in the CT-generated image arises because of differential tissue absorption of X-rays. The main advantages of CT imaging are high spatial resolution (0.5–2.0 mm), fast acquisition time, simplicity, availability, and excellent hard-tissue imaging. CT imaging is being combined with PET, where it provides an anatomical context to the relatively low-resolution PET image. In the clinic, the fusion of X-ray CT and PET images has led to improvements in tumor detection.

Radionuclide Imaging

Radionuclide molecular imaging mainly includes positron-emitting tomography (PET) and single-positron emission CT (SPECT) imaging. Due to their high sensitivity and quantitative nature of acquiring images, radionuclide molecular imaging has played a significant role in advancing the preclinical and clinical studies [14]. We highlight some preclinical and clinical studies that have confirmed the feasibility of using radionuclide molecular imaging in cancer [15, 16].

PET and SPECT

Positron-emitting tomography (PET) and single-positron emission CT (SPECT) imaging are radionuclide-imaging techniques, which provide relatively low-resolution images of injected probe molecules that have been labeled with positron-emitting (PET) or γ-emitting isotopes (SPECT). The sensitivity of PET is in the picomolar range, facilitating investigation of biological processes without any adverse pharmacological effects from the labeled probe molecule, namely, ^{11}C, ^{15}O, ^{18}F, and ^{124}I [17]. PET can accurately assess the functional and biochemical processes of the body's tissues, before any detectable anatomical or structural changes have occurred. In the clinic, PET has been crucial for cancer detection and staging, as well as evaluation of response to therapy. An important advantage of PET over SPECT is that positron-emitting isotopes can be substituted for naturally occurring atoms in the probe compound without any effect on probe function. Over the past decade, with the progress of molecular biology and radiochemistry, a variety of PET tracers have been developed with high specificities and affinities. Several PET tracers have been characterized for their application in functional imaging of tumors preclinically and clinically. Among several PET radiotracers used for cancer imaging, ^{18}F-FDG is the most widely used and acceptable PET tracer. PET imaging lacks anatomical parameters to identify molecular events with accurate correlation to anatomical findings, and this disadvantage has been compensated by merging PET imaging with either CT or MR. PET/CT imaging can help to differentiate neoplastic areas with hypermetabolic activity within the surrounding normal tissue (Fig. 5.1) [18]. PET has become extremely useful to delineate the GTV for radiotherapy planning and monitoring treatment response.

Like PET, SPECT has also been extensively employed in the clinic. In general, SPECT isotopes have long half-lives, whereas PET isotopes have relatively short half-lives. Commonly used isotopes for SPECT imaging include [^{111}In] indium and [^{177}Lu] lutetium. Most importantly, SPECT can distinguish among different radioisotopes based on the isotope-specific energies of the emitted photons. Therefore, it is possible to image different targets simultaneously using SPECT [19]. In recent times, application of SPECT imaging in the clinic is less compared to MRI, PET, and ultrasound.

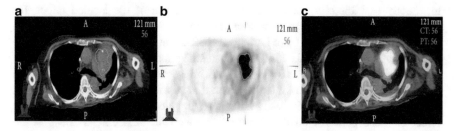

Fig. 5.1 PET images differentiate neoplastic areas with hypermetabolic activity from within the surrounding normal tissue. (**a**) CT image, (**b**) PET image, and (**c**) fused PET/CT image. The teal color marks the gross tumor volume (GTV) as determined from PET image. *Modified and adapted with permission* [18]

MRI

In modern times, magnetic resonance imaging (MRI) has become a highly versatile imaging and diagnostic tool [20]. The technique was developed in the early 1970s and led to a Nobel Prize in Physiology and Medicine to Paul Lauterbur and Peter Mansfield in 2003. MRI involves the detection of nuclear spin reorientation in an applied magnetic field [21]. Compared to CT imaging, MRI has several advantages, such as high temporal and spatial resolution, excellent tissue contrast and tissue penetration, no ionizing radiation, capability of serial studies, and simultaneous acquisition of anatomical structure and physiological function [22]. The intensity of the MR image depends mainly on four parameters: nuclear density; two relaxation times, called T1 (T1 relaxation time is a time constant in which the nuclei align in a given magnetic field) and T2 (T2 is the time constant for loss of phase coherence of excited spins); and motion of the nuclei within the region of interest (ROI). As the nuclear density increases, increasing numbers of nuclei align with the magnetic field, producing a proportionately intense MR signal [21]. Abnormal soft tissue can be better differentiated through measurement of these four parameters compared to any other previous described techniques. MRI-based high soft-tissue contrast allows the assessment of extent and spread of disease, which ultimately can influence radiation treatment volumes [23]. In addition, spatial orientation of the MR image can be performed in any plane, because of the feasibility of manipulating the magnetic field gradients. These inherent advantages of MRI make it a useful imaging method for the evaluation of neurological, musculoskeletal structures, cancer diagnosis, and radiotherapy treatment planning [24–28]. For brain metastases, MRI is much more sensitive than CT, particularly at identifying small lesions (≤0.5 cm) [29]. The ability to visualize tiny lesions prevents patients from aggressive definitive-intent local therapies and allows these lesions to be targeted by stereotactic radiosurgery, which can be delivered with submillimeter accuracy. Additionally, MRI is used for treatment planning in gastrointestinal [30], genitourinary [31, 32], head and neck [33], gynecologic [34], and sarcomatous tumors [23]. By attaching paramagnetic labels to appropriate targeting ligands, MR signal intensity and contrast can be modulated to directly or indirectly obtain functional information of the labeled target, for example, ^{1}H MRI of tissue water protons can be used to indirectly image membrane receptors, such as ERBB 2 (also known as HER-2) on breast cancer cells [35], the integrin $\alpha v\beta 3$ on endothelial cells [36–38], and the phospholipid phosphatidylserine on the surface of apoptotic cells [39, 40]. MR image resolution in vivo at the single cell level is currently not possible; however, it is possible to image the presence of single cells using iron oxide-based nanometer or micrometer-sized particles. The effect of these particles on the surrounding magnetic field extends beyond the boundaries of the cell enabling imaging of single cell [41]. This technique has been used to track implanted stem cells in the brain and spinal cord [42, 43], to monitor T-cell trafficking in immunogenic tumors [44, 45], and to image the location of implanted dendritic cells in the clinic [46].

Imaging of Tumor Metabolism

In recent years, molecular imaging of tumor metabolism has gained considerable interest. Several preclinical studies have indicated relationship between activation of various oncogenes and alterations in cellular metabolism, now considered as one of the hallmarks of cancer [47, 48]. In normal mammalian cells under aerobic conditions, mitochondria oxidize pyruvate to CO_2 and H_2O while generating energy equivalents. Conversion of glucose to lactic acid even in the presence of oxygen is termed as aerobic glycolysis and frequently noticed in malignant cells. Otto Warburg first reported this phenomenon at the beginning of the twentieth century as a specific metabolic abnormality of cancer cells, commonly known as "Warburg effect." He hypothesized that cancer arises from a defect in mitochondrial metabolism leading to aerobic glycolysis [49]. Over time studies conducted in human and rodent glioma cells exhibited high or moderate susceptibility to inhibitors of oxidative phosphorylation, and glioma cells exhibiting high glycolytic phenotype oxidized pyruvate and glutamine even when glucose levels were found to be low [50]. These experimental data suggested that a mitochondrial defect is not a prerequisite for the genesis of cancer and in a strict sense disproved Warburg's hypothesis. Nevertheless, several studies have confirmed frequent overexpression of glucose transporters and glycolytic enzymes in malignant tumors including brain, head and neck, breast, and prostate cancer indicating altered glucose metabolism [51, 52].

^{18}F-FDG PET/CT

^{18}F-fluorodeoxyglucose (FDG) is the most commonly used and the only oncologic PET tracer approved by the Food and Drug Administration (FDA) for routine clinical monitoring of tumor glucose metabolism. More than 90 % of oncologic PET imaging is performed by FDG-PET due to the increased metabolism of glucose by most of the solid tumors including the lung, colorectal, esophageal, stomach, head and neck, cervical, ovarian, breast, melanoma, and most types of lymphomas. In addition to diagnosis, staging, restaging, and monitoring response to cancer treatment, FDG-PET can be useful for selection or delineation of radiotherapy target volumes. FDG-PET has been used as a dose-painting target for sub-volume boosting and thus guiding radiotherapy planning. The use of FDG-PET for radiotherapy planning purposes has shown increasing importance, as more and more radiation oncologists believe that target volume selection and delineation can be adequately performed using FDG-PET in certain cancer types such as non-small cell lung carcinoma (NSCLC) stage N2-N3 patients [53]. In head and neck squamous cell carcinoma (HNSCC), methodological studies have shown that the use of pre-radiotherapy using FDG-PET led to a better estimate of the exact tumor volume, as defined by the pathologic specimens, compared with CT and MRI. Interestingly, when validated segmentation tools were used, the mean FDG-PET-based GTV was consistently smaller than the GTV defined from morphologic imaging in all investigated tumor locations and at all-time points during radiotherapy (Fig. 5.2a) [12, 56, 57]. ^{18}F-FDG PET/CT is also increasingly used for monitoring tumor response after completion of therapy as demonstrated for malignant lymphoma lung, colon, and breast cancer [58]. An example from a lymphoma patient shown in Fig. 5.2b demonstrates that high metabolic activity (measured by high uptake of FDG) of the tumor before the therapy had reduced after the therapy (indicated by reduced FDG uptake), indicating the efficacy of the treatment [54]. Persistently increased FDG uptake after treatment is also associated in predicting a high risk for early disease recurrence and poor prognosis. In patients with Hodgkin's disease and aggressive non-Hodgkin's lymphoma, ^{18}F-FDG PET showed very promising results for assessing tumor response early in the course of therapy. This study included 260 patients with Hodgkin's lymphoma and utilized ^{18}F-FDG PET before and after two cycles of chemotherapy to monitor tumor response. The 2-year progression-free survival for patients with positive PET results after two cycles of chemotherapy was 13%, whereas it was 95% for patients with a negative PET scan. In a univariate analysis, the treatment outcome was significantly associated with PET response after two cycles of chemotherapy and various well-known clinical prognostic factors such as stage and the international prognostic score (IPS). In multivariate analyses, however, only positive PET results after two cycles of chemotherapy turned out to be significantly correlated with patient survival ($P < 0.0001$). These data indicated that tumor response in ^{18}F-FDG PET after two cycles of chemotherapy is a stronger predictor of patient outcome than the IPS and other well-established clinical prognostic factors [59]. The results from this study concluded that ^{18}F-FDG PET appears to be the single most important tool for risk-adapted treatment in Hodgkin's lymphoma [59]. The ability of ^{18}F-FDG PET to predict tumor response early in the course of therapy as in the case of Hodgkin's lymphoma offers the opportunity to intensify treatment in patients who are unlikely to respond to first-line chemotherapy. Conversely, treatment could be shortened in patients who show a favorable response after two cycles of chemotherapy. This is of particular interest in Hodgkin's lymphoma, since chemotherapy combined with radiotherapy can cure most of the

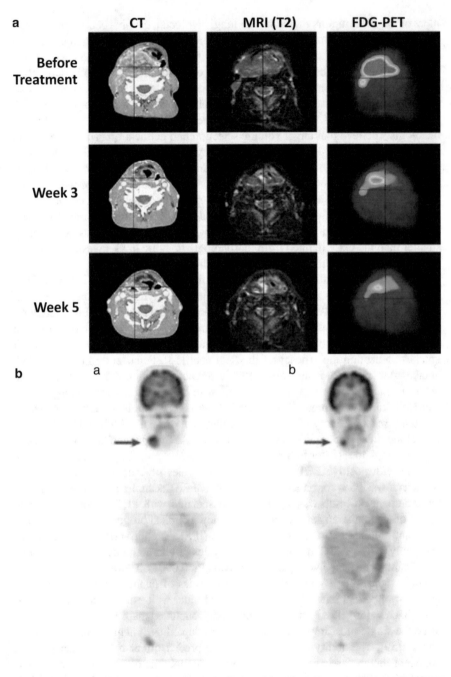

Fig. 5.2 (**a**) An example showing application of FDG-PET over conventional CT and MRI (T2-weighted sequence). A patient with right-sided hypopharyngeal squamous cell carcinoma received concomitant chemoradiotherapy. Images were obtained using intravenous contrast CT, MRI (T2-weighted sequence), and FDG-PET before treatment (*upper panel*) and at the end of weeks 3 and 5 of 30 Gy and 50 Gy radiation dose, respectively (*lower two panels*).

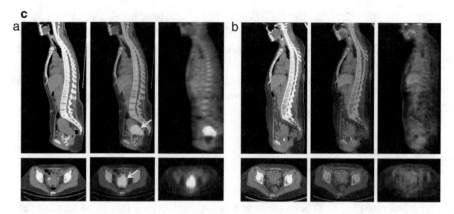

Fig. 5.2 (continued) FDG-PET imaging depicted the most pronounced decrease in tumor volume post therapy compared to CT or MRI. Modified and adapted with permission from [12]. (**b**) FDG-PET-based imaging to determine response to chemotherapy. (*a*) High FDG-PET uptake of 2-[¹⁸F] fluoro-2-deoxy-D-glucose (FDG) in a patient with lymphoma arrowed before (*a*) and reduced uptake after (*b*) drug chemotherapy, seen in the tumor and brain. Modified and adapted with permission from [54]. (**c**) Application of ¹⁸F-FDG-PET to assess complete metabolic response. PET/CT image of 52-year-old women diagnosed with stage IVA squamous cell cancer of the cervix. (*a*) Sagittal (*top*) and transaxial (*bottom*) CT (*left*), fused PET/CT (*middle*), and PET (*right*) images taken at the initial stage demonstrate high ¹⁸F-FDG uptake within the cervical mass. (*b*) Sagittal (*top*) and transaxial (*bottom*) CT image (*left*), fused PET/CT (*middle*) image, and PET (*right*) image taken 3 months after concurrent radiotherapy clearly showing resolution of cervical mass with mild or diffuse uptake of ¹⁸F-FDG within the cervix, depicting complete metabolic response. Adapted with permission from [55]

patients but also puts them at increased risk for secondary malignancies and other serious long-term complications, such as infertility and cardiopulmonary toxicity. Focal ¹⁸F-FDG uptake after chemo- or radiotherapy has been shown to be a strong prognostic factor. In one of the largest prospective studies published so far, Schwarz et al. [55, 60] prospectively performed ¹⁸F-FDG PET in patients with cervical cancer treated by chemoradiotherapy. Post therapy ¹⁸F-FDG PET (2–4 months later) showed a complete metabolic response (Fig. 5.2c) in 70 % of the patients, a partial metabolic response in 16 %, and progressive disease in 13 % of patients. The 3-year progression-free survival rates of these patient subgroups were estimated to be 78 %, 33 %, and 0 %, respectively ($P < 0.001$) [55, 60]. Another application of ¹⁸F-FDG PET could be in deciding sub-volumes within tumor or lymph nodes that demonstrate high metabolic activity and therefore represent high-risk lesions to be selectively treated with an increased radiation dose. Several studies in rectal and lung cancer have shown that FDG-PET allows selective boosting of hypermetabolic areas. For example, in a study conducted in patients with small-cell lung cancer, FDG-PET-based radiation planning for mediastinal lymph nodes changed the radiotherapy field in 24 % of the patients [61]. In patients with head and neck cancer, the radiation boost dose was markedly elevated and directed at the tumors with the highest FDG-avidity, and the adverse treatment-related effects remained limited [62].

Despite its great clinical utility, FDG-PET has a few limitations. The technique has lower sensitivity for slow growing, metabolically less active tumors (such as prostate, thyroid, and neuroendocrine tumors), and high levels of uptake in some normal tissues, such as the brain, that can make quantification of tumor uptake specifically difficult. Accumulation of PET tracers in infiltrating inflammatory cells, which also show high glycolysis, might give false-positive results and limit the sensitivity of the technique for detecting tumor response to treatment [63].

Hyperpolarized Metabolic MR

Hyperpolarized ^{13}C MRI is an emerging molecular imaging technique that can provide unprecedented gain in amplifying signal intensity. This technique can be used to monitor uptake and metabolism of ^{13}C-labeled endogenous biomolecules such as glucose, pyruvate, fumarate, etc. [64, 65]. The degree and magnitude of the increase in sensitivity of biomolecules depend on the extent of polarization achieved, the T1 relaxation time of the agent, the delivery time, and the MR imaging methods employed. The polarization of ^{13}C at a magnetic field strength of 3 T is calculated to be 2.5 ppm. Consequently, biological molecules enriched with ^{13}C suffer from poor sensitivity because of a lower magnetic moment, lower polarization, and reduced concentrations compared to tissue water proton (in range of a few mM versus 80 M for water ^{1}H). As a result of these differences, ~ four orders of sensitivity difference for ^{13}C-containing molecules compared to water protons need to be bridged to implement metabolic imaging using endogenous organic molecules. Increasing the polarization (fraction of molecules with nuclear spins emitting signal) needs to be increased significantly. Among the various methods used to enhance the polarization of nuclei, dynamic nuclear polarization (DNP) technique has so far been the most successful for in vivo applications [64–66]. In DNP, the higher polarization of a molecule with an unpaired electron spin is transferred to nuclei such as ^{1}H, ^{13}C, ^{15}N and ^{19}F, etc. Firstly, for a molecule to be sufficiently polarized with long signal decay, it should possess a carbon site with long intrinsic T1 that can be enriched in ^{13}C (e.g., carbonyl or carboxylic acid). Introducing deuterium in aliphatic carbons has been shown to be very amenable. Secondly, the molecule should be able to form a homogenous glassy solid formulation with the paramagnetic agent as when frozen it must ensure polarization transfer from the electrons to nuclei. Thirdly, upon dissolution the loss of polarization should be marginal and not significantly high. Fourthly, the chemical shifts of the injected molecule and products should be clearly distinct. Lastly, the molecule should not exhibit any associated side effects when injected as a bolus at the required doses (typically approx. 0.1 mmol/kg body weight). Pyruvate labeled with ^{13}C in the C-1 position satisfies all the prerequisite conditions listed above for a polarized agent. Hyperpolarization of pyruvate is achieved by mixing ^{13}C-labeled compounds with an electron paramagnetic agent (EPA), e.g., OXO-63. The mixed entity is then placed in a 3.35-T magnetic field, cooled to ~1 K, and microwaves are used to transfer polarization from the electron

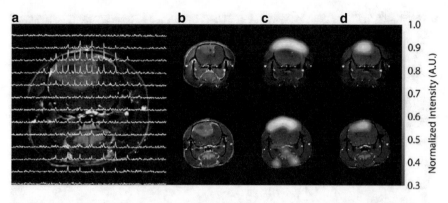

Fig. 5.3 Representative images of hyperpolarized ^{13}C pyruvate (**c**) and lactate (**d**) in a C6 glioma-bearing animal before (*top*) and 96 h after radiotherapy (*bottom*). ACSI dataset is shown in (**a**). The chemical shift images were superimposed on grayscale T1-weighted proton images (**b**) for anatomical reference. The lactate signals, in the false color images, were normalized to the maximum pyruvate signal in each dataset. The lactate signal was reduced following exposure to 15-Gy radiation [67]. *CSI* chemical shift imaging

spin of the EPA to the ^{13}C nuclei of the biomolecule [66]. Once the polarization is achieved, the sample is rapidly dissolved with hot, sterile water and neutralized to physiological pH, temperature, and osmolality. Hyperpolarized ^{13}C pyruvate can be intravenously injected where it metabolized in tissues to various metabolites such as bicarbonate, lactate, and alanine depending on the dominant metabolic pathway in the tissue of interest in vivo. The conversion of pyruvate to each of these metabolites can be imaged using chemical shift MRI or MR spectroscopic imaging (MRSI). The data acquisition utilizing hyperpolarized pyruvate is very rapid, approximately 60 s for [1-^{13}C] pyruvate at 3 T. Several studies have shown the preclinical application of using hyperpolarized pyruvate [64, 65]. Studies examined hyperpolarized ^{13}C pyruvate and lactate in a C6 glioma-bearing animal before radiotherapy (Fig. 5.3b–d, top) and 96 h after radiotherapy (Fig. 5.3b–d, bottom). Comparison of spectra from tumor voxels with those on the contralateral side of the brain indicated high lactate signal in the tumor than in the brain (Fig. 5.3a). ^{13}C chemical shift images acquired following intravenous injection of hyperpolarized [1-^{13}C] pyruvate into rats with implanted C6 gliomas showed significant labeling of lactate within the tumors but comparatively low levels in the surrounding brain. Labeled pyruvate signal was observed at high levels in blood vessels above the brain and from other major vessels elsewhere but was detected at only low levels in the tumor and in the brain [67, 68]. The ratio of hyperpolarized ^{13}C label in tumor lactate compared with the maximum pyruvate signal in the blood vessels was decreased from 0.38 to 0.23 (a reduction of 34 %) by 72 h following whole-brain irradiation with 15 Gy (Fig. 5.3) [67]. Further studies in a transgenic adenocarcinoma of the mouse prostate (TRAMP) model demonstrated elevated levels of hyperpolarized [1-^{13}C] lactate in tumor, with the ratio of [1-^{13}C] lactate/[1-^{13}C] pyruvate being increased in high-grade tumors and decreased after successful treatment (Fig. 5.4) [69]. The preclinical studies using

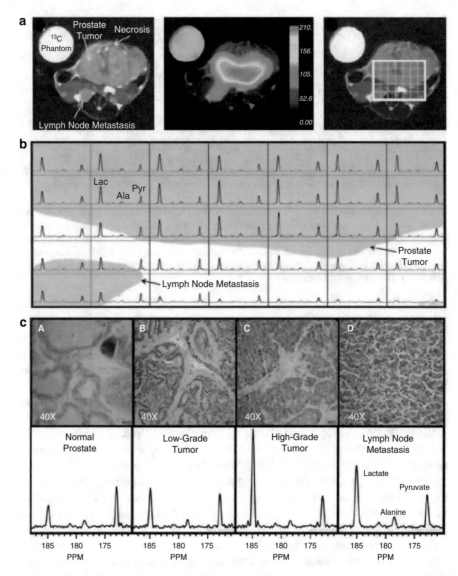

Fig. 5.4 Hyperpolarized ^{13}C metabolic images of a TRAMP mouse. *Upper*: representative anatomical image (**a**) and hyperpolarized ^{13}C lactate image (**b**) following the injection of hyperpolarized [1-^{13}C] pyruvate, overlaid on T2-weighted ^{1}H image. *Middle*: hyperpolarized ^{13}C spectra of primary prostrate and metastatic tumor regions. (**c**) *Lower*: 3D MRSI depicting markedly elevated lactate in the high-grade primary tumor compared with the low-grade tumor. This study demonstrated application of hyperpolarized MRSI imaging of lactate-pyruvate ratio as a biomarker for the assessment of radiation therapy response [67]. *Ala* alanine, *Lac* lactate, *Pyr* pyruvate

hyperpolarization of pyruvate has now advanced to human clinical trials. The first human translation of hyperpolarized technology was successfully demonstrated in patients with prostate tumor [70]. In brief, the study imaged 31 untreated patients diagnosed with localized prostate cancer, where 23 patients had Gleason score of 6, 6 patients with Gleason score 7, and 2 patients with Gleason score 8. The initial phase 1 of the study evaluated the safety, feasibility, and tolerability of injected hyperpolarized [1-^{13}C] pyruvate. The study indicated no dose-limiting toxicities associated with hyperpolarized [1-^{13}C] pyruvate. In addition, the median time taken for the dissolution of the agent to delivery into patient was 66 s. The ^{1}D dynamic MRSI data obtained showed higher [1-^{13}C] lactate signal coming from tumor, and no detectable [1-^{13}C] lactate signal came from the area which did not had tumor. The study confirmed correlation between the high lactate signals with prostate cancer grade. In conclusion, the study successfully demonstrated safety, tolerability, kinetics of hyperpolarized pyruvate delivery, and imaging hyperpolarized ^{13}C metabolism (Fig. 5.5). In the future, more studies will be designed utilizing hyperpolarized [1-^{13}C] pyruvate in larger cohorts of patients with different tumor types to firmly acknowledge the correlation with tumor grade and changes with therapy.

Imaging Cellular Proliferation

Measures of tumor cell proliferation can help to assess the degree of tumor aggressiveness. Several in vitro biomarkers and assays have been developed to estimate tumor proliferation correlating its aggressiveness and stage. However, conventional anatomic pathology is limited in its ability to quantify the rate of cellular proliferation and requires invasive biopsies making it difficult to obtain over time from different metastatic lesions of the patient. Therefore, efforts have been taken to develop imaging modalities to noninvasively measure and quantify the rate of cell proliferation. Noninvasive imaging to estimate the rate of tumor cell proliferation has focused on the application of PET in conjunction with tracers for the thymidine salvage pathway of DNA synthesis. A tracer of thymidine has great implications, as it is the only pyrimidine or purine base unique to DNA, thereby measuring only the DNA synthesis. In the clinics, 3-deoxy-3-[^{18}F]fluorothymidine (FLT) is the most widely used PET tracer to noninvasively measure tumor proliferation. The principles and application of FLT/PET imaging-based radiotherapy planning and tumor response are covered comprehensively in the section on clinical imaging and radiotherapy (see Chap. 9). Here we discuss application of spectroscopy-based imaging involving magnetic resonance spectroscopy imaging (MRSI) to measure cellular proliferation and its application in radiotherapy.

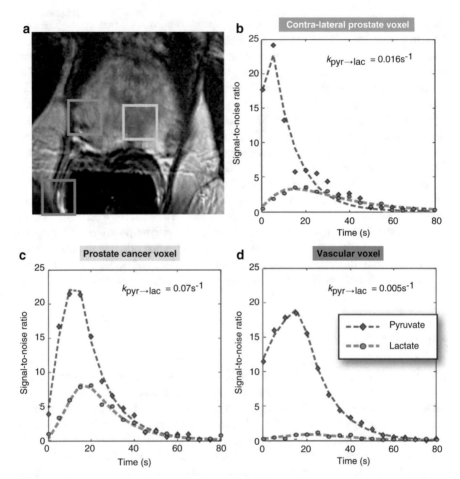

Fig. 5.5 Representative image showing 2D ^{13}C dynamic MRSI data. Images are from a representative patient with a current PSA of 3.6 ng/ml, who had biopsy-proven prostate cancer in the left apex (Gleason grade 3+4) and received the highest dose of hyperpolarized [1-^{13}C] pyruvate (0.43 ml/kg). (**a**) A focus of mild hypo-intensity can be seen on the T2-weighted image, which was consistent with the biopsy findings. (**b–d**) 2D localized dynamic hyperpolarized [1-^{13}C] pyruvate and [1-^{13}C] lactate from spectral data that were acquired every 5 s from voxels overlapping the contralateral region of the prostate (*turquoise*), a region of prostate cancer (*yellow*), and a vessel outside the prostate (*green*). The dynamic data were fit as described previously [71]. Data taken with permission from [70]

MRSI

MRSI combines the ability of spectroscopy to acquire a large volume of metabolic information, with the ability of imaging to localize information spatially. Although phosphorus (^{31}P) and carbon (^{13}C) MRSI are possible, proton (^{1}H) MRSI is the technique most often used in clinical settings. On ^{1}H MRSI, tumor spectra contain resonances from metabolites such as taurine, total choline (choline, phosphocholine, and glycerophosphocholine), total creatine (phosphocreatine and creatine), pyruvate, and lactate.

Among the hallmarks of cancer described by Hanahan and Weinberg, elevated choline metabolism resulting in the accumulation of choline containing compounds such as choline, phosphocholine, and glycerophosphocholine (together represented as tCho) is recognized as an important hallmark, which is amenable for in vivo detection, by MRSI. Studies have shown that malignant transformation rather than just rapid proliferation as the reason for the increased accumulation of tCho is making this a very specific MRI-based imaging biomarker for proliferation [72, 73]. Tumor microenvironmental features such as hypoxia and acidotic extracellular conditions have also been associated with elevated tCho [74]. Several clinical studies already support the strength of monitoring tCho in detecting malignancies and predicting survival. Numerous multi-institutional clinical studies are examining the utility of MRS to detect tCho to aid in the diagnosis and treatment response monitoring.

Imaging Tumor Microenvironment

Tumors survive obtaining oxygen and nutrients passively up to a size of ~2–3 mm^3. For further growth, they invoke neo-angiogenesis to grow new blood vessel network, commonly known as tumor vasculature. While in normal tissue, the angiogenesis processes are tightly regulated resulting in a physically robust vascular network functioning well to deliver oxygen and nutrients, the tumor vascular network is aberrant and not well organized and functions abnormally resulting in a marked heterogeneity in perfusion. As a consequence, tumors exhibit hypoxia and acidotic environments. These are two common features characterizing the tumor microenvironment. Imaging techniques, which can obtain information pertaining to the tumor microenvironment, such as tumor oxygen status, perfusion, and tumor pH, will be useful in both diagnoses and treatment planning.

Development of hypoxia in the tumor microenvironment is highly dynamic process resulting in alterations in cellular metabolism and proliferation. Typically, focal areas of hypoxia are observed in many solid tumors (mainly in the core of the tumor). Tumors exhibit high proliferation ability, and one of the direct consequences of unregulated cellular growth results in a greater demand of oxygen (as well as other nutrients) for energy metabolism. However, unlike normal cells, tumor cells rapidly adapt to hypoxic microenvironment by slowing their growth rate, inhibiting apoptosis, switching mitochondria respiration to glycolysis, stimulating growth of new vasculature (neo-angiogenesis), and promoting metastatic spread. Several preclinical and clinical studies have shown that hypoxic tumors also have elevated expression of key transcription factors notably hypoxia-inducible factor (HIF) expression [75]. A number of hypoxia-related genes, downstream transcription factors, and signaling molecules are also found to be responsible for the genomic changes within the tumor. Some of the most commonly associated molecular changes associated with tumor hypoxia include elevated expression of endothelial cytokines such as vascular endothelial growth factor (VEGF) and signaling molecules such as IL-1, tumor necrosis factor alpha (TNF-α), transforming growth factor beta (TGF-β), and loss of p53 expression [76]. Increased glycolysis observed in most hypoxic cells leads to accumulation of lactate in the microenvironment resulting in reduced glycolytic activity and increased acidosis (reduced pH) [77]. These changes arising from hypoxia create an environment conducive for tumor progression and development of metastases as well as therapy-resistant clones [77, 78]. Most chemotherapeutic drugs act by inhibiting tumor growth, but when a tumor becomes hypoxic, cells enter a resting phase in their cell cycle and tend to become refractory to these cytotoxic agents. The hypoxia-induced metastatic phenotype is also a contributing factor for the disappointing success of much acclaimed anti-angiogenic therapy. Ionizing radiation is an alternative and effective strategy for killing proliferating cells because the radiation field is homogenous and the killing effect of radiation is independent of vascular delivery. However, radiobiologists have long recognized negative influence of hypoxia on response to radiation therapy as the cytotoxicity of ionizing radiation depends on the level of intracellular O_2. Gray made this observation over 50 years ago that about a three times higher dose of radiation is required to kill hypoxic cells over well-oxygenated cells. Thus, the presence of tumor hypoxia can compromise the effectiveness of radiation treatment.

Another key characteristic of tumor hypoxia is that it is heterogeneously distributed and its dynamics keeps changing over time and with therapy [79]. The blood supply of a malignant tumor is thought to be suboptimal as its vasculature network is immature, leaky, and randomly distributed making it chaotic. This chaotic microvasculature of tumor tissue leads to two types of hypoxia, which can be defined as either diffusion limited or perfusion limited. The first, also known as chronic hypoxia, is the consequence of proliferating cells exceeding the oxygen capacity of the newly formed vascular network. This is because the newly synthesized microvasculature is often insufficient in providing the normoxic microenvironment in the distant tumor areas resulting in diffusion-limited hypoxia [78]. Tumor cells exposed to acute hypoxia have easier access to the blood circulatory system, as they are thought to be nearer the blood vessels. These tumor cells may therefore have greater perfusion limited hypoxia or acute hypoxia, resulting from the structural and functional abnormalities in the newly formed vasculature with poor or insufficient blood supply. Subsequently, this leads to an unstable blood supply to the core of proliferating tumor cells producing intermittent hypoxia. This form of hypoxia is often characterized by rapidly fluctuating oxygen concentration [78]. The relevance of cycling hypoxia in tumor radiobiology and/or conferring radio resistance has been studied using animal models [80, 81]. There are few studies showing evidence of the existence of cycling hypoxia in human tumors. One such study conducted by Pigott et al. examined blood flow in various superficial human tumors, using implanted laser Doppler flow probe. In around 50 % of the lesions examined, fluctuations in the flux of red blood cells were observed to be more than a factor of 1.5 correlative to cycling hypoxia measured in animal models [82]. Another study conducted by Janssen et al. in head and neck cancer patients detected cycling hypoxia by immunohistochemistry [83]. However, all these indirect approaches to assess cycling hypoxia in human tumors are invasive and could not firmly establish any correlation between the overall oxygenation state of the tumors and the incidence of cycling hypoxia.

Methods for Evaluating Hypoxia

Clearly, the ability to identify and quantify tumor oxygenation status and energy metabolism has far-reaching implications in a wide range of medical settings. Most importantly, a clinically useful assay to measure hypoxia, firstly, must be able to distinguish normoxic regions from the ones that are hypoxic at a level relevant to tumor oxygen partial pressure (pO_2) falling in the range of 5–15 mmHg. The ability to simultaneously image tumor oxygenation and metabolic profile can profoundly guide future therapies involving inclusion of radiosensitizers, hypoxia-directed cytotoxins, oxygen-enhanced gas mixtures such as carbogen (a mixture consisting of 95 % oxygen and 5 % carbon dioxide) [84], and hypoxia-activated prodrugs. Non-toxic prodrugs that generate active species in hypoxic tissue by selective bioreduction have now reached advanced clinical trials. Such hypoxia prodrugs mainly include tirapazamine [85], PR104 [86], and TH-302 [87]. In the early 1990s, hypoxia measurements were achieved by implanting properly calibrated, oxygen-sensitive electrodes (Eppendorf pO_2 histograph) which directly measured pO_2 in units of mmHg [88]. This technique had several practical disadvantages. It is limited to tumors that the probe can be easily accessed, and its invasive nature can cause tissue damage. However, this approach is still in use in the clinic. Other approaches such as immunohistochemistry of tumor tissue using extrinsic hypoxia-specific biomarker such as pimonidazole and intrinsic hypoxia biomarker such as carbonic anhydrase IX (CAIX), VEGF receptor expression, and glucose transporter 1 (Glut1) are utilized to measure hypoxia [89]. These biomarker signatures show poor prognosis and are correlative to the extent of tumor hypoxia. However, the drawback of this approach is that it requires a biopsy, which is challenging and sometimes is not possible. Serum markers have also been evaluated to measure tumor hypoxia but with less success [90, 91]. Furthermore, sampled biomarkers are not able to evaluate spatial heterogeneity, which is often relevant to overall response and is essential for defining a radiation treatment field. Notably, all the above methods do not provide the longitudinal monitoring of hypoxia as the measurement is restricted to only a smaller sub-volume of a tumor. Noninvasive approaches have been instrumental in allowing serial imaging of hypoxia quantitatively and provide valuable information about cycling nature of hypoxia in both space and time. PET hypoxia imaging is noninvasive and routinely used in clinic. Due to the clinical significance of hypoxia imaging, an increasing number of hypoxia PET tracers are available and are being evaluated in the clinical setting. The first radionuclide detection of hypoxia in tumors was reported using ^{14}C-misonidazole autoradiography [92]. Subsequently, two main tracer classes have been developed to specifically study hypoxia with PET. These tracers are ^{18}F-labeled 2-nitroimidazole derivatives, such as [^{18}F]-fluoromisonidazole ([^{18}F]-FMISO), [18F]-azomycinarabinoside [^{18}F]-FAZA, [18F]-fluoroerythronitroimidazole [^{18}F]-FETNIM, and Cu-labeled diacetyl-bis (N^4-methylthiosemicarbazone) analogues. Among all these tracers, ^{18}F-FMISO is the lead candidate and most extensively studied 2-nitroimidazole-based radiopharmaceutical PET tracer in the clinics. Clinical application of ^{18}F-FMISO in radiotherapy planning and dose painting of different solid tumors is well described in Chap. 9. Despite its potential clinical application, ^{18}F-FMISO imaging in rectal cancer was shown to be compromised by high nonspecific tracer accumulation in normoxic tissue [93]. Several other techniques to measure tumor hypoxia quantitatively and noninvasively are in preclinical development, namely, Overhauser MRI (OMRI), electron paramagnetic resonance imaging (EPRI), and ^{19}F MRI. Electron paramagnetic resonance (EPR) predominantly measures interstitial hypoxia. We describe here highly promising hypoxia imaging modalities that have gained immense attention in both preclinical and clinical setting.

DCE-MRI

Dynamic contrast-enhanced MRI is a powerful MRI technique to examine tissue perfusion profiles. It involves collecting a series of images rapidly following a bolus intravenous administration of the T1 contrast agents, typically gadolinium complexes. Following the bolus administration, these agents localize in the extravascular-extracellular space and are gradually cleared. The time-intensity features from these rapidly acquired sequences of images allow the determination of the microvasculature of the tumors. DCE-MRI has been applied for over a decade to extract functional information regarding the peripheral vascular system such as blood volume, blood flow, vascular permeability, as well as distribution volume and available interstitial space for the contrast agent. DCE-MRI acquires serial MR images before, during, and after the administration of an intravenous contrast agent such as low molecular weight, gadolinium-based (Gd-DTPA) contrast medium. DCE-MRI has grown with the development of anti-angiogenic and neoadjuvant strategies for treating cancer. Angiogenic inhibitors are known to reduce both the number of vessels (particularly non-functional vessels) and their permeability, which can be quantitatively imaged using DCE-MRI. In cervical cancer, DCE-MRI was shown to measure tumor hypoxia in good correlation to Eppendorf oxygen electrode and was an independent predictor of tumor recurrence and death than clinically accepted prognostic factors (e.g., stage, lymph node status, and histology) [94]. Newbold et al. demonstrated a statistically significant correlation between various dynamic contrast-enhanced MR imaging parameters [95], particularly K^{trans} (which represents the permeability of blood vessels) and pimonidazole staining (an exogenous marker for hypoxia). DCE-MR imaging of head and neck squamous cell carcinoma and rectal cancer also has been used to successfully predict treatment response to chemoradiation therapy [96, 97]. DCE imaging also offers an exciting opportunity to predict the extent of normal tissue function post radiation. Radiation treatment can lead to vascular damage such as vessel dilation, endothelial cell death and apoptosis, microvessel hemorrhage, and eventually vessel occlusion affecting organs such as the brain, liver, and rectum [98–100]. Risk of damaging the normal tissue thereby hinders increasing the radiation dose for better tumor control or even cure. DCE-MRI can be used for early monitoring of vascular response to radiation treatments and predict the outcome of organ function after therapy, thereby selecting the patient who is resistant to radiation for higher dose, potentially leading to a better chance of tumor local control and better overall therapeutic outcome. DCE-MRI/CT thus offers promise of early assessment of tumor response to radiation therapy, opening a window for adaptively optimizing radiation therapy based upon functional alterations that occur earlier than morphological changes and enhancing radiotherapy therapeutic ratio. Although holding great promise, to date DCE-MRI and CT have yet to qualify to be a surrogate endpoint for radiation therapy assessment or for modifying treatment strategies in any prospective phase III clinical trial for any tumor site.

BOLD-MRI

The primary form of functional MRI that uses the blood-oxygen-level dependent (BOLD) contrast was discovered by Seiji Ogawa. In BOLD-MRI hypoxia imaging, the primary source of contrast in images is contributed by the endogenous, paramagnetic deoxyhemoglobin. This technique relies on the delivery of red blood cells to the tissue of interest to provide information about the tissue oxygenation. When hemoglobin becomes saturated with increasing oxygen concentrations, the iron within the heme subunit changes from a paramagnetic high spin state (under hypoxia) to a diamagnetic low spin state (under normoxia). Hoskin et al. evaluated BOLD-MRI sequences to measure regional hypoxia in normal prostate gland and in 20 prostate cancer patients. They validated the reliability and reproducibility of BOLD-MRI with pimonidazole staining of the excised tissues from the same patients [101]. Recently, clinical and preclinical correlations between BOLD-MRI radiotherapy and chemotherapy treatment response have been established. Tissue oxygenation-level-dependent contrast MRI has been shown to corroborate tumor growth delay after irradiation supplemented with hyperoxic breathing in rat prostate tumors [102]. Another pilot study was conducted using BOLD-MRI approach to evaluate response to neoadjuvant chemotherapy in patients with advanced breast cancer [103]. Significantly, higher BOLD response to oxygen breathing was observed in patients who exhibited complete pathological response. These findings establish the effectiveness of BOLD-MRI as a convenient and noninvasive imaging modality in identification of hypoxic subregions within a tumor and providing predictive capabilities for estimating the therapeutic response. Functional MRI (fMRI) has gained unprecedented applications in mapping neural activity of brain in resting and active state. This technique has dominated brain-mapping research since the early 1950s as it does not require subjects to undergo injections and surgery, or to ingest substances, or be exposed to radiation, etc. However, more studies in future are required to characterize the clinical utility of BOLD-MRI in mapping tumor hypoxia in various types of solid tumors.

EPRI and OMRI

Overhauser-enhanced MRI (OMRI) is a proton-electron double resonance imaging technique that provides anatomically co-registered quantitative pO_2 maps. It uses the enhanced paramagnetic resonance (EPR) transition of the injected paramagnetic agent to enhance the intensity of the tissue water protons. The enhancement is dependent inversely on the tissue oxygen content allowing the determination of pO_2. Briefly, the object to be imaged is placed in a resonator assembly whose resonance frequency has been tuned to the frequencies of both paramagnetic agent and water ^1H when placed in a magnetic field of ~ 10 mT. By saturating the electron spin of paramagnetic oxygen-sensitive contrast agent, water protons in tissue become hyperpolarized via dynamic nuclear polarization (DNP). The resultant images reflect both the concentration of the contrast agent and local oxygen concentration. However, limitations with this technique made translation to human studies not possible. However, direct imaging of the paramagnetic agent OXO-63 by EPRI has provided advantages over OMRI allowing improved spatial, temporal resolutions and allow dynamic [104, 105] and longitudinal [106] of tumor oxygenation. In principle, EPR is a noninvasive and quantitative imaging technique to measure the pO_2. It is based on the principle where species with unpaired electron exhibiting paramagnetic properties, for example, transition metal complex and free radicals, can be detected. Notably, oxygen exhibits paramagnetic properties and can influence the relaxation rates of the exogenous paramagnetic agent. EPRI is highly sensitive in the detection of changes in oxygen concentrations [107–110]. However, EPR cannot be used to estimate directly the dissolved molecular oxygen. Instead EPR can determine tumor oximetry repeatedly by measuring average tumor pO_2 with minimal perturbation to the microenvironment [111]. Studies have indicated that multisite EPR oximetry is achieved by applying gradient of magnetic field [107, 112, 113]. This approach can simultaneously measure pO_2 at multiple sites in a given tissue of interest. Generally, to obtain EPR image, an exogenous paramagnetic agent is injected to capture the signal. Therefore, an appropriate EPR tracer/agent must meet the indicated criteria: (1) it must be able to generate simple EPR spectra, (2) should have longer pharmacological half-life than the imaging time, and (3) should not confer by itself any associated toxicity. One such agent for EPRI is triarylmethyl radical, OXO-63, used to study tissue oxygen in live animals. The collision interaction between OXO-63 and O_2 broadens the spectral line of OXO-63 in direct proportion to oxygen concentration, thereby enabling a quantitative measure of tissue pO_2 in vivo [114]. The EPRI pO_2 mapping can be co-registered with the host of related physiologic and metabolic information. In a study from our group, we demonstrated that tumor region with higher pO_2 (22.8 mmHg) contained clearly high

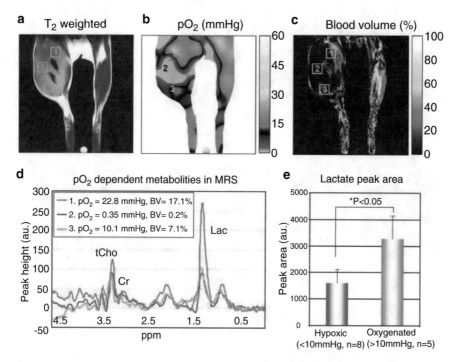

Fig. 5.6 Co-registration of EPRI and MRS/MRI to simultaneously monitor pO₂ distribution and metabolite levels in same tumors. (**a**) T2-weighted anatomical MRI image of SCC tumor-bearing mouse and ROI locations for MRS. (**b**) EPRI pO₂ map of the same animal and the corresponding ROIs chosen for MRS. (**c**) Blood volume image of the slice using USPIO and the corresponding ROIs for MRS. Numbers 1–3 in **a**–**c** correspond with numbers 1–3 in **d**. (**d**) Representative MRS spectra obtained from three different tumor regions selected with different pO₂ and blood volume levels. (**e**) Averaged lactate peak area of MRS spectra obtained from radiobiological hypoxic (<10 mmHg) and normoxic (>10 mmHg) regions. High level of lactate production was detected even in the well-oxygenated tumor region. *BV* blood volume, *MRS* magnetic resonance spectroscopy, *Cr* creatine, *Lac* lactate, *tCho* total choline [111]

levels of lactate (visualized by MRI/MRS) indicating the predominance of aerobic glycolytic process in normoxic tumor regions. In contrary, the averaged lactate peak area observed in radiobiologically oxygenated region (>10 mmHg) was significantly higher than that in hypoxic region (<10 mmHg). The difference in lactate content was attributed to limited blood supply and nutrient supply, as estimated from the blood volume differences in these regions (Fig. 5.6) [111]. With advancement in image formation and reconstitution strategies, it is possible to obtain three-dimensional (3D) maps of pO₂ within 3 min in tumor-bearing mice to enable monitoring of intermittent hypoxia. Studies from our group have shown a successful visualization of dynamic changes of tumor oxygenation over a 30 min time frame using EPRI, where the images were imaged every 3 min, and 3D reconstruction of pO₂, (Fig. 5.7) [67] was achieved. EPRI has also been useful in studying tumor responses to therapy with regard to oxygenation. In another study, changes in

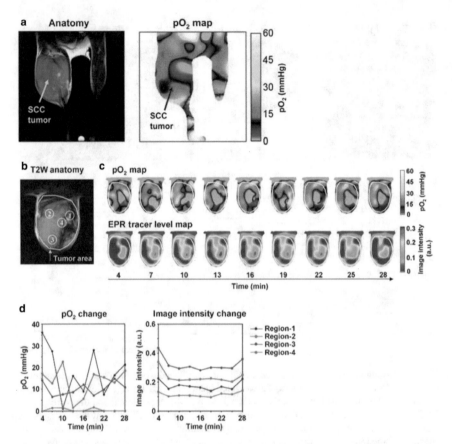

Fig. 5.7 Representative EPRI oxygen image monitoring temporal and spatial dynamics of cycling and chronic hypoxia. (**a**) An EPR oxygen imaging of tumor-bearing mice. The EPRI method allows the pO$_2$ map from the deep tissue of healthy mouse to be obtained. (**b**) T2-weighted anatomical image of a representative SCCVII tumor-bearing mouse. The large yellow line indicates the tumor region. The four ROIs that are indicated by the small white lines were chosen for tracing fluctuations of pO$_2$ and spin intensity with time. (**c**) Corresponding pO$_2$ maps (*top*) and the tracer level maps (*bottom*) were obtained from EPRI. The white line indicates the tumor region. Time increased from *left* to *right* from 4 to 28 min. (**d**) The values of pO$_2$ and the tracer level in each ROI, described in (b), were quantified and plotted as a function of time. *SCCVII* squamous cell carcinoma VII [67]

chronic and cycling tumor hypoxia were imaged before and 1 day after radiation in an SCCVII murine model (Fig. 5.8). In this study, two regions of cycling and chronic hypoxia were imaged using EPRI. Interestingly, the study indicated that despite no significant changes in tumor volume before or 1 day after radiation, visible changes in cycling and chronic hypoxia were observed. The region of cycling hypoxia showed a decrease, whereas chronic hypoxia regions in the tumor exhibited a significant increase in response to radiation treatment. Matsumoto et al. used EPRI and MRI approaches to demonstrate vascular renormalization in tumor-bearing mice by obtaining longitudinal mapping of tumor pO$_2$ and microvessel density during

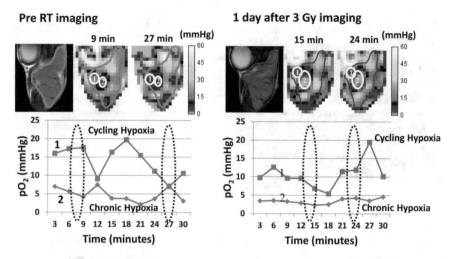

Fig. 5.8 Three-dimensional-EPR oxygen images monitoring the spatial and temporal dynamics of chronic and cycling hypoxia in response to radiation. EPR images obtained from subcutaneous SCCVII tumors in mice before RT and 1 day after irradiation (3 Gy). 1 and 2 marked within white circle represent region of interest (ROI) selected to monitor changes in pO_2 dynamics every 3 min over 30 min time period. ROI 1 represents cycling hypoxia (median $pO_2 > 10$ mmHg during 30 min duration) and ROI 2 represents chronic hypoxia (median $pO_2 < 10$ mmHg during 30 min duration). Representative images and EPR images captured during 9 min and 27 min before RT and at 15 min and 24 min after RT are shown. *EPR* electron paramagnetic resonance, *pO_2* partial pressure of O_2, *ROI* region of interest (Personal communication to Murali C. Krishna)

treatment with the multi-tyrosine inhibitor, sunitinib (Fig. 5.9). This study demonstrated that radiation treatment during the period of improved oxygenation by anti-angiogenic therapy resulted in a synergistic delay in tumor growth. Most importantly, sunitinib treatment suppressed cycling tumor hypoxia [106]. These preclinical results demonstrate a potential of noninvasive monitoring of tumor pO_2 enabling identification of a window of vascular renormalization to maximize the effects of radiation in combination therapy such as anti-angiogenic drugs. Subsequently noninvasive imaging modality can be useful in uncovering the dynamics of functional heterogeneity such as tumor pO_2 associated during and after the response to therapy. Despite its great clinical potential, EPRI is currently available only for preclinical applications. Efforts from radiation biologists, radiation oncologists, and imaging experts are needed to conduct studies toward designing clinical trials and strengthening the application of EPRI, fostering the advancements of this technology for clinical use.

Conclusion

The ultimate aim of molecular and functional imaging approaches in clinical oncology is to improvise cancer diagnosis and treatment. These imaging approaches aid clinicians to visualize tumors and their response to treatments. Research focused on

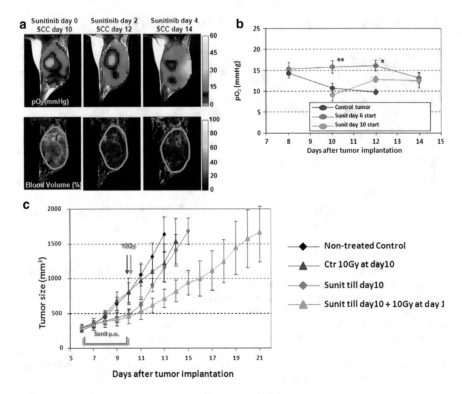

Fig. 5.9 EPRI imaging of tumor pO₂ and blood volume for monitoring chemoradiation response. (**a**) Administration of anti-angiogenic agent sunitinib treatment at later stage of tumor development improved tumor oxygenation (*upper panel*) and reduced tumor blood volume (*lower panel*) without significant change in tumor size. (**b**) Quantification of tumor pO₂ changes in sunitinib-treated mice and vehicle control mice. *P<0.05, *P<0.01. (**c**) Transient increase in tumor oxygenation with sunitinib treatment enhances outcome of radiation therapy. The tumor growth kinetic shown for untreated control mice (*black*), mice treated with a single10-Gy radiation at SCC day 10 (*blue*), mice treated for 4 days with sunitinib during 6–10 days after SCC implantation (*red*), and mice treated for 4 days with sunitinib followed by a single 10 Gy radiation (*green*). *SCC* squamous cell carcinoma. Data taken from [106]

cancer molecular genetics and epigenetics has contributed a number of targeted therapies, whose clinical utility can be successfully characterized using molecular imaging. Future discoveries identifying novel imaging biomarkers will accelerate and improve drug development by helping to determine if the drug under investigation is hitting the desired target and causing the intended effect to tumors. Molecular imaging-based targeted therapy has great potential in making personalized medicine a reality. Collectively, image-guided targeted therapies are the only noninvasive approach that provides real-time intervention rather than facing endpoint failures in cancer management. So far two major tumor characteristics have been well exploited using molecular imaging approaches. These include the altered tumor metabolism and changes in tumor microenvironment such as hypoxia.

Tumor glucose metabolism has been highly successful in monitoring, staging, and early assessment of targeted therapies including radiotherapy in the clinics. The utility of ^{18}F-FDG with PET and MRSI will remain the cornerstone of imaging metabolism in the near future. More advancement in better PET tracers along with our current understanding of altered tumor metabolism and key factors influencing tumor microenvironment will impact future management of cancer patient diagnosis, tumor staging, radiation treatment planning, and monitoring of tumor response to therapy. Tumor hypoxia is another well-characterized biological phenomenon that is prevalent in various solid tumors. Hypoxic tumors tend to be more resistant to radiation-induced death. Years of research have shed light on the cyclic and chronic hypoxia present in solid tumors which is heterogeneously dispersed and is independent of size, stage, grade, or histology of any given tumor. Therefore, noninvasive measurement of tumor hypoxia is of paramount importance in clinical management with radiotherapy. It has been observed that tumors can overcome hypoxia by several different survival mechanisms, including loss of apoptotic potential, increased proliferative potential, and formation of new blood vessels that encourage the evolutionary selection for a more malignant phenotype. Noninvasive techniques such as DCE-MRI and BOLD-MRI have shown some promise in measuring hypoxia noninvasively. Currently, EPRI seems to the highly sensitive technique to measure hypoxia quantitatively. Still, in its infancy, future work needs to be done to make this technique applicable in a clinical setting. Incorporating EPRI/MRSI in radiotherapy will help advance its application in targeting deep-seated, surgically unresolved tumors. The assessment of tumor hypoxia by noninvasive means will be of immense value to radiation oncologists, medical oncologists, and pharmaceutical companies to develop and test hypoxia-based therapies or other combinatorial treatment strategies. Multimodality or hybrid imaging will play a major role in the clinical assessment in the near future. This trend has already been set by the replacement of separate PET and CT by hybrid PET/CT technology and will continue with the establishment of integrated MRI/PET. In summary, application of integrated imaging tools for detecting tumor physiology has tremendous potential in oncology and can improve the effectiveness of radiation therapy.

Future Perspective

A number of promising molecular imaging platforms are emerging to provide radiation oncologists with biochemical and physiological information of tumor and normal tissues before, during, and after treatment. This information has the potential to aid clinicians in diagnosis and perhaps rapid assessment of treatment response. With respect to tumor metabolism, FDG has been and will continue to be useful in diagnosis and monitoring treatment responses. Future, emerging multimodalities for metabolic imaging using hyperpolarized biochemical substrates such as *hyper-PET* may provide better specificity of metabolic processes. This technique utilizes simultaneous in vivo PET combined with hyperpolarized MRI. The first example

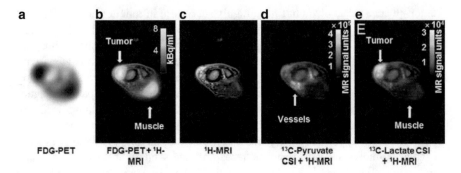

Fig. 5.10 *Hyper-PET* showing sensitivity of ¹³C-hyperpolarized pyruvate over ¹⁸F-FDG to measure tumor glucose metabolism. Image showing right front leg of canine patient with liposarcoma. High uptake of ¹⁸F-FDG in muscle (marked in *arrow*, panel **b**, ¹⁸F-FDG-PET + ¹H-MRI) and of ¹³C pyruvate in the large vessels (marked in *arrow*, panel **d**, ¹³C-Pyruvate CSI + ¹H-MRI). (**a**) ¹⁸F-FDG-PET. (**b**) ¹⁸F-FDG-PET + ¹H-MRI. (**c**) ¹H-MRI. (**d**) ¹³C-pyruvate CSI + ¹H-MRI. (**e**) ¹³C-lactate CSI + ¹H-MRI. Data taken with permission from [115]

demonstrating the application of *hyper-PET* has recently been tested in canine liposarcoma model [115]. In this study, ¹³C-hyperpolarized pyruvate was combined with ¹⁸F-FDG-PET and MRI to assess the feasibility and specificity of glucose uptake by tumor over normal muscle tissue. Interestingly, the muscle forepaw of the subject indicated significantly high ¹⁸F-FDG uptake compared to ¹³C-hyperpolarized pyruvate. High ¹⁸F-FDG in the normal muscle tissue was attributed to high activity of these muscles before anesthesia. However, real-time conversion of ¹³C-pyruvate into ¹³C-lactate corresponding to high ¹⁸F-FDG was observed in the tumor tissue (Fig. 5.10). This study confirms the sensitivity and specificity of ¹³C-hyperpolarized pyruvate for the diagnosis of cancer. Such cross comparison and application of emerging imaging platforms will be necessary to choose and optimize the most accurate functional imaging approach. Lastly, imaging with specific hyperpolarized biochemical substrates may be useful in delineating tumors with specific mutations in metabolic pathways.

The ongoing identification of a variety of tumor specific markers that can be incorporated into imaging platforms will further enhance the clinician's ability to diagnose and monitor treatment response. Imaging that reports on physiological and microenvironmental processes such as diffusion, perfusion, proliferation, and hypoxia, which are known to be important in tumor growth and treatment response, will further enhance the information base. There will also be a need to evaluate many of the new imaging modalities not only for tumor but also for normal tissues within the radiation field. Establishing a therapeutic ratio of radiation and/or chemoradiation cancer treatment is not always straightforward. It is anticipated that the newer molecular imaging approaches will complement and perhaps hybridize with existing imaging platforms to yield more information, particularly at the biochemical/molecular level that might be used to more precisely derive a therapeutic ratio for various treatment strategies.

References

1. Bedard PL, Hansen AR, Ratain MJ, Siu LL (2013) Tumour heterogeneity in the clinic. Nature 501:355–364
2. Junttila MR, de Sauvage FJ (2013) Influence of tumour micro-environment heterogeneity on therapeutic response. Nature 501:346–354
3. Cardenas-Navia LI, Mace D, Richardson RA, Wilson DF, Shan S, Dewhirst MW (2008) The pervasive presence of fluctuating oxygenation in tumors. Cancer Res 68:5812–5819
4. Schroeder T, Yuan H, Viglianti BL, Peltz C, Asopa S, Vujaskovic Z, Dewhirst MW (2005) Spatial heterogeneity and oxygen dependence of glucose consumption in R3230Ac and fibro-sarcomas of the Fischer 344 rat. Cancer Res 65:5163–5171
5. Serganova I, Doubrovin M, Vider J, Ponomarev V, Soghomonyan S, Beresten T, Ageyeva L, Serganov A, Cai S, Balatoni J, Blasberg R, Gelovani J (2004) Molecular imaging of temporal dynamics and spatial heterogeneity of hypoxia-inducible factor-1 signal transduction activity in tumors in living mice. Cancer Res 64:6101–6108
6. Eskey CJ, Koretsky AP, Domach MM, Jain RK (1992) 2H-nuclear magnetic resonance imaging of tumor blood flow: spatial and temporal heterogeneity in a tissue-isolated mammary adenocarcinoma. Cancer Res 52:6010–6019
7. Hamberg LM, Kristjansen PE, Hunter GJ, Wolf GL, Jain RK (1994) Spatial heterogeneity in tumor perfusion measured with functional computed tomography at 0.05 microliter resolution. Cancer Res 54:6032–6036
8. Degani H, Gusis V, Weinstein D, Fields S, Strano S (1997) Mapping pathophysiological features of breast tumors by MRI at high spatial resolution. Nat Med 3:780–782
9. Choi YP, Shim HS, Gao MQ, Kang S, Cho NH (2011) Molecular portraits of intratumoral heterogeneity in human ovarian cancer. Cancer Lett 307:62–71
10. Gatenby RA, Silva AS, Gillies RJ, Frieden BR (2009) Adaptive therapy. Cancer Res 69:4894–4903
11. Ling CC, Humm J, Larson S, Amols H, Fuks Z, Leibel S, Koutcher JA (2000) Towards multidimensional radiotherapy (MD-CRT): biological imaging and biological conformality. Int J Radiat Oncol Biol Phys 47:551–560
12. Bentzen SM, Gregoire V (2011) Molecular imaging-based dose painting: a novel paradigm for radiation therapy prescription. Semin Radiat Oncol 21:101–110
13. Chen ZY, Wang YX, Lin Y, Zhang JS, Yang F, Zhou QL, Liao YY (2014) Advance of molecular imaging technology and targeted imaging agent in imaging and therapy. BioMed Res Int 2014:819324
14. Anderson CJ, Ferdani R (2009) Copper-64 radiopharmaceuticals for PET imaging of cancer: advances in preclinical and clinical research. Cancer Biother Radiopharm 24:379–393
15. Phelps ME (2000) Positron emission tomography provides molecular imaging of biological processes. Proc Natl Acad Sci U S A 97:9226–9233
16. Zhu A, Lee D, Shim H (2011) Metabolic positron emission tomography imaging in cancer detection and therapy response. Semin Oncol 38:55–69
17. Gambhir SS (2002) Molecular imaging of cancer with positron emission tomography. Nat Rev Cancer 2:683–693
18. Pereira GC, Traughber M, Muzic RF Jr (2014) The role of imaging in radiation therapy planning: past, present, and future. BioMed Res Int 2014:231090
19. Hijnen NM, de Vries A, Nicolay K, Grull H (2012) Dual-isotope 111In/177Lu SPECT imaging as a tool in molecular imaging tracer design. Contrast Media Mol Imaging 7:214–222
20. Blamire AM (2008) The technology of MRI–the next 10 years? Br J Radiol 81:601–617
21. Scherzinger AL, Hendee WR (1985) Basic principles of magnetic resonance imaging–an update. West J Med 143:782–792
22. Gore JC, Manning HC, Quarles CC, Waddell KW, Yankeelov TE (2011) Magnetic resonance in the era of molecular imaging of cancer. Magn Reson Imaging 29:587–600

23. Khoo VS (2000) MRI–"magic radiotherapy imaging" for treatment planning? Br J Radiol 73:229–233
24. Anderson SA, Frank JA (2007) MRI of mouse models of neurological disorders. NMR Biomed 20:200–215
25. Kerkhof EM, Balter JM, Vineberg K, Raaymakers BW (2010) Treatment plan adaptation for MRI-guided radiotherapy using solely MRI data: a CT-based simulation study. Phys Med Biol 55:N433–N440
26. Klostergaard J, Parga K, Raptis RG (2010) Current and future applications of magnetic resonance imaging (MRI) to breast and ovarian cancer patient management. P R Health Sci J 29:223–231
27. Lee DJ, Ahmed HU, Moore CM, Emberton M, Ehdaie B (2014) Multiparametric magnetic resonance imaging in the management and diagnosis of prostate cancer: current applications and strategies. Curr Urol Rep 15:390
28. Schulze M, Kotter I, Ernemann U, Fenchel M, Tzaribatchev N, Claussen CD, Horger M (2009) MRI findings in inflammatory muscle diseases and their noninflammatory mimics. AJR Am J Roentgenol 192:1708–1716
29. Akeson P, Larsson EM, Kristoffersen DT, Jonsson E, Holtas S (1995) Brain metastases–comparison of gadodiamide injection-enhanced MR imaging at standard and high dose, contrast-enhanced CT and non-contrast-enhanced MR imaging. Acta Radiol 36:300–306
30. O'Neill BD, Salerno G, Thomas K, Tait DM, Brown G (2009) MR vs CT imaging: low rectal cancer tumour delineation for three-dimensional conformal radiotherapy. Br J Radiol 82:509–513
31. Chen L, Price RA Jr, Wang L, Li J, Qin L, Mcneeley S, Ma CM, Freedman GM, Pollack A (2004) MRI-based treatment planning for radiotherapy: dosimetric verification for prostate IMRT. Int J Radiat Oncol Biol Phys 60:636–647
32. O'Connor JP, Tofts PS, Miles KA, Parkes LM, Thompson G, Jackson A (2011) Dynamic contrast-enhanced imaging techniques: CT and MRI. Br J Radiol 84:S112–S120
33. Newbold K, Partridge M, Cook G, Sohaib SA, Charles-Edwards E, Rhys-Evans P, Harrington K, Nutting C (2006) Advanced imaging applied to radiotherapy planning in head and neck cancer: a clinical review. Br J Radiol 79:554–561
34. Barillot I, Reynaud-Bougnoux A (2006) The use of MRI in planning radiotherapy for gynaecological tumours. Cancer Imaging 6:100–106
35. Artemov D, Mori N, Ravi R, Bhujwalla ZM (2003) Magnetic resonance molecular imaging of the HER-2/neu receptor. Cancer Res 63:2723–2727
36. Debergh I, van Damme N, de Naeyer D, Smeets P, Demetter P, Robert P, Carme S, Pattyn P, Ceelen W (2014) Molecular imaging of tumor-associated angiogenesis using a novel magnetic resonance imaging contrast agent targeting alphavbeta 3 integrin. Ann Surg Oncol 21:2097–2104
37. Schnell O, Krebs B, Carlsen J, Miederer I, Goetz C, Goldbrunner RH, Wester HJ, Haubner R, Popperl G, Holtmannspotter M, Kretzschmar HA, Kessler H, Tonn JC, Schwaiger M, Beer AJ (2009) Imaging of integrin alpha(v)beta(3) expression in patients with malignant glioma by [18F] Galacto-RGD positron emission tomography. Neuro Oncol 11:861–870
38. Sipkins DA, Cheresh DA, Kazemi MR, Nevin LM, Bednarski MD, Li KC (1998) Detection of tumor angiogenesis in vivo by alphaVbeta3-targeted magnetic resonance imaging. Nat Med 4:623–626
39. Blankenberg FG (2008) In vivo imaging of apoptosis. Cancer Biol Ther 7:1525–1532
40. Maiseyeu A, Mihai G, Kampfrath T, Simonetti OP, Sen CK, Roy S, Rajagopalan S, Parthasarathy S (2009) Gadolinium-containing phosphatidylserine liposomes for molecular imaging of atherosclerosis. J Lipid Res 50:2157–2163
41. Dodd SJ, Williams M, Suhan JP, Williams DS, Koretsky AP, Ho C (1999) Detection of single mammalian cells by high-resolution magnetic resonance imaging. Biophys J 76:103–109
42. Bulte JW, Zhang S, van Gelderen P, Herynek V, Jordan EK, Duncan ID, Frank JA (1999) Neurotransplantation of magnetically labeled oligodendrocyte progenitors: magnetic resonance tracking of cell migration and myelination. Proc Natl Acad Sci U S A 96:15256–15261

43. Franklin RJ, Blaschuk KL, Bearchell MC, Prestoz LL, Setzu A, Brindle KM, ffrench-Constant C (1999) Magnetic resonance imaging of transplanted oligodendrocyte precursors in the rat brain. Neuroreport 10:3961–3965
44. Hu DE, Kettunen MI, Brindle KM (2005) Monitoring T-lymphocyte trafficking in tumors undergoing immune rejection. Magn Reson Med 54:1473–1479
45. Kircher MF, Allport JR, Graves EE, Love V, Josephson L, Lichtman AH, Weissleder R (2003) In vivo high resolution three-dimensional imaging of antigen-specific cytotoxic T-lymphocyte trafficking to tumors. Cancer Res 63:6838–6846
46. de Vries IJ, Lesterhuis WJ, Barentsz JO, Verdijk P, van Krieken JH, Boerman OC, Oyen WJ, Bonenkamp JJ, Boezeman JB, Adema GJ, Bulte JW, Scheenen TW, Punt CJ, Heerschap A, Figdor CG (2005) Magnetic resonance tracking of dendritic cells in melanoma patients for monitoring of cellular therapy. Nat Biotechnol 23:1407–1413
47. Dang CV (2012) Links between metabolism and cancer. Genes Dev 26:877–890
48. Hanahan D, Weinberg RA (2011) Hallmarks of cancer: the next generation. Cell 144: 646–674
49. Warburg O (1956) On respiratory impairment in cancer cells. Science 124:269–270
50. Griguer CE, Oliva CR, Gillespie GY (2005) Glucose metabolism heterogeneity in human and mouse malignant glioma cell lines. J Neurooncol 74:123–133
51. Carvalho KC, Cunha IW, Rocha RM, Ayala FR, Cajaiba MM, Begnami MD, Vilela RS, Paiva GR, Andrade RG, Soares FA (2011) GLUT1 expression in malignant tumors and its use as an immunodiagnostic marker. Clinics (Sao Paulo) 66:965–972
52. Macheda ML, Rogers S, Best JD (2005) Molecular and cellular regulation of glucose transporter (GLUT) proteins in cancer. J Cell Physiol 202:654–662
53. van Der Wel A, Nijsten S, Hochstenbag M, Lamers R, Boersma L, Wanders R, Lutgens L, Zimny M, Bentzen SM, Wouters B, Lambin P, De Ruysscher D (2005) Increased therapeutic ratio by 18FDG-PET CT planning in patients with clinical CT stage N2-N3M0 non-small-cell lung cancer: a modeling study. Int J Radiat Oncol Biol Phys 61:649–655
54. Brindle K (2008) New approaches for imaging tumour responses to treatment. Nat Rev Cancer 8:94–107
55. Schwarz JK, Siegel BA, Dehdashti F, Grigsby PW (2007) Association of posttherapy positron emission tomography with tumor response and survival in cervical carcinoma. JAMA 298:2289–2295
56. Daisne JF, Duprez T, Weynand B, Lonneux M, Hamoir M, Reychler H, Gregoire V (2004) Tumor volume in pharyngolaryngeal squamous cell carcinoma: comparison at CT, MR imaging, and FDG PET and validation with surgical specimen. Radiology 233:93–100
57. Geets X, Lee JA, Bol A, Lonneux M, Gregoire V (2007) A gradient-based method for segmenting FDG-PET images: methodology and validation. Eur J Nucl Med Mol Imaging 34:1427–1438
58. Kostakoglu L, Goldsmith SJ (2003) 18F-FDG PET evaluation of the response to therapy for lymphoma and for breast, lung, and colorectal carcinoma. J Nucl Med 44:224–239
59. Gallamini A, Hutchings M, Rigacci L, Specht L, Merli F, Hansen M, Patti C, Loft A, Di Raimondo F, D'amore F, Biggi A, Vitolo U, Stelitano C, Sancetta R, Trentin L, Luminari S, Iannitto E, Viviani S, Pierri I, Levis A (2007) Early interim 2-[18F]fluoro-2-deoxy-D-glucose positron emission tomography is prognostically superior to international prognostic score in advanced-stage Hodgkin's lymphoma: a report from a joint Italian-Danish study. J Clin Oncol 25:3746–3752
60. Schwarz JK, Grigsby PW, Dehdashti F, Delbeke D (2009) The role of 18F-FDG PET in assessing therapy response in cancer of the cervix and ovaries. J Nucl Med 50(Suppl 1): 64S–73S
61. van Loon J, Offermann C, Bosmans G, Wanders R, Dekker A, Borger J, Oellers M, Dingemans AM, van Baardwijk A, Teule J, Snoep G, Hochstenbag M, Houben R, Lambin P, De Ruysscher D (2008) 18FDG-PET based radiation planning of mediastinal lymph nodes in limited disease small cell lung cancer changes radiotherapy fields: a planning study. Radiother Oncol 87:49–54

62. Madani I, Duthoy W, Derie C, De Gersem W, Boterberg T, Saerens M, Jacobs F, Gregoire V, Lonneux M, Vakaet L, Vanderstraeten B, Bauters W, Bonte K, Thierens H, De Neve W (2007) Positron emission tomography-guided, focal-dose escalation using intensity-modulated radiotherapy for head and neck cancer. Int J Radiat Oncol Biol Phys 68:126–135

63. Juweid ME, Cheson BD (2006) Positron-emission tomography and assessment of cancer therapy. N Engl J Med 354:496–507

64. Golman K, Ardenkjaer-Larsen JH, Petersson JS, Mansson S, Leunbach I (2003) Molecular imaging with endogenous substances. Proc Natl Acad Sci U S A 100:10435–10439

65. Golman K, Olsson LE, Axelsson O, Mansson S, Karlsson M, Petersson JS (2003) Molecular imaging using hyperpolarized 13C. Br J Radiol 76:S118–S127

66. Ardenkjaer-Larsen JH, Fridlund B, Gram A, Hansson G, Hansson L, Lerche MH, Servin R, Thaning M, Golman K (2003) Increase in signal-to-noise ratio of > 10,000 times in liquid-state NMR. Proc Natl Acad Sci U S A 100:10158–10163

67. Matsuo M, Matsumoto S, Mitchell JB, Krishna MC, Camphausen K (2014) Magnetic resonance imaging of the tumor microenvironment in radiotherapy: perfusion, hypoxia, and metabolism. Semin Radiat Oncol 24:210–217

68. Day SE, Kettunen MI, Cherukuri MK, Mitchell JB, Lizak MJ, Morris HD, Matsumoto S, Koretsky AP, Brindle KM (2011) Detecting response of rat C6 glioma tumors to radiotherapy using hyperpolarized [1- 13C]pyruvate and 13C magnetic resonance spectroscopic imaging. Magn Reson Med 65:557–563

69. Albers MJ, Bok R, Chen AP, Cunningham CH, Zierhut ML, Zhang VY, Kohler SJ, Tropp J, Hurd RE, Yen YF, Nelson SJ, Vigneron DB, Kurhanewicz J (2008) Hyperpolarized 13C lactate, pyruvate, and alanine: noninvasive biomarkers for prostate cancer detection and grading. Cancer Res 68:8607–8615

70. Nelson SJ, Kurhanewicz J, Vigneron DB, Larson PE, Harzstark AL, Ferrone M, van Criekinge M, Chang JW, Bok R, Park I, Reed G, Carvajal L, Small EJ, Munster P, Weinberg VK, Ardenkjaer-Larsen JH, Chen AP, Hurd RE, Odegardstuen LI, Robb FJ, Tropp J, Murray JA (2013) Metabolic imaging of patients with prostate cancer using hyperpolarized [1-(1)(3)C] pyruvate. Sci Transl Med 5:198ra108

71. Zierhut ML, Yen YF, Chen AP, Bok R, Albers MJ, Zhang V, Tropp J, Park I, Vigneron DB, Kurhanewicz J, Hurd RE, Nelson SJ (2010) Kinetic modeling of hyperpolarized 13C1-pyruvate metabolism in normal rats and TRAMP mice. J Magn Reson 202:85–92

72. Aboagye EO, Bhujwalla ZM (1999) Malignant transformation alters membrane choline phospholipid metabolism of human mammary epithelial cells. Cancer Res 59:80–84

73. Glunde K, Bhujwalla ZM, Ronen SM (2011) Choline metabolism in malignant transformation. Nat Rev Cancer 11:835–848

74. van Sluis R, Bhujwalla ZM, Raghunand N, Ballesteros P, Alvarez J, Cerdan S, Galons JP, Gillies RJ (1999) In vivo imaging of extracellular pH using 1H MRSI. Magn Reson Med 41:743–750

75. Semenza GL (2012) Hypoxia-inducible factors: mediators of cancer progression and targets for cancer therapy. Trends Pharmacol Sci 33:207–214

76. Wilson WR, Hay MP (2011) Targeting hypoxia in cancer therapy. Nat Rev Cancer 11:393–410

77. Subarsky P, Hill RP (2003) The hypoxic tumour microenvironment and metastatic progression. Clin Exp Metastasis 20:237–250

78. Chaudary N, Hill RP (2007) Hypoxia and metastasis. Clin Cancer Res 13:1947–1949

79. Vaupel P, Kallinowski F, Okunieff P (1989) Blood flow, oxygen and nutrient supply, and metabolic microenvironment of human tumors: a review. Cancer Res 49:6449–6465

80. Lanzen J, Braun RD, Klitzman B, Brizel D, Secomb TW, Dewhirst MW (2006) Direct demonstration of instabilities in oxygen concentrations within the extravascular compartment of an experimental tumor. Cancer Res 66:2219–2223

81. Martinive P, Defresne F, Bouzin C, Saliez J, Lair F, Gregoire V, Michiels C, Dessy C, Feron O (2006) Preconditioning of the tumor vasculature and tumor cells by intermittent hypoxia: implications for anticancer therapies. Cancer Res 66:11736–11744

82. Pigott KH, Hill SA, Chaplin DJ, Saunders MI (1996) Microregional fluctuations in perfusion within human tumours detected using laser Doppler flowmetry. Radiother Oncol 40:45–50

83. Janssen HL, Ljungkvist AS, Rijken PF, Sprong D, Bussink J, van der Kogel AJ, Haustermans KM, Begg AC (2005) Thymidine analogues to assess microperfusion in human tumors. Int J Radiat Oncol Biol Phys 62:1169–1175

84. Nordsmark M, Bentzen SM, Rudat V, Brizel D, Lartigau E, Stadler P, Becker A, Adam M, Molls M, Dunst J, Terris DJ, Overgaard J (2005) Prognostic value of tumor oxygenation in 397 head and neck tumors after primary radiation therapy. An international multi-center study. Radiother Oncol 77:18–24

85. Peters KB, Brown JM (2002) Tirapazamine: a hypoxia-activated topoisomerase II poison. Cancer Res 62:5248–5253

86. Houghton PJ, Lock R, Carol H, Morton CL, Phelps D, Gorlick R, Kolb EA, Keir ST, Reynolds CP, Kang MH, Maris JM, Wozniak AW, Gu Y, Wilson WR, Smith MA (2011) Initial testing of the hypoxia-activated prodrug PR-104 by the pediatric preclinical testing program. Pediatr Blood Cancer 57:443–453

87. Wojtkowiak JW, Cornnell HC, Matsumoto S, Saito K, Takakusagi Y, Dutta P, Kim M, Zhang X, Leos R, Bailey KM, Martinez G, Lloyd MC, Weber C, Mitchell JB, Lynch RM, Baker AF, Gatenby RA, Rejniak KA, Hart C, Krishna MC, Gillies RJ (2015) Pyruvate sensitizes pancreatic tumors to hypoxia-activated prodrug TH-302. Cancer Metab 3:2

88. Kavanagh MC, Sun A, Hu Q, Hill RP (1996) Comparing techniques of measuring tumor hypoxia in different murine tumors: Eppendorf pO_2 Histograph, [3H]misonidazole binding and paired survival assay. Radiat Res 145:491–500

89. Hockel M, Vaupel P (2001) Tumor hypoxia: definitions and current clinical, biologic, and molecular aspects. J Natl Cancer Inst 93:266–276

90. Drevs J (2003) Soluble markers for the detection of hypoxia under antiangiogenic treatment. Anticancer Res 23:1159–1161

91. Le QT, Courter D (2008) Clinical biomarkers for hypoxia targeting. Cancer Metastasis Rev 27:351–362

92. Chapman JD (1979) Hypoxic sensitizers–implications for radiation therapy. N Engl J Med 301:1429–1432

93. Roels S, Slagmolen P, Nuyts J, Lee JA, Loeckx D, Maes F, Stroobants S, Penninckx F, Haustermans K (2008) Biological image-guided radiotherapy in rectal cancer: is there a role for FMISO or FLT, next to FDG? Acta Oncol 47:1237–1248

94. Mayr NA, Yuh WT, Jajoura D, Wang JZ, Lo SS, Montebello JF, Porter K, Zhang D, Mcmeekin DS, Buatti JM (2010) Ultra-early predictive assay for treatment failure using functional magnetic resonance imaging and clinical prognostic parameters in cervical cancer. Cancer 116:903–912

95. Newbold K, Castellano I, Charles-Edwards E, Mears D, Sohaib A, Leach M, Rhys-Evans P, Clarke P, Fisher C, Harrington K, Nutting C (2009) An exploratory study into the role of dynamic contrast-enhanced magnetic resonance imaging or perfusion computed tomography for detection of intratumoral hypoxia in head-and-neck cancer. Int J Radiat Oncol Biol Phys 74:29–37

96. de Bree R (2013) Functional imaging to predict treatment response after (chemo) radiotherapy of head and neck squamous cell carcinoma. Quant Imaging Med Surg 3:231–234

97. Tong T, Sun Y, Gollub MJ, Peng W, Cai S, Zhang Z, Gu Y (2015) Dynamic contrast-enhanced MRI: Use in predicting pathological complete response to neoadjuvant chemoradiation in locally advanced rectal cancer. J Magn Reson Imaging 42(3):673–680

98. Lawrence TS, Robertson JM, Anscher MS, Jirtle RL, Ensminger WD, Fajardo LF (1995) Hepatic toxicity resulting from cancer treatment. Int J Radiat Oncol Biol Phys 31:1237–1248

99. Michalski JM, Gay H, Jackson A, Tucker SL, Deasy JO (2010) Radiation dose-volume effects in radiation-induced rectal injury. Int J Radiat Oncol Biol Phys 76:S123–S129

100. Sundgren PC, Cao Y (2009) Brain irradiation: effects on normal brain parenchyma and radiation injury. Neuroimaging Clin N Am 19:657–668

101. Hoskin PJ, Carnell DM, Taylor NJ, Smith RE, Stirling JJ, Daley FM, Saunders MI, Bentzen SM, Collins DJ, D'arcy JA, Padhani AP (2007) Hypoxia in prostate cancer: correlation of BOLD-MRI with pimonidazole immunohistochemistry-initial observations. Int J Radiat Oncol Biol Phys 68:1065–1071

102. Hallac RR, Zhou H, Pidikiti R, Song K, Stojadinovic S, Zhao D, Solberg T, Peschke P, Mason RP (2014) Correlations of noninvasive BOLD and TOLD MRI with pO_2 and relevance to tumor radiation response. Magn Reson Med 71:1863–1873

103. Jiang L, Weatherall PT, Mccoll RW, Tripathy D, Mason RP (2013) Blood oxygenation level-dependent (BOLD) contrast magnetic resonance imaging (MRI) for prediction of breast cancer chemotherapy response: a pilot study. J Magn Reson Imaging 37:1083–1092

104. Matsumoto A, Matsumoto K, Matsumoto S, Hyodo F, Sowers AL, Koscielniak JW, Devasahayam N, Subramanian S, Mitchell JB, Krishna MC (2011) Intracellular hypoxia of tumor tissue estimated by noninvasive electron paramagnetic resonance oximetry technique using paramagnetic probes. Biol Pharm Bull 34:142–145

105. Yasui H, Matsumoto S, Devasahayam N, Munasinghe JP, Choudhuri R, Saito K, Subramanian S, Mitchell JB, Krishna MC (2010) Low-field magnetic resonance imaging to visualize chronic and cycling hypoxia in tumor-bearing mice. Cancer Res 70:6427–6436

106. Matsumoto S, Batra S, Saito K, Yasui H, Choudhuri R, Gadisetti C, Subramanian S, Devasahayam N, Munasinghe JP, Mitchell JB, Krishna MC (2011) Antiangiogenic agent sunitinib transiently increases tumor oxygenation and suppresses cycling hypoxia. Cancer Res 71:6350–6359

107. Hou H, Dong R, Lariviere JP, Mupparaju SP, Swartz HM, Khan N (2011) Synergistic combination of hyperoxygenation and radiotherapy by repeated assessments of tumor pO_2 with EPR oximetry. J Radiat Res 52:568–574

108. Krishna MC, Matsumoto S, Yasui H, Saito K, Devasahayam N, Subramanian S, Mitchell JB (2012) Electron paramagnetic resonance imaging of tumor pO(2). Radiat Res 177:376–386

109. Matsumoto K, Subramanian S, Devasahayam N, Aravalluvan T, Murugesan R, Cook JA, Mitchell JB, Krishna MC (2006) Electron paramagnetic resonance imaging of tumor hypoxia: enhanced spatial and temporal resolution for in vivo pO_2 determination. Magn Reson Med 55:1157–1163

110. Subramanian S, Devasahayam N, Mcmillan A, Matsumoto S, Munasinghe JP, Saito K, Mitchell JB, Chandramouli GV, Krishna MC (2012) Reporting of quantitative oxygen mapping in EPR imaging. J Magn Reson 214:244–251

111. Matsumoto S, Hyodo F, Subramanian S, Devasahayam N, Munasinghe J, Hyodo E, Gadisetti C, Cook JA, Mitchell JB, Krishna MC (2008) Low-field paramagnetic resonance imaging of tumor oxygenation and glycolytic activity in mice. J Clin Invest 118:1965–1973

112. Hou H, Abramovic Z, Lariviere JP, Sentjurc M, Swartz H, Khan N (2010) Effect of a topical vasodilator on tumor hypoxia and tumor oxygen guided radiotherapy using EPR oximetry. Radiat Res 173:651–658

113. Hou H, Lariviere JP, Demidenko E, Gladstone D, Swartz H, Khan N (2009) Repeated tumor pO(2) measurements by multi-site EPR oximetry as a prognostic marker for enhanced therapeutic efficacy of fractionated radiotherapy. Radiother Oncol 91:126–131

114. Matsumoto K, English S, Yoo J, Yamada K, Devasahayam N, Cook JA, Mitchell JB, Subramanian S, Krishna MC (2004) Pharmacokinetics of a triarylmethyl-type paramagnetic spin probe used in EPR oximetry. Magn Reson Med 52:885–892

115. Gutte H, Hansen AE, Henriksen ST, Johannesen HH, Ardenkjaer-Larsen J, Vignaud A, Borresen B, Klausen TL, Wittekind AM, Gillings N, Kristensen AT, Clemmensen A, Hojgaard L, Kjaer A (2015) Simultaneous hyperpolarized (13)C-pyruvate MRI and (18) F-FDG-PET in cancer (hyperPET): feasibility of a new imaging concept using a clinical PET/ MRI scanner. Am J Nucl Med Mol Imaging 5:38–45

Chapter 6
Remodeling the Irradiated Tumor Microenvironment: The Fifth R of Radiobiology?

Mary Helen Barcellos-Hoff

Abstract With the recognition that the host and tumor are inextricably intertwined as a malignant system, the tumor microenvironment (TME) is now considered to be an important target in cancer therapy. A long-standing objective to improve the therapeutic ratio of radiotherapy has been to manipulate microenvironmental factors that impede cancer cell radiosensitivity, most notably hypoxia. A more recent idea is to eradicate or reeducate the components of TME that support and sustain cancer in order to better control the local tumor and prevent metastatic disease. The TME includes the vasculature, stromal cells, and immune cells, each of which is locally corrupted by the presence of cancer, which itself influences distant tissue and cell behaviors. The biology of the irradiated TME provides robust targets to augment local tumor control and intersect with immunological mechanisms that can eliminate distant disease. Transforming growth factor β (TGFβ) is an example of a critical mediator of the irradiated TME. TGFβ inhibition in the context of radiotherapy is predicated on understanding its mechanistic opposition to therapeutic benefit. Therapeutic strategies to biologically augment radiotherapy by preventing the reestablishment of a functional TME could motivate the addition to the classic "Rs" of radiation biology in oncology: repair, reoxygenation, repopulation, redistribution, and now, remodeling the TME.

Keywords Tumor microenvironment • TGFβ • Extracellular matrix • Radiotherapy • Cancer

M.H. Barcellos-Hoff (✉)
Department of Radiation Oncology, Helen Diller Family Comprehensive Cancer Center,
University of California, 2340 Sutter Street, San Francisco, CA 94147, USA
e-mail: mary.barcellos-hoff@ucsf.edu

© Springer International Publishing Switzerland 2017   135
P.J. Tofilon, K. Camphausen (eds.), *Increasing the Therapeutic
Ratio of Radiotherapy*, Cancer Drug Discovery and Development,
DOI 10.1007/978-3-319-40854-5_6

Introduction

At least one course of radiation therapy is prescribed to more than half of all patients with solid tumors. The therapeutic efficacy of radiation is generally considered to be mediated by its capacity to directly kill cancer cells, encouraging dose escalation strategies and combinations with chemotherapy to enhance its antitumor effect. The basis for radiation therapy is often described in terms of the 4 Rs of radiobiology: repair, reoxygenation, repopulation, and redistribution. Double-strand DNA breaks cause a molecular response that results in cell cycle arrest and repair or cell death by diverse processes ranging from apoptosis to senescence [1]. Accordingly, efforts to understand and improve the therapeutic efficacy of radiotherapy have largely concentrated on the molecular mechanisms of DNA damage recognition and repair.

When cancer is treated with radiation, death of tumor cells is coupled with tumor microenvironment (TME) changes that accompany tumor regression. The radiation response of tumor cells has been far better characterized than that of the TME, with the major exception of hypoxia which is a critical barrier to tumor control [2]. Radiation oncology principles thus incorporate the vascular response as a concomitant therapeutic target and resultant effects of radiation on hypoxia (i.e., reoxygenation). However, it is becoming increasingly clear that additional aspects of the TME can contribute to tumor control and even determine radiation sensitivity.

The growing appreciation that TME complexity is inextricably intertwined with tumor growth, metastasis, and response to therapy has engendered clinical strategies to target the TME [3]. Here, we focus on the potential of knowledge about the TME response to radiotherapy. Understanding TME dynamics in response to radiation provides a view of the tumor as an adaptive "organ." This area of investigation is in an exponential growth phase as evidenced by the number of research papers on which radiotherapy and microenvironment are keywords, from 11 in 2000 to 250 in 2015, but is still relatively understudied, particularly as a function of fractionation. One might thus propose the addition of *remodeling* of the TME to the "Rs" of radiobiology.

The Tumor Microenvironment

The cellular component of the TME is comprised of inflammatory cells, innate and adaptive immune cells, including natural killer cells, T cells, and B cells, and cancer-associated fibroblasts [4]. These cells collectively create a stromal environment that promotes tumor progression by providing growth factors, pro-angiogenic factors, proteases, and adhesion molecules that facilitate tumor cell proliferation, angiogenesis, invasion, and metastasis [5, 6]. The dynamic changes in the TME also provides a selective pressure for tumor cell variants that may promote genomic instability, genomic heterogeneity, and epigenetic alteration [7].

In order for cancer to evolve from early dysplastic lesions into invasive cancer, further changes in both the epithelium and the stroma are required to establish the tumor. When initiated cells activate oncogenic signaling pathways that promote growth, motility, and resistance to apoptosis, they also activate the stroma, leading to further recruitment of inflammatory cells and reprogramming of the stromal niche [8]. For example, many of the key downstream targets of mutant *Kras* are cytokines and chemokines that promote progression to dysplasia in a large part through activation and remodeling of stromal cells [9]. Thus, initiated cells begin to "educate" the niche cells to provide greater growth signals and immune suppression. Moreover, these stromal educating signals are not confined simply to the local microenvironment, but are in fact systemic signals. Recent data indicate that as carcinogenesis progresses to the stage of dysplasia, there are systemic signals sent out that lead to profound reprogramming of the bone marrow stroma, with increased production of bone marrow myofibroblasts and recruitment of mesenchymal stem cells into the blood stream and then into the tumor site [10]. The education of the bone marrow by the tumor is likely to be a critical step in cancer progression. The nature of these signals is not fully defined but could include TGFβ, SDF-1, and possibly exosomes. Prior to metastatic spread of cancer, activation and generation of distant "niches" provide a suitable environment for the growth and spread of the tumor [11, 12]. Early-stage tumors are able to generate these "pre-metastatic niches" in a systemic fashion, and these niches are likely a major factor determining metastatic spread [13]. Indeed, the ability to metastasize is probably acquired early on by many cancer cells, and individual tumor cells are likely released frequently into the circulation. However, in the absence of suitable niche cells, these cancer may remain localized for years.

With respect to treatment of established cancer, emerging evidence supports the idea that the stromal niche contributes substantially to chemoresistance and to the inability to eradicate cancer [14]. This could be due in part to the role of stroma as a barrier to drug delivery, via high interstitial pressure [15], but likely the stroma also contributes positively to signaling pathways that sustain cancer cells and/or inhibit apoptosis and cell death. Thus, additional efforts to understand the TME, and to target key pathways or cellular components, may be important to improve therapies for many solid tumors.

Most epithelial-derived tumors are characterized by the recruitment of mesenchymal-derived stromal cells, including intratumoral and peritumoral fibroblasts, often designated as cancer-associated fibroblasts (CAF), that mediate tumor growth, angiogenesis, invasion, and metastasis [16, 17]. CAF are often described as being in an "activated" state, as might occur in wound healing, which is phenotypically distinct from normal fibroblasts. Although their heterogeneity is yet to be fully explored, a subset of CAF has characteristics similar to myofibroblasts based, for example, on expression of α-smooth muscle actin. The mechanism of fibroblast activation in cancer is not completely understood. In adult tissues, differentiation from resident stromal fibroblasts into activated myofibroblasts occurs through paracrine signaling by TGFβ generated by damaged or inflamed tissues [18–20]. Both TGFβ and interleukin-1β induce differentiation of quiescent fibroblasts into activated myofibroblasts, but TGFβ is considered the predominate inducer [21]. Radiation-induced TGFβ-mediated activation of fibroblasts is evident in culture

[22] and may occur in tumors. The origins of activated fibroblasts in tumors are also incompletely described. Although the majority of CAF are thought to arise from the activation of resident fibroblasts, activated fibroblasts can also originate from pericytes, vascular smooth muscle cells, bone marrow-derived mesenchymal cells, and epithelial to mesenchymal cell transition [23].

Prognostic significance of CAF-associated gene-expression signature has been reported in multiple independent cohorts of non-small cell lung cancer (NSCLC) patients [24]. When compared with normal fibroblasts, CAF significantly increase the invasiveness of co-cultured lung cancer cells and enhance tumorigenicity in vivo. Genes differentially expressed by CAF compared to normal fibroblasts include signal transduction, response to stress, cell adhesion, and angiogenesis [24].

The ability of tumor cells to induce new blood vessel formation is essential for progressive tumor growth and blood-borne metastasis. Angiogenesis is the formation of new capillaries from pre-existing vessels which is of fundamental importance in development, normal organ maintenance, and homeostasis. Tumor angiogenesis relies on many of the same processes as those involved in physiological angiogenesis. Ischemia and hypoxic conditions, which initiate a cascade of highly coordinated cellular functions resulting in the establishment of new blood vessels and oxygen and nutrient supply, are major drivers of both physiological and tumor angiogenesis. This complex process requires interaction between different cell types, the extracellular matrix, and several cytokines and growth factors.

Under physiological conditions, the chain of events leading to changes in cellular function and composition recedes following vascular perfusion. In contrast, during tumor angiogenesis, the angiogenic cascade is persistent and unresolved, fueled in part by tumor-secreted factors and areas of transient tumor hypoxia due to tortuous vasculature. Angiogenesis contributes to the progression of cancer from a dormant in situ lesion to life-threatening invasive disease.

Inflammatory cells are components of the microenvironment of normal tissues and organs, regulating various processes during development, including epithelial growth and branching and clearance of apoptotic cells [25]. The progressive change in both inflammation and antitumor immunity with tumor stage is important in that a balance toward anti-tumor immunity initially suppresses cancer cell growth, but eventually tumor cells escape this control and elicit inflammation that is more conducive to tumor progression [26].

Of particular importance are myeloid-derived suppressor cells (MDSC) which are a heterogeneous population of immature macrophages, granulocytes, and other myeloid cells in early stages of differentiation and have properties similar to those that have been described for M2 macrophages. More MDSC, marked by CD11b+/CD14+/CD15+/CD33+, are present in the peripheral blood of advanced-stage NSCLC patients compared with healthy controls [27]. MDSC oppose the actions of cytotoxic T cells. Cytotoxic T lymphocytes (CTL), mostly CD8+, are associated with prolonged survival in squamous cell NSCLC [28]. Stromal CD4+ T cell and co-localization of stromal CD8+ T cells and CD4+ T cell are associated with improved NSCLC survival [29, 30]. In a study of stage I compared to III NSCLC, immunosuppressive tumor-infiltrating Foxp3+ Treg cells were associated with increased tumor recurrence [31]. Anti-tumor tumor-associated macrophages (TAM) are classified as M1 phenotype. M1 accumulate intratumorally, whereas pro-tumor M2 phenotype accumulates in the stroma and expresses interleukin-8 (IL-8) and IL-10 and triggers TREM-1, a receptor expressed on myeloid cells.

IL-8 is an angiogenic factor, and the angiogenic role of TAM in cancer has been shown by correlating macrophage density with intratumor microvessel counts and poor NSCLC patient outcomes [32]. IL-10 is an immunosuppressive cytokine, and its expression by TAM has been observed more commonly in late-stage NSCLC, which correlates with decreased overall survival. Furthermore, increased levels of TREM-1 high TAM in resected specimens was an independent predictor of shorter overall survival in stage I to III NSCLC patients [33].

In late-stage tumor development, TAM and MDSC also activate TGFβ and are classically involved in cancer progression and metastasis [34]. It is likely that TGFβ acts in an autocrine manner to convert TAM from an M1 to M2 phenotype and that TAM contribute to the general immunosuppressive TME in turn by producing large amounts of TGFβ. MDSC are polarized toward immunosuppression that impedes the ongoing immune and inflammatory response to cancer. Such polarized MDSC suppresses T cells and natural killer cells, as well as antigen-presenting cells, abrogating the antitumor immune response. Thus, the presence of MDSC in cancer poses a serious obstacle to therapies that attempt to stimulate antitumor immune responses. The expansion of MDSC population in the circulation of cancer patients may be useful as a biomarker of TGFβ inhibition. One study reports that polymorphisms in TGFβ pathway members are associated with dramatically different median survival times of 45.39 versus 13.55 months and 18.02 versus 5.89 months for high- and low-risk populations of NSCLC patients as a function of chemoradiation and chemotherapy, respectively [35].

A canonical target of TGFβ is the extracellular matrix (ECM), which is actively remodeled during tumor development and in response to therapy. The composition of the ECM is tissue specific, e.g., collagen rich in epithelial organs in which it provides a "skeleton" to support the parenchyma versus hyaluronic acid rich in the brain supportive of neuronal networks. The ECM composition also differs across cancers and is often a hallmark as in the dense collagen of breast and pancreatic desmoplastic cancers. Matrix metalloproteinases, commonly produced by activated macrophages recruited by TGFβ, degrade ECM components can release TGFβ, VEGF, and other sequestered factors of TME remodeling [36].

TGFβ in Cancer and Radiation Biology

TGFβ biology warrants further exploration in the TME and particularly in the context of therapy. Although TGFβ is a canonical tumor suppressor due to inhibiting epithelial proliferation and inducing apoptosis, loss of response to TGFβ as a growth inhibitor and increased expression of TGFβ is nearly universal in cancer [37]. Increased TGFβ activity in tumors can act in a variety of ways to promote neoplastic progression. Production of TGFβ in malignant cells acts on the host to suppress antitumor immune responses, to enhance extracellular matrix production, and to augment angiogenesis (reviewed in [38]). These activities resemble those induced by TGFβ during wound healing and may create a "permissive" microenvironment that promotes malignant growth by acting on the host.

TGFβ ligands are enriched in the TME where their production by stroma or tumor cells varies according to tumor phenotype [39]. TGFβ activity is controlled by production as a latent complex that requires extracellular modification to initiate ligand binding to ubiquitous receptors; TGFβ activation is efficiently induced by radiation, in part due to the presence of a redox-sensitive motif in the latency-associated peptide (reviewed in [40]). TGFβ is a canonical tumor suppressor due to inhibiting epithelial proliferation and inducing apoptosis [37]. Loss of response to TGFβ as a growth inhibitor and increased expression of TGFβ have been associated with malignant conversion and progression in breast, gastric, endometrial, ovarian, and cervical cancers, as well as glioblastoma and melanoma [37]. Inactivation of the Smad4 gene through homozygous deletion or intragenic mutation occurs frequently in association with malignant progression in pancreatic and colorectal cancer [41]. However, mutation of the TGFβ pathway genes occurs only occasionally in many human cancers. For example, Reiss and colleagues showed that 92% of more than 500 breast cancers were positive for nuclear, phosphorylated Smad2, indicating activation of the TGFβ pathway [42]. Indeed, many TGFβ transcriptional responses are intact, while cancer cells have escaped the control of proliferation.

The conundrum of why tumors maintain TGFβ expression and signaling when it is an extremely potent growth inhibitor becomes less perplexing when control of the DNA damage response is incorporated. Cancer cells that have high genomic instability fail to progress; indeed invasive breast tumors are more stable than ductal carcinoma in situ [43]. Genomic instability is a less well-recognized consequence of TGFβ loss, yet deletion of *Tgfb1* greatly increases genomic instability in murine epithelial cells [44]. Using cultured keratinocytes isolated from newborn *Tgfb1* null, heterozygote, and wild-type mice, Yuspa and colleagues found that *Tgfb1* null cells spontaneously immortalized more readily than TGFβ competent cells. Compared to wild-type cells, *Tgfb1* null cells gave rise to 1000-fold more mutant clones resistant to a chemical, which requires amplification of the dihydrofolate reductase gene. This unexpected phenotype was difficult to place within the pathways controlled by TGFβ.

Following up on this finding, inhibition of TGFβ signaling in non-malignant human epithelial cells using a small-molecule inhibitor of the TGFβ type I receptor kinase increased frequency of centrosome aberrations, chromosomal instability, and spontaneous DNA damage [45]. Moreover, *Tgfb1* heterozygote mammary epithelium, which expresses only 10–30% of wild-type protein levels, exhibits genomic instability at a level comparable to *Trp53* heterozygote epithelium. Proteomic profiling of TGFβ-treated mink lung epithelial cells suggests that TGFβ can inhibit DNA repair genes by causing downregulation through ubiquitylation and proteosomal degradation of Rad51, an essential component of the DNA-DSB repair machinery, in a Smad-dependent manner [46]. Rad51 fails to form nuclear foci in TGFβ-treated cells, which results in more DNA fragmentation in response to double-strand breaks compared to untreated controls [46].

Given that epithelial tissues of *Tgfb1* null embryos fail to undergo apoptosis or cell cycle arrest in response to high-dose (5Gy) radiation [47], this suggested major defects in the DNA damage pathway; studies in mouse and human epithelial cells demonstrated that TGFβ is necessary for ATM kinase activity elicited by DNA damage [48]. ATM is a phosphoinositide 3-kinase-related serine/threonine kinase that mediates DNA damage responses to initiate, recruit, and activate a complex program of checkpoints for cell cycle, apoptosis, and genomic integrity. Mutations in human ATM lead to ataxia-telangiectasia, a genetic disease characterized by cellular radiosensitivity and high levels of chromosome aberrations [49]. ATM is activated in response to DNA damage caused by IR and, in turn, phosphorylates numerous substrates, thereby modulating cell fate decisions. ATM precisely controls its downstream pathways, often by approaching the same DNA damage process from several different directions, e.g., the cell cycle checkpoints, each of which is governed by several ATM-mediated pathways [50]. Notably, in addition to ATM's versatility as a protein kinase with numerous substrates, the ATM nexus contains protein kinases that are themselves capable of targeting several downstream effectors simultaneously and thereby concomitantly control subsets of pathways (e.g., the Chk1 and Chk2 kinases). A prototypic example is ATM-mediated phosphorylation and subsequent stabilization of the p53 protein, a major player both in the G1/S cell cycle checkpoint and in damage-induced apoptosis [51].

Tgfb1 depletion by genetic knockout in mouse cells, or inhibition of TGFβ signaling in human cells, compromises ATM kinase activity and autophosphorylation, leading to reduced phosphorylation of critical DNA damage transducers, abrogation of the cell cycle block, and increased radiosensitivity [47, 48]. The ability of exogenous TGFβ to restore these responses indicates that the effect is both cell intrinsic and distal to TGFβ signaling. Radiation induces TGFβ activity in vitro and in vivo both in normal and cancer cells [52–58]. Inhibiting TGFβ signaling in irradiated human cells phenocopies the molecular and cellular consequences of genetic deletion in mouse cells [48]. Consistent with reduced ATM activity, TGFβ genetic deletion in murine cells or signaling inhibition in human cells increases radiosensitivity. The requirement for TGFβ in the genotoxic stress program provides an understudied avenue by which TGFβ acts as a tumor suppressor, whereby its loss would prime genomic instability and cancer progression.

Many TGFβ transcriptional responses are intact, while cancer cells have escaped TGFβ's control of proliferation. The necessity for TGFβ signaling to maintain genomic stability and the recognition that TGFβ regulates ATM kinase suggests the following: TGFβ acts to initially suppress cancer by ensuring genomic integrity and yet protects malignant cells both by limiting the level of genomic instability and by enabling recovery from DNA damage induced by radiation and other therapies.

TGFβ Inhibition in Radiation Therapy

Studies spanning two decades have identified TGFβ as a key extracellular signal in irradiated tissues and tumors. Among all radiation-induced cytokines, TGFβ arguably elicits the most complex and far-reaching effects in determining outcome. Testing clinically viable TGFβ inhibitors in oncology is motivated by its pleomorphic consequences in cancer, including regulating the DNA damage response, facilitating the mechanism of metastasis, and compromising antitumor immunity [59].

Execution of DNA damage response is compromised by blocking TGFβ activity in the context of RT, which increases both tumor cell radiosensitivity in vitro and tumor growth delay in vivo [60, 61]. Most cancer cell lines treated with a small-molecule inhibitor of TGFβ type I receptor kinase are more radiation sensitive, i.e., 10–70% less dose is needed to reduce survival to 10% as measured by clonogenic cell kill. Consistent with deficient ATM activity, ATM autophosphorylation and γH2AX foci formation are decreased. Irradiation of tumors in mice treated with preclinical pan-neutralizing TGFβ antibodies shows reduced γH2AX foci and increased tumor growth delay. Inhibiting TGFβ enhances tumor control by radiation in preclinical brain, breast, and lung cancer models. Thus, epithelial tumors appear to rely on TGFβ to effectively mount the DDR, even though most are resistant to TGFβ growth control. These data provide a strong rationale for TGFβ inhibitors as a means to increase tumor response to radiation across a range of cancers [62].

Of particular interest is glioblastoma multiforme (GBM), which is characterized by a high degree of radioresistance and inevitable local and/or disseminated recurrence. Several clinical trials are underway combining TGFβ inhibition with cancer RT and chemotherapy, including a phase II trial in glioblastoma. The addition of TGFβ inhibitors improves radiation response in preclinical models of GBM [63, 64]. Zhang et al. specifically reported that the addition of the small-molecule inhibitor of TGFβ receptor type I and II kinase, LY2109761, to the current standard of care treatment (radiation and the oral alkylating agent temozolomide) provided benefit. In addition to radiosensitization and tumor growth delay, TGFβ signaling blockade had antiangiogenic and anti-migration effects as well. Mengxian et al. similarly reported radiosensitization, tumor growth delay, and improved survival with the addition of the same small-molecule inhibitor of TGFβ, LY2109761, without combining with temozolomide. They further demonstrated that either TGFβ inhibition or radiation decreased self-renewal of glioma stemlike cells in a neurosphere assay and a greater decrease when these were combined.

Our studies have also added significantly to the growing body of evidence that TGFβ is a therapeutic target in GBM [61]. First, we showed that autocrine TGFβ potentiates an effective molecular DNA damage response and that radiation-induced TGFβ mediates self-renewal signals in glioma-initiating cells (GIC). Second, the magnitude of radiosensitization (dose-enhancement ratio (DER) ~1.25 by clonogenic assay) is similar to that treated with temozolomide (DER 1.32) [65]. Considering that the addition of temozolomide to radiation therapy in the treatment of GBM was one of the largest breakthroughs in this disease in decades and is now considered the standard of care, radiosensitization of this magnitude reported here must be considered significant, particularly since the radiation sensitivity of GIC increased nearly threefold. Last, GIC produce more TGFβ, which actually enables more effective execution of the DDR and increases self-renewal signals that together ensure survival following radiation exposure [61].

Recent studies in murine triple-negative breast cancer models also suggest that TGFβ inhibition during RT can also drastically reduce metastasis and promote anti-tumor immunity [66]. It is clear that increased TGFβ in cancer can act in a variety of ways to promote neoplastic progression. Production of TGFβ in malignant cells acts on the host to suppress antitumor immune responses, to enhance extracellular matrix production, and to augment angiogenesis (reviewed in [38]). These activities resemble those induced by TGFβ during wound healing and may create a "permissive" microenvironment that promotes malignant growth by acting on the host. The excellent safety profiles demonstrated in clinical trials [59], as well as the possibility of protection from late normal tissue complications [67], provide further motivation for assessing TGFβ inhibitors as a means to augment response to radiation therapy.

Targeting the Irradiated TME

Ionizing radiation induces modifications of the TME that profoundly impact tumor biology and also influence tumor responses to subsequent exposures to radiation, thus providing novel routes for manipulating the response to radiotherapy [3, 40]. Preclinical tumor models that shed light on the importance of the tumor microenvironment in modulating the tumor response to radiotherapy suggest opportunities for the development of novel therapeutic strategies to synergize with radiotherapy. Thus, strategies to improve radiotherapy can be envisioned that change "molecular" regulatory cancer cell intrinsic sensitivity to targeting of the "microenvironment."

Tumor vascular endothelium plays a crucial role in tumor radiation response. In irradiated tumors, endothelial cell apoptosis precedes tumor cell apoptosis by 3–5 days, suggesting that tumor cells are dependent on endothelial cells for survival [68]. Paris et al. suggested that early-phase microvascular endothelial apoptosis is mandatory for tumor cure [69]. Recent data indicate that radiation-induced endothelial cell apoptosis can lead to vascular destruction [70] and secondary tumor cell death [71].

Of high clinical and biological relevance is the growing evidence that the profound radiation resistance of GBM is mediated by the TME. Rich and colleagues showed that glioblastoma stem-like cells appear to be intrinsically resistant to radiation [72]. Additional studies in model systems support the critical role of the microenvironment in the radioresistance of GBM. First, intracranial tumors are more resistant than the same cells grown in subcutaneous tumors [73]. Second, human glioblastoma stem-like cells grown in co-culture with human astrocytes showed significantly decreased the radiosensitivity of glioblastoma stem-like cells compared to standard culture conditions via a paracrine-based mechanism [74]. The cytokine milieu resulting from cell-cell interactions of glioblastoma stem-like cells grown in neurosphere-type conditions makes them more resistant than those cells in standard culture as measured by secondary neurosphere-forming capacity and DNA damage foci [61]. Notably the cells grown in neurosphere conditions make five-fold more TGFβ, which enables efficient activation of the DDR. These data suggest that both autocrine and paracrine signals may create the "perfect storm" for radioresistance that is clinically evident in GBM.

Brown and colleagues provided compelling evidence that ionizing radiation induces recruitment of tumor-protective myeloid cells that promote blood vessel formation sufficient to support the growth of recurring tumors postirradiation [75]. Suppression with antibodies against an immature myeloid cell surface marker, CD11b, greatly enhanced tumor radiation response in a preclinical GBM model. Blockade of either SDF-1 or CSF1 achieved the same effect in both transplantable GBM and spontaneous glioma by blocking signals that motivate myeloid cells [76–78]. Notably, inhibiting tissue-resident macrophages before radiotherapy also protected radiation-induced normal tissue damage significantly [79, 80]. CAF promote further cell recruitment through secretion of chemokines such as SDF-1 that in turn enhances the recruitment of bone marrow-derived cells involved in tumor vasculogenesis [81].

In the era of personalized medicine, it is imperative to stratify patients for modern trials to identify optimal candidates for testing biological therapies to be used in conjunction with radiotherapy. Radiation dose delivery and fractionation schedules have rapidly changed because of gains in technology, particularly imaging, that motivate renewed interest in specialized regimens that include hypofractionation and radiosurgery [82]. Additional motivation comes from re-examination of the cell biology that underlies tumor and normal tissue response to ionizing radiation. Ultimately, better understanding of the biology of irradiated tissues and tumors means new opportunities to optimize radiotherapy for particular tumors, specific regimes, and individual patients. The subversion of normal cells that constitute the TME provides the lifeline for cancer cell growth, a barrier to the immune system, and can promote extrinsic mechanisms of resistance during treatment. Thus, deconstruction of the irradiated TME could also improve outcomes, for example, in combination with immunotherapy by removing exogenous immune system breaks like TGFβ. Targeting radiation delivery to the tumor provides unequivocal patient benefit by eliminating tumors cells and hobbling the supporting stroma and vasculature. Substantial potential for augmenting that success could be achieved by preventing TME remodeling, which reestablishes the support network that enables regrowth of cancer cells.

References

1. Begg AC, Stewart FA, Vens C (2011) Strategies to improve radiotherapy with targeted drugs. Nat Rev Cancer 11:239–253
2. Harris AL (2002) Hypoxia–a key regulatory factor in tumour growth. Nat Rev Cancer 2:38–47
3. Russell JS, Brown JM (2013) The irradiated tumor microenvironment: role of tumor-associated macrophages in vascular recovery. Front Physiol 4:157
4. Yang L, Pang Y, Moses HL (2010) TGF-beta and immune cells: an important regulatory axis in the tumor microenvironment and progression. Trends Immunol 31:220–227
5. Balkwill F, Coussens LM (2004) Cancer: an inflammatory link. Nature 431:405–406
6. Du R, Lu KV, Petritsch C, Liu P, Ganss R, Passegué E, Song H, Vandenberg S, Johnson RS, Werb Z, Bergers G (2008) HIF1alpha induces the recruitment of bone marrow-derived vascular modulatory cells to regulate tumor angiogenesis and invasion. Cancer Cell 13:206–220
7. Bristow RG, Hill RP (2008) Hypoxia and metabolism. Hypoxia, DNA repair and genetic instability. Nat Rev Cancer 8:180–192
8. Barcellos-Hoff MH, Lyden D, Wang TC (2013) The evolution of the cancer niche during multistage carcinogenesis. Nat Rev Cancer 13:511–518
9. Ji H, Houghton AM, Mariani TJ, Perera S, Kim CB, Padera R, Tonon G, McNamara K, Marconcini LA, Hezel A, El-Bardeesy N, Bronson RT, Sugarbaker D, Maser RS, Shapiro SD, Wong KK (2006) K-ras activation generates an inflammatory response in lung tumors. Oncogene 25:2105–2112
10. Casbon AJ, Reynaud D, Park C, Khuc E, Gan DD, Schepers K, Passegue E, Werb Z (2015) Invasive breast cancer reprograms early myeloid differentiation in the bone marrow to generate immunosuppressive neutrophils. Proc Natl Acad Sci U S A 112:E566–E575
11. Jin DK, Shido K, Kopp H-G, Petit I, Shmelkov SV, Young LM, Hooper AT, Amano H, Avecilla ST, Heissig B, Hattori K, Zhang F, Hicklin DJ, Wu Y, Zhu Z, Dunn A, Salari H, Werb Z, Hackett NR, Crystal RG, Lyden D, Rafii S (2006) Cytokine-mediated deployment of SDF-1 induces revascularization through recruitment of CXCR4+ hemangiocytes. Nat Med 12:557–567
12. Kaplan RN, Riba RD, Zacharoulis S, Bramley AH, Vincent L, Costa C, MacDonald DD, Jin DK, Shido K, Kerns SA, Zhu Z, Hicklin D, Wu Y, Port JL, Altorki N, Port ER, Ruggero D, Shmelkov SV, Jensen KK, Rafii S, Lyden D (2005) VEGFR1-positive haematopoietic bone marrow progenitors initiate the pre-metastatic niche. Nature 438:820–827
13. Kaplan RN, Rafii S, Lyden D (2006) Preparing the soil: the premetastatic niche. Cancer Res 66:11089–11093
14. Sun Y, Campisi J, Higano C, Beer TM, Porter P, Coleman I, True L, Nelson PS (2012) Treatment-induced damage to the tumor microenvironment promotes prostate cancer therapy resistance through WNT16B. Nat Med 18:1359–1368
15. Munson JM, Bellamkonda RV, Swartz MA (2013) Interstitial flow in a 3D microenvironment increases glioma invasion by a CXCR4-dependent mechanism. Cancer Res 73:1536–1546
16. Gaggioli C, Hooper S, Hidalgo-Carcedo C, Grosse R, Marshall JF, Harrington K, Sahai E (2007) Fibroblast-led collective invasion of carcinoma cells with differing roles for RhoGTPases in leading and following cells. Nat Cell Biol 9:1392–1400
17. Schor SL, Ellis IR, Jones SJ, Baillie R, Seneviratne K, Clausen J, Motegi K, Vojtesek B, Kankova K, Furrie E, Sales MJ, Schor AM, Kay RA (2003) Migration-stimulating factor: a genetically truncated onco-fetal fibronectin isoform expressed by carcinoma and tumor-associated stromal cells. Cancer Res 63:8827–8836
18. De Wever O, Demetter P, Mareel M, Bracke M (2008) Stromal myofibroblasts are drivers of invasive cancer growth. Int J Cancer 123:2229–2238
19. Rønnov-Jessen L, Petersen OW (1993) Induction of alpha-smooth muscle actin by transforming growth factor-beta 1 in quiescent human breast gland fibroblasts. Implications for myofibroblast generation in breast neoplasia. Lab Invest 68(6):696–707

20. Tuxhorn JA, McAlhany SJ, Yang F, Dang TD, Rowley DR (2002) Inhibition of transforming growth factor-beta activity decreases angiogenesis in a human prostate cancer-reactive stroma xenograft model. Cancer Res 62:6021–6025

21. Chen H, Yang WW, Wen QT, Xu L, Chen M (2009) TGF-beta induces fibroblast activation protein expression; fibroblast activation protein expression increases the proliferation, adhesion, and migration of HO-8910PM. Exp Mol Pathol 87:189–194

22. Herskind C, Rodemann HP (2000) Spontaneous and radiation-induced differentiation of fibroblasts. Exp Gerontol 35:747–755

23. Quante M, Tu SP, Tomita H, Gonda T, Wang SS, Takashi S, Baik GH, Shibata W, Diprete B, Betz KS, Friedman R, Varro A, Tycko B, Wang TC (2011) Bone marrow-derived myofibroblasts contribute to the mesenchymal stem cell niche and promote tumor growth. Cancer Cell 19:257–272

24. Navab R, Strumpf D, Bandarchi B, Zhu CQ, Pintilie M, Ramnarine VR, Ibrahimov E, Radulovich N, Leung L, Barczyk M, Panchal D, To C, Yun JJ, Der S, Shepherd FA, Jurisica I, Tsao MS (2011) Prognostic gene-expression signature of carcinoma-associated fibroblasts in non-small cell lung cancer. Proc Natl Acad Sci U S A 108:7160–7165

25. Pollard JW (2009) Trophic macrophages in development and disease. Nat Rev Immunol 9:259–270

26. Andreu P, Johansson M, Affara NI, Pucci F, Tan T, Junankar S, Korets L, Lam J, Tawfik D, DeNardo DG, Naldini L, de Visser KE, De Palma M, Coussens LM (2010) FcRgamma activation regulates inflammation-associated squamous carcinogenesis. Cancer Cell 17: 121–134

27. Liu CY, Wang YM, Wang CL, Feng PH, Ko HW, Liu YH, Wu YC, Chu Y, Chung FT, Kuo CH, Lee KY, Lin SM, Lin HC, Wang CH, Yu CT, Kuo HP (2010) Population alterations of L-arginase- and inducible nitric oxide synthase-expressed CD11b+/CD14−/CD15+/CD33+ myeloid-derived suppressor cells and CD8+ T lymphocytes in patients with advanced-stage non-small cell lung cancer. J Cancer Res Clin Oncol 136:35–45

28. Ruffini E, Asioli S, Filosso PL, Lyberis P, Bruna MC, Macrì L, Daniele L, Oliaro A (2009) Clinical significance of tumor-infiltrating lymphocytes in lung neoplasms. Ann Thorac Surg 87:365–371

29. Al-Shibli KI, Donnem T, Al-Saad S, Persson M, Bremnes RM, Busund LT (2008) Prognostic effect of epithelial and stromal lymphocyte infiltration in non-small cell lung cancer. Clin Cancer Res 14:5220–5227

30. Hiraoka K, Miyamoto M, Cho Y, Suzuoki M, Oshikiri T, Nakakubo Y, Itoh T, Ohbuchi T, Kondo S, Katoh H (2006) Concurrent infiltration by CD8+ T cells and CD4+ T cells is a favourable prognostic factor in non-small-cell lung carcinoma. Br J Cancer 94:275–280

31. Shimizu K, Nakata M, Hirami Y, Yukawa T, Maeda A, Tanemoto K (2010) Tumor-infiltrating Foxp3+ regulatory T cells are correlated with cyclooxygenase-2 expression and are associated with recurrence in resected non-small cell lung cancer. J Thorac Oncol 5:585–590

32. Chen JJ, Yao PL, Yuan A, Hong TM, Shun CT, Kuo ML, Lee YC, Yang PC (2003) Up-regulation of tumor interleukin-8 expression by infiltrating macrophages: its correlation with tumor angiogenesis and patient survival in non-small cell lung cancer. Clin Cancer Res 9:729–737

33. Ho CC, Liao WY, Wang CY, Lu YH, Huang HY, Chen HY, Chan WK, Chen HW, Yang PC (2008) TREM-1 expression in tumor-associated macrophages and clinical outcome in lung cancer. Am J Respir Crit Care Med 177:763–770

34. Ruffell B, Affara NI, Coussens LM (2012) Differential macrophage programming in the tumor microenvironment. Trends Immunol 33:119–126

35. Lin M, Stewart DJ, Spitz MR, Hildebrandt MA, Lu C, Lin J, Gu J, Huang M, Lippman SM, Wu X (2011) Genetic variations in the transforming growth factor-beta pathway as predictors of survival in advanced non-small cell lung cancer. Carcinogenesis 32:1050–1056

36. Kessenbrock K, Plaks V, Werb Z (2010) Matrix metalloproteinases: regulators of the tumor microenvironment. Cell 141:52–67

37. Derynck R, Akhurst RJ, Balmain A (2001) TGF-β signaling in tumor suppression and cancer progression. Nat Genet 29:117–129

38. Akhurst RJ (2002) TGF-{beta} antagonists: why suppress a tumor suppressor? J Clin Invest 109:1533–1536
39. Bierie B, Moses HL (2006) Tumour microenvironment: TGFbeta: the molecular Jekyll and Hyde of cancer. Nat Rev Cancer 6:506–520
40. Du S, Barcellos-Hoff MH (2013) Biologically augmenting radiation therapy by inhibiting TGFβ actions in carcinomas. Semin Radiat Oncol 23:242–251
41. Miyaki M, Kuroki T (2003) Role of Smad4 (DPC4) inactivation in human cancer. Biochem Biophys Res Commun 306:799–804
42. Xie W, Mertens JC, Reiss DJ, Rimm DL, Camp RL, Haffty BG, Reiss M (2002) Alterations of Smad signaling in human breast carcinoma are associated with poor outcome: a tissue micro-array study. Cancer Res 62:497–505
43. Chin K, de Solorzano CO, Knowles D, Jones A, Chou W, Rodriguez EG, Kuo WL, Ljung BM, Chew K, Myambo K, Miranda M, Krig S, Garbe J, Stampfer M, Yaswen P, Gray JW, Lockett SJ (2004) In situ analyses of genome instability in breast cancer. Nat Genet 36:984–988
44. Glick AB, Weinberg WC, Wu IH, Quan W, Yuspa SH (1996) Transforming growth factor beta 1 suppresses genomic instability independent of a G1 arrest, p53, and Rb. Cancer Res 56:3645–3650
45. Maxwell CA, Fleisch MC, Costes SV, Erickson AC, Boissiere A, Gupta R, Ravani SA, Parvin B, Barcellos-Hoff MH (2008) Targeted and nontargeted effects of ionizing radiation that impact genomic instability. Cancer Res 68:8304–8311
46. Kanamoto T, Hellman U, Heldin CH, Souchelnytskyi S (2002) Functional proteomics of trans-forming growth factor-beta1-stimulated Mv1Lu epithelial cells: Rad51 as a target of TGFbeta1-dependent regulation of DNA repair. EMBO J 21:1219–1230
47. Ewan KB, Henshall-Powell RL, Ravani SA, Pajares MJ, Arteaga CL, Warters RL, Akhurst RJ, Barcellos-Hoff MH (2002) Transforming growth factor-β1 mediates cellular response to DNA damage in situ. Cancer Res 62:5627–5631
48. Kirshner J, Jobling MF, Pajares MJ, Ravani SA, Glick A, Lavin M, Koslov S, Shiloh Y, Barcellos-Hoff MH (2006) Inhibition of TGFβ1 signaling attenuates ATM activity in response to genotoxic stress. Cancer Res 66:10861–10868
49. Shiloh Y, Lehmann AR (2004) Maintaining integrity. Nat Cell Biol 6:923–928
50. Shiloh Y (2003) ATM and related protein kinases: safeguarding genome integrity. Nat Rev Cancer 3:155–168
51. Meek DW (2004) The p53 response to DNA damage. DNA Repair (Amst) 3:1049–1056
52. Barcellos-Hoff MH (1993) Radiation-induced transforming growth factor β and subsequent extracellular matrix reorganization in murine mammary gland. Cancer Res 53:3880–3886
53. Becker KA, Lu S, Dickinson ES, Dunphy KA, Mathews L, Schneider SS, Jerry DJ (2005) Estrogen and progesterone regulate radiation-induced p53 activity in mammary epithelium through TGF-beta-dependent pathways., Oncogene
54. Ehrhart EJ, Carroll A, Segarini P, Tsang ML-S, Barcellos-Hoff MH (1997) Latent transform-ing growth factor-β activation in situ: quantitative and functional evidence following low dose irradiation. FASEB J 11:991–1002
55. Hauer-Jensen M, Richter KK, Wang J, Abe E, Sung CC, Hardin JW (1998) Changes in trans-forming growth factor beta1 gene expression and immunoreactivity levels during development of chronic radiation enteropathy. Radiat Res 150:673–680
56. Milliat F, Francois A, Isoir M, Deutsch E, Tamarat R, Tarlet G, Atfi A, Validire P, Bourhis J, Sabourin JC, Benderitter M (2006) Influence of endothelial cells on vascular smooth muscle cells phenotype after irradiation: implication in radiation-induced vascular damages. Am J Pathol 169:1484–1495
57. Tabatabai G, Frank B, Mohle R, Weller M, Wick W (2006) Irradiation and hypoxia promote homing of haematopoietic progenitor cells towards gliomas by TGF-beta-dependent HIF-1alpha-mediated induction of CXCL12. Brain 129:2426–2435
58. Wang J, Zheng H, Sung C-C, Richter KK, Hauer-Jensen M (1998) Cellular sources of trans-forming growth factor-ß isoforms in early and chronic radiation enteropathy. Am J Pathol 153:1531–1540

59. Akhurst RJ, Hata A (2012) Targeting the TGF[beta] signalling pathway in disease. Nat Rev Drug Discov 11:790–811
60. Bouquet SF, Pal A, Pilones KA, Demaria S, Hann B, Akhurst RJ, Babb JS, Lonning SM, DeWyngaert JK, Formenti S, Barcellos-Hoff MH (2011) Transforming growth factor ®1 inhibition increases the radiosensitivity of breast cancer cells in vitro and promotes tumor control by radiation in vivo. Clin Cancer Res 17:6754–6765
61. Hardee ME, Marciscano AE, Medina-Ramirez CM, Zagzag D, Narayana A, Lonning SM, Barcellos-Hoff MH (2012) Resistance of glioblastoma-initiating cells to radiation mediated by the tumor microenvironment can be abolished by inhibiting transforming growth factor-β. Cancer Res 72:4119–4129
62. Barcellos-Hoff MH, Cucinotta FA (2014) New tricks for an old fox: impact of TGFbeta on the DNA damage response and genomic stability. Sci Signal 7:re5
63. Zhang M, Herion TW, Timke C, Han N, Hauser K, Weber KJ, Peschke P, Wirkner U, Lahn M, Huber PE (2011) Trimodal glioblastoma treatment consisting of concurrent radiotherapy, temozolomide, and the novel TGF-β receptor I kinase inhibitor LY2109761. Neoplasia 13:537–549
64. Zhang M, Kleber S, Rohrich M, Timke C, Han N, Tuettenberg J, Martin-Villalba A, Debus J, Peschke P, Wirkner U, Lahn M, Huber PE (2011) Blockade of TGF-beta signaling by the TGFbetaR-I kinase inhibitor LY2109761 enhances radiation response and prolongs survival in glioblastoma. Cancer Res 71:7155–7167
65. Kil WJ, Cerna D, Burgan WE, Beam K, Carter D, Steeg PS, Tofilon PJ, Camphausen K (2008) In vitro and in vivo radiosensitization induced by the DNA methylating agent temozolomide. Clin Cancer Res 14:931–938
66. Vanpouille-Box C, Diamond J, Pilones KA, Zavadil J, Babb JS, Formenti SC, Barcellos-Hoff MH, Demaria S (2015) Transforming growth factor (TGF) β is a master regulator of radiotherapy-induced anti-tumor immunity. Cancer Res 75:2232–2242
67. Anscher MS, Thrasher B, Zgonjanin L, Rabbani ZN, Corbley MJ, Fu K, Sun L, Lee W-C, Ling LE, Vujaskovic Z (2008) Small molecular inhibitor of transforming growth factor-[beta] protects against development of radiation-induced lung injury. Int J Radiat Oncol Biol Phys 71:829–837
68. Browder BC, Butterfield CE, Kräling BM, Shi B, Marshall B, O'Reilly MS, Folkman J (2000) Antiangiogenic scheduling of chemotherapy improves efficacy against experimental drug-resistant cancer. Cancer Res 60:1878–1886
69. Paris F, Fuks Z, Kang A, Capodieci P, Juan G, Ehleiter D, Haimovitz-Friedman A, Cordon-Cardo C, Kolesnick R (2001) Endothelial apoptosis as the primary lesion initiating intestinal radiation damage in mice. Science 293:293–297
70. Czarnota GJ, Karshafian R, Burns PN, Wong S, Al Mahrouki A, Lee JW, Caissie A, Tran W, Kim C, Furukawa M, Wong E, Giles A (2012) Tumor radiation response enhancement by acoustical stimulation of the vasculature. Proc Natl Acad Sci U S A 109:E2033–E2041
71. Garcia-Barros M, Paris F, Cordon-Cardo C, Lyden D, Rafii S, Haimovitz-Friedman A, Fuks Z, Kolesnick R (2003) Tumor response to radiotherapy regulated by endothelial cell apoptosis. Science 300:1155–1159
72. Bao S, Wu Q, McLendon RE, Hao Y, Shi Q, Hjelmeland AB, Dewhirst MW, Bigner DD, Rich JN (2006) Glioma stem cells promote radioresistance by preferential activation of the DNA damage response. Nature 444:756–760
73. Jamal M, Rath BH, Williams ES, Camphausen K, Tofilon PJ (2010) Microenvironmental regulation of glioblastoma radioresponse. Clin Cancer Res 16:6049–6059
74. Rath BH, Wahba A, Camphausen K, Tofilon PJ (2015) Coculture with astrocytes reduces the radiosensitivity of glioblastoma stem-like cells and identifies additional targets for radiosensitization. Cancer Med 4:1705–1716
75. Kioi M, Vogel H, Schultz G, Hoffman RM, Harsh GR, Brown JM (2010) Inhibition of vasculogenesis, but not angiogenesis, prevents the recurrence of glioblastoma after irradiation in mice. J Clin Invest 120:694–705

76. Liu SC, Alomran R, Chernikova SB, Lartey F, Stafford J, Jang T, Merchant M, Zboralski D, Zollner S, Kruschinski A, Klussmann S, Recht L, Brown JM (2014) Blockade of SDF-1 after irradiation inhibits tumor recurrences of autochthonous brain tumors in rats. Neuro Oncol 16:21–28

77. Stafford JH, Hirai T, Deng L, Chernikova SB, Urata K, West BL, Brown JM (2015) Colony stimulating factor 1 receptor inhibition delays recurrence of glioblastoma after radiation by altering myeloid cell recruitment and polarization., Neuro-oncology

78. Walters MJ, Ebsworth K, Berahovich RD, Penfold ME, Liu SC, Al Omran R, Kioi M, Chernikova SB, Tseng D, Mulkearns-Hubert EE, Sinyuk M, Ransohoff RM, Lathia JD, Karamchandani J, Kohrt HE, Zhang P, Powers JP, Jaen JC, Schall TJ, Merchant M, Recht L, Brown JM (2014) Inhibition of CXCR7 extends survival following irradiation of brain tumours in mice and rats. Br J Cancer 110:1179–1188

79. Du SS, Qiang M, Zeng ZC, Ke AW, Ji Y, Zhang ZY, Zeng HY, Liu Z (2010) Inactivation of kupffer cells by gadolinium chloride protects murine liver from radiation-induced apoptosis. Int J Radiat Oncol Biol Phys 76:1225–1234

80. Epperly MW, Shields D, Niu Y, Carlos T, Greenberger JS (2006) Bone marrow from CD18-/- (MAC-1-/-) homozygous deletion recombinant negative mice demonstrates increased longevity in long-term bone marrow culture and decreased contribution to irradiation pulmonary damage. In vivo (Athens, Greece) 20:431–438

81. Orimo A, Gupta PB, Sgroi DC, Arenzana-Seisdedos F, Delaunay T, Naeem R, Carey VJ, Richardson AL, Weinberg RA (2005) Stromal fibroblasts present in invasive human breast carcinomas promote tumor growth and angiogenesis through elevated SDF-1/CXCL12 secretion. Cell 121:335–348

82. Lo SS, Fakiris AJ, Chang EL, Mayr NA, Wang JZ, Papiez L, Teh BS, McGarry RC, Cardenes HR, Timmerman RD (2010) Stereotactic body radiation therapy: a novel treatment modality. Nat Rev Clin Oncol 7:44–54

Chapter 7
Combining Radiotherapy and Immunotherapy: Emerging Preclinical Observations of Lymphocyte Costimulatory and Inhibitory Receptor Modulation

Robert M. Samstein, Sadna Budhu, Taha Mergoub, and Christopher A. Barker

Abstract A greater understanding of immune system biology has translated into more effective cancer immunotherapeutics. This has prompted exploration of the combination of these agents with other cancer treatments such as radiotherapy, which has also been shown to promote antitumor immunity independently. This review will present data from reports of immune modulators and radiotherapy and will discuss common themes and observations. Costimulatory molecules including CD40 and CD134/OX40; glucocorticoid-induced tumor necrosis factor receptor family-related gene (GITR), CD137/4-1BB; and inhibitory molecules CD152/ cytotoxic T lymphocyte-associated protein 4 (CTLA4), lymphocyte activation gene 3 (LAG3), programmed death 1 (PD-1)/programmed death ligand 1 (PD-L1), and T cell immunoglobulin and mucin domain 3 (TIM-3) will be discussed. Observations regarding radiotherapy sequencing, dose, and fractionation will also be addressed. We conclude that a strategy combining immune modulation and radiotherapy is rational and holds promise for future successful translation in clinical trials.

Keywords Radiotherapy • Radiation • Immunotherapy • Immune checkpoint • CTLA4 • PD-1 • PD-L1 • Abscopal effect • Checkpoint blockade

R.M. Samstein • C.A. Barker (✉)
Department of Radiation Oncology, Memorial Sloan Kettering Cancer Center,
275 York Avenue, New York, NY 10065, USA
e-mail: samsteir@mskcc.org; barkerc@mskcc.org

S. Budhu • T. Mergoub
Ludwig Collaborative and Swim Across America Laboratory, Department of Medicine,
Memorial Sloan Kettering Cancer Center, 1275 York Avenue, New York, NY 10065, USA
e-mail: budhus@mskcc.org; merghout@mskcc.org

© Springer International Publishing Switzerland 2017
P.J. Tofilon, K. Camphausen (eds.), *Increasing the Therapeutic Ratio of Radiotherapy*, Cancer Drug Discovery and Development,
DOI 10.1007/978-3-319-40854-5_7

Introduction

A greater understanding of immune system biology has translated into more effective cancer immunotherapeutics. This has prompted exploration of the combination of these agents with other cancer treatments such as radiotherapy, which has also been shown to promote antitumor immunity independently. This review will present data from reports of immune modulators and radiotherapy and will discuss common themes and observations. Costimulatory molecules including CD40 and CD134/OX40; glucocorticoid-induced tumor necrosis factor receptor family-related gene (GITR), CD137/4-1BB; and inhibitory molecules CD152/cytotoxic T lymphocyte-associated protein 4 (CTLA4), lymphocyte activation gene 3 (LAG3), programmed death 1 (PD-1)/programmed death ligand 1 (PD-L1), and T cell immunoglobulin and mucin domain 3 (TIM-3) will be discussed. Observations regarding radiotherapy sequencing, dose, and fractionation will also be addressed.

Cancer Immunity and Radiation Response

In order to generate a robust and sustained immune response to a pathogen or cancer, several key elements are required. These include the presence of an immunogenic antigen at sufficient quantities to be picked up, processed, and presented by antigen-presenting cells (APCs) such as dendritic cells (DCs) for T cell recognition. Antigen presentation by APCs in the context of MHC molecules and subsequent recognition by the TCR complex on a T cells are a critical first step for mounting an immune response. In order for the APC-T cell interaction to result in activation of the T cell and subsequent immune response, a second costimulatory signal is required either directly from the APC or from the surrounding microenvironment to promote T cell maturation. The immune response can also be modulated by the presence of inhibitory molecules on the surface of the dendritic cell, T cell, or target cancer cell. In addition, the microenvironment can dramatically affect the degree and type of immune response via circulating cytokines and chemokines as well as direct cell-cell interactions. Suppressor cells such as regulatory T (Treg) cells and myeloid-derived suppressor cells (MDSCs) can promote an anti-inflammatory milieu and thus curtail the antitumor immune response. All these factors contribute to the activation, efficacy, and duration of an antigen-specific immune response, and cancers have thus developed mechanisms to modulate these pathways in order to subvert anticancer immunity.

The interplay of radiotherapy and the local and systemic immune response has been demonstrated in numerous preclinical studies. The efficacy of RT is severely reduced in the absence of an immune response in nude mice, which are deficient in B and T cells, and is significantly dependent on local CD8 T cell infiltration [1]. The absence of an innate immune response also results in reduced efficacy of RT [2]. Radiation can promote tumor antigen availability and presentation via immunogenic cell death via cell apoptosis and modification of the microenvironment with upregulation of damage-associated molecular patterns (DAMPs) including calreticulin, secreted ATP, and HMGB1 [3–5]. Tumor irradiation also results in upregulation of major histocompatibility complex class I (MHC-1) expression [6] and chemokine and cytokine secretion promoting an inflammatory infiltrate within the tumor as well as draining lymph node [7, 8]. Of note, tumor irradiation has been shown to induce some immunosuppressive properties such as increased proportion of Treg cells and promotion of inhibitory factors such as TGF-beta and PD-L1 expression which can be overcome with some of the immunotherapeutics discussed [9].

Cancer cells have thus been shown to evade recognition and elimination by the immune system via a variety of mechanisms including antigen variation or editing, downregulation of MHC, immunosuppressive cytokines, recruitment of regulatory cells, and overexpression of inhibitory ligands. Irradiation of the tumor can result in reversal or neutralization of many of these mechanisms supporting its potential synergy in attempts to promote tumor immunity via systemic immunotherapy.

Modulation of Lymphocyte Costimulatory or Inhibitory Receptors and Experimental Methods

A variety of cell surface receptors are present on lymphocytes and are critical to function of the immune system [10]. These are generally grouped into costimulatory or inhibitory receptors, with corresponding ligands (see Table 7.1). Recently, therapeutic strategies have evolved to antagonize inhibitory molecules or agonize costimulatory molecules with monoclonal antibodies independently or in combination. Some of these lymphocyte receptor modulators are used in clinical practice, while others are still undergoing preclinical development. Importantly, the therapeutic target of these agents is the lymphocyte signaling process, not the cancer cell itself. In addition, modulating some of these targets can also lead to activation of the innate immune system.

Several investigations combining radiotherapy and lymphocyte receptor modulators in preclinical models have been reported. Many of these studies use similar immunologic experimental methods. For readers unfamiliar with these methods, they are explained briefly here. The reader is also referred to several recent reviews on the immunologic effects of radiation therapy for further understanding of the effect of radiation on the immune system, in the absence of lymphocyte receptor modulators [11, 12].

As the target for experimental manipulation is the immune system, most studies are performed in vivo, rather than in vitro. For this reason, the models must use immunocompetent syngeneic species-specific (often murine) tumor grafts, rather than xenografts from human tumors in immunocompromised hosts. Investigators have studied tumor grafts placed subcutaneously or intradermally (on the flank or hind limb) and orthotopically (in the organ of tissue origin, such as the breast, brain,

Table 7.1 Costimulatory and inhibitor lymphocyte receptors and ligands. Representative costimulatory and inhibitory lymphocyte receptors and ligands studied in combination with radiotherapy are presented, with example agonistic and antagonistic therapies listed

	Cell surface receptor	Cell surface receptor ligand	Therapeutic agonist/antagonist examples
Costimulatory	CD40	CD40L	CP-870,893 (Pfizer), dacetuzumab (Seattle Genetics)
	CD134/OX40	CD252/OX40L	MEDI0562, MEDI6469, MEDI6383 (AstraZeneca)
	GITR	GITRL	TRX518 (GITR Incorporated)
	CD137/4-1BB	CD137L	PF-05082566 (Pfizer), lipocalin (Pieris Pharmaceuticals), urelumab (Bristol-Myers Squibb)
Inhibitory	CD152/CTLA4	CD80, CD86	Ipilimumab (Bristol-Myers Squibb), tremelimumab (AstraZeneca)
	LAG3	MHC II	BMS-986016 (Bristol-Myers Squibb), IMP321 (Immuntep)
	PD-1	PD-L1, PD-L2	Nivolumab (Bristol-Myers Squibb), pembrolizumab (Merck), pidilizumab (Cure Tech), AMP-224, AMP-514 (Amplimmune)
	TIM-3	Galectin-9, HMGB1, PS, CEACAM-1	Anti-TIM-3 (Tesaro)

GITR glucocorticoid-induced TNFR family-related gene, *CTLA4* cytotoxic T lymphocyte-associated protein 4, *LAG3* lymphocyte activation gene 3, *PD-1* programmed death 1, *PD-L1* programmed death ligand 1, *PD-L2* programmed death ligand 2, *TIM-3* T cell immunoglobulin and mucin domain 3, *HMGB1* high-mobility group box 1, *PS* phosphatidylserine, *CECAM-1* carcinoembryonic antigen-related cell adhesion molecule 1

or skin). Tumor size, tumor growth delay, tumor response, metastasis, and overall survival are often the simplest measures of treatment effect. To demonstrate immune-mediated response to cancer distant from the radiotherapy target, some models incorporate two tumors, where one is irradiated and the other is not irradiated. This allows for demonstration of an abscopal effect (effect of radiation away from the target of radiotherapy) [13].

Immunologic response to tumor, radiotherapy, and lymphocyte receptor modulation can also be characterized at the treated tumor or in the peripheral lymphoid organs. Often immune cell populations (lymphocytes, myeloid cells, macrophages) are characterized based on cell surface markers (of differentiation, activation, exhaustion, etc.) in different anatomic compartments (infiltrating the tumor, draining the lymph node basin, spleen, etc.). The dependency of the treatment effect on specific immune cell populations can be interrogated by performing experiments in animal models deficient for immune function (through genetic knockout) or through depletion of immune cell populations by neutralizing monoclonal antibodies against cell surface markers (CD4, CD8, etc.) and ligands (PD-L1, TIM-3, etc.). Determining whether immune cells recognize tumor-specific antigens can be carried out using ex vivo assays to determine if lymphocytes can kill tumor cells or if they elaborate cytokines such as interferon gamma in response to tumor antigens. Finally, immunologic memory can be tested after complete tumor regression by rechallenging the host with the tumor graft and assessing for the presence or absence of tumor growth. Similarly, immune cells from hosts with complete tumor regression can be adoptively transferred to naïve, tumor-bearing animals to assess for antitumor properties of the transferred immune cells.

Combinations of Costimulatory Receptor Modulation and Radiotherapy

CD137/4-1BB

CD137 or 4-1BB is a member of the tumor necrosis factor receptor (TNFR) superfamily and is expressed on T cells and other immune subsets following activation. Ligation of the receptor via its ligand or agonist antibodies results in enhanced T cell proliferation and production of cytokines. CD137 activation has also been shown to provide a strong survival signal for CD8 T cells via upregulation of anti-apoptotic pathways [14]. In 2006, investigators first reported on the combination of 4-1BB agonism (with a monoclonal antibody, BMS-469492) and radiotherapy (5–15 Gy/1 fraction or 40 Gy/10 fractions) in a preclinical breast (EMT6) and lung (M109) cancer model. The authors found that 4-1BB agonism could effectively delay the growth of tumors in the breast cancer model, but not the lung cancer model. In the breast cancer model, when treated with the combination of single-dose or fractionated radiotherapy followed by 4-1BB agonism, investigators observed a delay in tumor growth significantly longer than either therapy when given alone. In the lung cancer model, only the highest single dose of radiotherapy (15 Gy), but not fractionated treatment, yielded a significant delay in tumor growth compared to either therapy given alone. The lung cancer cell line was found to have high basal expression of 4-1BBL which could not be increased by irradiation, while the breast cancer cell line had low basal expression of 4-1BBL, which could be increased by irradiation [15]. This suggests that the expression of 4-1BB ligand may be a good biomarker for combining RT with 4-1BB agonism.

In a preclinical orthotopic model of glioma using the GL261 cell line, investigators observed that the 4-1BB agonist antibody (BMS-469492) in combination with whole-head radiotherapy (8 Gy/2 fractions) yielded significantly longer survival rates than either treatment alone. Of the long-term survivors treated with radiotherapy alone ($n=2$) or in combination with BMS-469492 ($n=6$), 50 % and 83 % demonstrated no evidence of tumor regrowth after tumor rechallenge, respectively.

All had pathologic complete response in the brain. When examining the tumor-infiltrating lymphocytes, significantly higher numbers of CD8 and CD4 lymphocytes were noted in the group treated with radiotherapy alone compared to the untreated control group, and even higher numbers were observed in those treated with 4-1BB agonism and radiotherapy. Finally, the production of interferon gamma, indicative of T cell effector function, in a tumor-specific manner by splenocytes was greatest in the group treated with 4-1BB agonism and radiotherapy [16].

CD134/OX40

CD134 or OX40 is another member of the TNFR superfamily expressed on activated CD4 and CD8 T cells as well as neutrophils, DCs, and Treg cells. The natural ligand (OX40L) is found on APCs as well as activated T cells. Engagement of OX40 promotes T cell activation, maturation, survival, and cytokine production [17]. Investigators have also observed that single-dose radiotherapy (20 Gy) followed by OX40 agonism (with a monoclonal antibody clone OX86) increased the rate of cure in a preclinical lung (Lewis lung carcinoma) model, compared to either treatment alone. This effect was found to be dependent on CD8 lymphocytes, but not CD4 lymphocytes or natural killer cells. The combination of OX40 agonism and radiotherapy significantly increased the proportion of CD8 lymphocytes in the draining lymph node compared to either treatment alone. The CD8 lymphocytes had the ability to kill the lung cancer cell line in an antigen-specific manner. Finally, the combination of OX40 agonism and radiotherapy was found to yield immunologic memory and tumor rejection after rechallenge, compared to animals not previously treated [18].

Other investigators found that in a preclinical model of lung cancer (Lewis lung carcinoma, LLC), radiotherapy (60 Gy/3 fractions) followed by OX40 agonism (starting one day after the first fraction of radiotherapy) yielded significantly longer survival compared to either treatment alone. Tumor rechallenge after combination radiotherapy and OX40 agonism demonstrated immunologic memory [19].

GITR

Glucocorticoid-induced TNFR family-related (GITR) gene is expressed on CD4 and CD8 T cells and is upregulated after activation. Similar to other TNFR family members, ligation with its natural ligand (GITRL) expressed on activated APCs and endothelial cells (EC) results in enhanced T cell proliferation, survival, and effector function [20]. Investigators explored the effect of radiotherapy (30 Gy/1 fraction) with or without GITR agonism using a monoclonal antibody (DTA-1) in a lung carcinoma (Lewis lung carcinoma, LLC) model. The authors observed that irradiation of LLC significantly delayed tumor growth and increased survival, compared to no irradiation. Depletion of CD8 lymphocytes significantly decreased the tumor growth delay and survival suggesting that the effect is CD8 dependent. When GITR agonism and radiotherapy were combined, there was a nonsignificant tumor growth delay greater than either treatment alone, but no association with longer survival [21].

CD40

CD40 is another member of the TNFR superfamily constitutively expressed on APCs, and its ligation results in promotion of functional maturation with enhanced antigen presentation and cytokine production resulting in increased activation of T cells [22]. In 2003, investigators reported on studies of two syngeneic models of B cell lymphoma (A31 and BCL1) treated with total body irradiation (TBI, 2–8 Gy/1 fraction) for systemic lymphoma and/or costimulation by CD40 agonist monoclonal antibody 4 h after irradiation. The investigators observed a significant increase in survival with the combination of TBI and CD40 agonism, compared to either treatment alone. However, the effect was dependent on the dose of TBI used; 5 Gy yielded the highest proportion of survivors, with higher or lower doses of radiation proving inferior. The authors found that a wide range of doses of the CD40 agonist were effective at promoting survival, but that other B cell-depleting antibodies (against CD19, MHC II, CD22) did not yield the same effect as the CD40 agonist suggesting that the CD40 antibody is not acting by simply depleting B cells. In vitro analyses of apoptosis and clonogenic survival suggest that CD40 agonism did not increase the cellular radiosensitivity of the lymphoma cell lines. Interestingly, in an experiment where variable numbers of lymphoma cells were inoculated, the authors observed that a minimum amount of lymphoma cells must be treated to yield long-term immunity, again suggesting that CD40 is not a general sensitizer to radiation. By tracking the number of lymphoma cells present after combination treatment, investigators found that TBI alone yielded a dose-dependent decrease in the number of lymphoma cells, which regrew in the absence of CD40 agonism. The combination of TBI and CD40 agonism led to a two-phase (early and late) pattern of lymphoma regression. Importantly, a significant increase in CD8 cells was noted in animals treated with 5 Gy of TBI and CD40 agonism compared to those given 5 Gy of TBI alone. However, this was not observed with higher (8 Gy) or lower (2 Gy) doses of radiation, or in animals not bearing lymphoma, or with the use of other monoclonal antibodies. The authors observed that CD8 cells in the group receiving CD40 agonism and TBI had a significantly greater lymphoma-specific cytotoxic activity. In addition, CD8, but not CD4, lymphocyte depletion abrogated the therapeutic effect of TBI and CD40 agonism. In long-term survivors of the CD40 agonism and TBI treatment, rechallenge with lymphoma cells demonstrated immunologic memory in 80% of the treated animals. Finally, adoptive transfer of T cells from survivors of the CD40 agonism and TBI combination to untreated lymphoma-bearing animals significantly increased the duration of survival in the recipient mice [23].

Combinations of Multiple Costimulatory Receptor Modulators and Radiotherapy

In 2012, investigators explored the combination of targeting multiple costimulation modulators in combination with radiotherapy in preclinical models. Using two triple-negative (estrogen/progesterone/Her-2/neu receptor negative) breast cancer cell (4T1.2 and AT-3) models, the authors explored the effect of 4-1BB and CD40 agonism alone, in combination, or immediately after radiotherapy (12 Gy/1 fraction). It was observed that 4-1BB agonism alone, or in combination with CD40 agonism, significantly delayed tumor growth compared to control. Notably, CD40 agonism alone did not significantly delay tumor growth. Likewise, when given radiotherapy, 4-1BB agonism alone, or in combination with CD40 agonism, significantly delayed tumor growth. This effect was not observed with CD40 agonism after radiotherapy. In the 4T1.2 cell line, tumor cure was observed with radiotherapy or in combination with CD40 and 4-1BB agonism; tumor cure occurred most often in the group receiving the combination of CD40 and 4-1BB agonism and radiotherapy. The antitumor effect was noted to be dependent on CD4, CD8, and natural killer cells. Moreover, rechallenge of the host with a tumor demonstrated immunologic memory. The authors hypothesized that the differences in response to the combination of immunotherapy and radiotherapy in the two cell lines were associated with 4T1.2 tumors supporting a necrotic core and undergoing an immunogenic, non-apoptotic death after radiotherapy, while AT-3 cells expressed PD-L1, possibly conferring resistance to the combination of costimulation and radiotherapy. The authors conducted further experiments to explore ways to overcome resistance (described further below) [24].

Combinations of Inhibitory Receptor Modulation and Radiotherapy

CTLA4

APCs present antigen in the context of MHC to a specific T cell receptor on the surface of T cells. However, for resulting T cell activation, costimulation is required by a variety of other cell surface receptors including CD28 on the T cell interacting with CD80/B7.1 and CD86 B7.2 on APCs. CTLA4 is a member of the CD28 family of receptors and is upregulated on activated T cells. CTLA4 has a higher affinity for CD80/CD86 than the costimulatory receptor CD28 and can therefore competitively bind ligand more avidly than CD28. Through this mechanism, it acts as a negative feedback loop for T cell activation after TCR stimulation. CTLA4 is also expressed constitutively at high levels on Treg cells and is important for their suppressive functions. The administration of anti-CTLA4 antibodies results in blockade of inhibitory signals as well as direct depletion of Treg cells resulting in immune activation [25].

In 2005, investigators reported on the effects of radiotherapy (12 Gy/1 fraction or 24 Gy/2 fractions 48 h apart) alone or followed by CTLA4 blockade with the antibody 9H10 in a breast cancer (4T1) model. The growth of implanted 4T1 tumors was significantly delayed only in animals treated with radiotherapy, with or without 9H10, compared to untreated controls. Treatment with 9H10 alone did not delay tumor growth. Moreover, radiotherapy or CTLA4 blockade did not significantly increase survival compared to the group that did not receive treatment. However, the combination of CTLA4 blockade and RT did significantly increase survival compared to the untreated control group. Compared to untreated controls, a significantly lower number of lung metastases were observed only with the combination of CTLA4 blockade and radiotherapy, but not either treatment alone. This effect was abrogated with CD8 lymphocyte depletion, but not CD4 lymphocyte depletion. The authors further demonstrated that a higher total dose of radiation (24 Gy/2 fractions) yielded a 57 % rate of complete regression of the primary tumor, which was not observed for the lower dose of radiation (12 Gy/1 fraction). Despite improvement in primary tumor control with a higher dose of radiation, similar to prior experiments, the combination of CTLA4 blockade with 9H10 and radiotherapy yielded significantly longer survival than either treatment alone or no treatment at all. In the group with long-term survival, tumor rechallenge demonstrated protective immunity with 4T1-specific cytolytic activity in the spleen [26].

A subsequent study from the same group investigated the effect of single-dose (20 Gy/1) or fractionated radiotherapy (30 Gy/5 fractions or 24 Gy/3 fractions) with or without concurrent or subsequent CTLA4 blockade with a monoclonal antibody (9H10) in breast cancer (TSA) or colon cancer (MCA38) models. Using a two-tumor model where tumors were implanted on each flank of the mice but only one tumor was irradiated (as illustrated in Fig. 7.1), the authors observed that 9H10

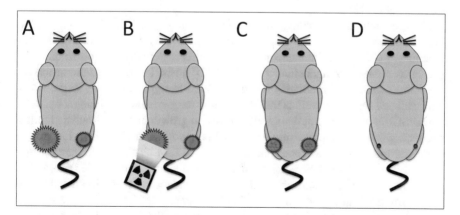

Fig. 7.1 Two-tumor model for the assessment of the abscopal effect. In this model, bilateral tumor grafts are placed, typically with one tumor being smaller than the other (**a**). Radiotherapy is administered to the larger of the two tumors (**b**), and the immune response in the tumors can be assessed after treatment (**c**). The unirradiated tumor is observed for abscopal response, or response away from the target of radiotherapy (**d**). This effect is thought to be immune mediated

alone had no effect on tumor growth compared to untreated controls. Radiotherapy alone caused tumor growth delay of the irradiated tumor of a similar magnitude across the three-dose schedules, but no growth delay in the unirradiated distant tumor. The combination of CTLA4 blockade and fractionated radiotherapy (but not single-dose radiotherapy) was associated with regression of both irradiated and unirradiated tumors demonstrating an abscopal effect. The effect was greatest in the 24 Gy/3 fraction regimen. The investigators further explored the effect of delaying the start of immunotherapy after initiating radiotherapy. They found that the longest delay between immunotherapy and radiotherapy was associated with the most rapid rate of tumor regression. Examination of the unirradiated tumors in the group receiving 9H10 and radiotherapy (24 Gy/3 fractions) demonstrated a significantly greater number of tumor-infiltrating CD4 and CD8 lymphocytes, compared to either treatment alone. Finally, the ex vivo tumor-specific production of interferon gamma by splenocytes was greatest in animals exhibiting rejection of the unirradiated tumor [27].

Another group of investigators examined the effects of combining radiotherapy (2–30 Gy/1 fraction) with or without CTLA4 blockade using a monoclonal antibody (9H10) in a lung carcinoma (Lewis lung carcinoma, LLC) model. The authors assessed secretion of HMGB1, a protein released after immunogenic cell death, after LLC cell irradiation in vitro. They noted no difference in HMGB1 levels between cells irradiated with 2 Gy and those not irradiated. However, cells irradiated with 6 or 30 Gy released threefold more HMGB1 than those not irradiated. The authors then carried out in vivo experiments, observing that radiotherapy (30 Gy/1 fraction) significantly delayed tumor growth and increased overall survival, compared to no radiotherapy. CD8 lymphocyte depletion significantly decreased the tumor growth delay and survival. CTLA4 blockade and radiotherapy significantly increased tumor growth delay and overall survival, compared to radiation or CTLA4 blockade alone [21].

Subsequently, other investigators studied radiotherapy (5–15 Gy/1–3 fractions) in combination with CTLA4 blockade with a monoclonal antibody in a mesothelioma model (AB12) in immunocompetent or immunodeficient (nonobese diabetic/severe combined immunodeficient, NOD/SCID) hosts. Using a two-tumor model, the authors found that irradiating one tumor leads to significant delay in growth of the irradiated tumor, as well as the unirradiated tumor. However, immunodeficient (NOD/SCID) hosts did not demonstrate delay in growth of the unirradiated tumor suggesting that the adaptive immune system is important in controlling the growth of the unirradiated tumors. The combination of CTLA4 blockade and radiotherapy delayed irradiated and unirradiated tumor growth significantly longer than either treatment alone. These same observations were made whether the irradiated tumor and unirradiated tumor were implanted synchronously or metachronously. Assessment of immune infiltrates in the tumor, draining lymph nodes, and spleen 10 days after treatment revealed significantly higher levels of activated (ICOS+) and proliferating (Ki67+) CD4 and CD8 lymphocytes, as well as dendritic cells in the draining lymph nodes (but not the spleen) of hosts with irradiated tumors, compared to control tumors. Significantly more CD8 T cells were noted in irradiated tumors in the group treated with CTLA4 blockade and radiotherapy, compared to those treated with either treatment alone. In the group treated with CTLA4 blockade and radiotherapy, a significant increase in the number of activated (but not total) CD4 and CD8 T cells in the spleen was observed compared to the group treated with radiotherapy alone. Finally, compared with irradiated or unirradiated tumors treated with radiotherapy alone, those treated with CTLA4 blockade and radiotherapy demonstrated an increase in the expression of pro-inflammatory markers including interferon gamma, perforin, IP-10, TNF alpha, granzyme B, ICOS, IL-4, IL-12, IL-12p70, IL-5, IL-6, IL-17A, and MCP-1 [28].

In a colon carcinoma (CT26) model, investigators studied the combination of radiotherapy (10 Gy/1 fraction) with intratumoral injection of immature dendritic cells (iDCs) with or without CTLA4 blockade (9H10). Using a two-tumor model, they observed a significantly longer delay in tumor growth, overall survival, and greater tumor-specific cytolytic T cell activity with the combination of radiotherapy and iDC injection with CTLA4 blockade, compared to either treatment alone [29].

PD-1/PD-L1

Programmed cell death protein-1 (PD-1) is a coinhibitory member of the CD28 superfamily expressed on activated T cells in a more delayed fashion than CTLA4 and thought to be involved in more chronic inflammation to induce T cell exhaustion or anergy. PD-1 binds to B7-family ligands PD-L1 and PD-L2 on APCs on other nonimmune cells which induce inhibitory signals within the T cells [30]. Tumor cells have been shown to dramatically upregulate PD-L1 to dampen the antitumor immune response [31]. Using two breast carcinoma (4T1 and AT3) models, investigators studied the effect of radiotherapy (12 Gy/1 fraction) followed by PD-1 blockade with a monoclonal antibody (RMP1-14). The investigators found that PD-L1 was not expressed on AT3 cells in vitro, but was present ex vivo whether taken from a subcutaneous or orthotopically grown tumor. Radiotherapy did not affect the expression of PD-L1 on explanted tumor cells. However, 12 h after radiotherapy, there was an enrichment of tumor-infiltrating CD8 cells that expressed high levels of PD-1 (PD-1^{High}) through the reduction of CD8 cells expressing low levels of PD-1 (PD-1^{Low}), with a resultant increase in the ratio of PD-1^{High} to PD-1^{Low} CD8 cells in treated AT3 tumors. In addition, 36 h after radiotherapy, tumor-infiltrating CD8 cells were noted to be actively proliferating and productive of interferon gamma, indicating preservation of functionality. Additional experiments confirmed these CD8 cells were tumor antigen specific. Finally, the combination of PD-1 blockade and radiotherapy in vivo did not delay tumor growth more than radiotherapy or PD-1 alone in the subcutaneous AT3 model. However, in the subcutaneous orthotopic AT3 model, the combination of radiotherapy and PD-1 blockade delayed tumor growth significantly longer than either treatment alone, with a long-term cure rate of 17 % [24].

Using an orthotopic glioblastoma model (GL261), other investigators tested stereotactic radiosurgery (10 Gy/1 fraction) with or without immediate PD-1 blockade with a monoclonal antibody (G4). In vitro, the investigators found that GL261 expressed PD-L1, a potential biomarker of the efficacy of PD-1 blockade. In addition, radiotherapy increased the surface expression of MHC I, ICAM1, and CXCL16 in vitro. In vivo, the investigators found that the combination of PD-1 blockade and radiotherapy yielded significantly longer overall survival than either treatment alone, or no treatment. Depletion of CD8 (more than CD4) was associated with abrogation of the survival benefit. In long-term survivors, tumor rechallenge demonstrated long-term immunity. On studying the brain immune infiltrates of mice treated with radiation or PD-1 blockade, investigators found that the combination significantly increased the number of CD8 cells, while radiation (with or without PD-1 blockade) seemed to decrease regulatory T cells. The net result was a significant increase in the ratio of CD8 to regulatory T cells in the group treated with PD-1 blockade and radiotherapy [32].

Other investigators subsequently reported on single-dose or fractionated radiotherapy (at various doses) and PD-1 blockade with an antibody in models of colorectal cancer (MC38-OVA), breast cancer (4T1-HA), and melanoma (B16-OVA). In vitro, they observed that radiotherapy (10–20 Gy/1 fraction) resulted in a dose-dependent increase in antigen presentation. In vivo, B16-OVA tumor growth delay was significantly longer with PD-1 blockade and radiotherapy, compared to either treatment alone. The investigators observe a significantly greater proportion of antigen-specific immune infiltrates in the spleen and draining lymph nodes after treatment with PD-1 blockade and radiotherapy, compared to either treatment alone. Adoptively transferred splenocytes from hosts treated with PD-1 blockade and radiotherapy significantly delayed tumor growth longer than splenocytes from untreated hosts, or hosts treated with PD-1 blockade alone. Greater numbers of tumor-infiltrating lymphocytes were noted after PD-1 blockade and radiotherapy, compared to radiotherapy alone. Greater numbers of CD4 and CD8 cells were noted to infiltrate irradiated tumors, compared to those not treated with radiotherapy. There was an increase in regulatory T cells in irradiated tumors (but not draining lymph nodes or spleens) not treated with PD-1 blockade. The combination of PD-1 blockade and radiotherapy yielded a significantly greater increase the CD8 to regulatory T cell ratio, compared to either treatment alone. The combination of PD-1 blockade and radiotherapy increased the frequency of effector memory T cells in the tumors to a greater extent than either treatment alone. Similar findings were observed in the 4T1-HA model [33].

Other investigators explored the effect of stereotactic ablative radiotherapy (15 Gy/1 fraction) and PD-1 blockade (G4) in breast cancer (4T1), renal cancer (RENCA), or melanoma (B16) in PD-1 wild-type or knockout mouse models. Using a two-tumor model, the authors observed that both irradiated and unirradiated tumors grew significantly slower in the PD-1 knockout model. Survival was also significantly longer in the PD-1 knockout model, compared to the wild-type model. In the wild-type model, the combination of PD-1 blockade and radiotherapy was associated with a significantly longer delay in irradiated and unirradiated tumor growth, compared to either treatment alone. The combination treatment was also associated with significantly longer survival than either treatment alone. The investigators went on to demonstrate that antitumor immune effect is antigen specific for the irradiated tumor. In a three tumor model, with two of the unirradiated tumors being of different origin (one 4T1, one RENCA), only the irradiated RENCA tumor and the unirradiated RENCA tumor responded to the combination of PD-1 blockade and radiotherapy; the 4T1 did not respond to treatment. In the two-tumor model, significantly more PD-1 expressing tumor-infiltrating reactive CD8 cells (CD11a^{High}) were present in irradiated or unirradiated tumors, compared to untreated controls. This population of cells was found to be tumor antigen specific and responsive. Moreover, PD-L1 expression on leukocytes (but not tumor cells) in the irradiated and unirradiated tumors significantly increased after irradiation. The expression of LAG3 and TIM-3 on tumor-infiltrating CD8 cells was not affected by irradiation. Finally, CD4, CD8, and CD11a depletion in vivo demonstrated dependence of unirradiated tumor regression on CD8 cells [34].

Investigators studied the combination of radiotherapy (12–20 Gy/1 fraction) and PD-L1 blockade (10F.9G2) in breast (TUBO) and colorectal cancer (MC38) models. The authors found that radiotherapy (12 Gy/1 fraction) increased PD-L1 expression on tumor cells and dendritic cells, but not on myeloid-derived suppressor cells or macrophages. PD-1 expression was slightly downregulated on CD8 (but not CD4) cells after radiotherapy. In vivo, the combination of PD-L1 blockade and radiotherapy delayed irradiated MC38 and TUBO tumor growth significantly longer than either treatment alone. In a two-tumor model, this combination also delayed the growth of an unirradiated TUBO tumor longer than either treatment alone. In the group with complete tumor regression after the combination of PD-L1 blockade and radiotherapy, tumor rechallenge experiments demonstrated long-lasting immunity. Depletion of CD8 cells was noted to abrogate the therapeutic effect of PD-L1 blockade and radiotherapy. The combination of PD-L1 blockade and radiotherapy was associated with tumor-specific T cell functionality that was greater than either treatment alone. On the investigation of the immune cells infiltrating the tumor and present in the spleen, the authors observed a significantly greater reduction in myeloid-derived suppressor cells (MDSCs) 10 days (but not 3 days) after PD-L1 blockade and radiotherapy, and this reduction was greater than those observed from either treatment alone. They noted that depletion of MDSCs could significantly delay tumor growth in animals treated with radiotherapy alone. Finally, the authors observed CD8 cells were in part responsible for the reduction in MDSCs, through the cytokine tumor necrosis factor alpha (TNFa). TNFa blockade abrogated the suppression of tumor growth in the combination of PD-L1 and radiotherapy [35].

Other investigators studied fractionated radiotherapy (10 Gy/5 fractions) and PD-1 or PD-L1 blockade with monoclonal antibodies in melanoma (4434), breast cancer (4T1), and colorectal cancer (CT26) models. The authors observed that PD-L1 expression increased on CT26 tumor cells, increased 1 day after in vivo tumor radiotherapy (10 Gy/5 fractions), reached a peak 3 days after radiotherapy, and declined significantly 7 days after radiotherapy. Subsequent experiments revealed that irradiation (2–10 Gy/1 fraction) of tumor cells in vitro had little effect on PD-L1 expression. In vivo, depletion of CD8 cells abrogated the increase in PD-L1 expression caused by radiotherapy. Depletion of natural killer cells had no effect on PD-L1 expression, while depletion of CD4 cells increased the expression of PD-L1 on tumor cells. In the absence of radiation, interferon gamma alone and in combination with tumor necrosis factor alpha (but not tumor necrosis factor alpha alone) increased PD-L1 expression on tumor cells in vitro. In addition, depletion of interferon gamma suppressed the overexpression of PD-L1 on irradiated cells. In vivo, local tumor control and overall survival were significantly greater in the group treated with the combination of PD-L1 or PD-1 blockade and radiotherapy, compared to either treatment alone. Combined PD-1 and PD-L1 blockade and radiotherapy were not associated with an improvement in the outcome of radiotherapy and PD-1 or PD-L1 blockade. In vitro, the authors found that the PD-1 and PD-L1 blocking monoclonal antibodies did not increase tumor cell radiosensitivity. Depletion of CD8 and natural killer cells abrogated the tumor growth delay provided by PD-L1 blockade and radiotherapy. Depletion of CD4 cells significantly increased tumor growth delay after PD-L1 blockade and radiotherapy, which the authors speculated may have been due to the presence of fewer regulatory T cells. Among the group with complete tumor regression after PD-L1 blockade and radiotherapy, tumor rechallenge demonstrated long-term antigen-specific immunity. In addition, the authors found that the scheduling of PD-L1 blockade and radiotherapy was important. The authors observed significantly longer survival in the groups initiating PD-L1 blockade on the first or last day of fractionated radiotherapy, compared to 7 days after the end of fractionated radiotherapy. Consistent with this time-dependent effect, the authors observed significantly higher PD-1 expression levels on CD4 and CD8 cells infiltrating the tumor 1 day after radiotherapy (compared to untreated controls), but not 7 days after radiotherapy [36].

Combinations of Multiple Inhibitory Receptor Modulators and Radiotherapy

Using a melanoma model (B16), investigators studied the effect of stereotactic ablative radiotherapy (15 Gy/1 fraction) and CTLA4 (9H10) and PD-1 (G4) blockade. Using a two-tumor model, they observed the greatest delay in tumor growth with the combination of CTLA4 blockade, PD-1 blockade, and radiotherapy, compared to CTLA4 or PD-1 blockade and radiotherapy. This effect was noted at the irradiated and unirradiated tumor, with the latter observation being statistically significant [34].

Using models of melanoma (B16-F10), breast cancer (TSA), and pancreas cancer (PDA.4662), investigators explored the effect of CTLA4 (9H10), PD-1 (RMP1-14), and PD-L1 (10F.9G2) blockade and radiotherapy (20 Gy/1 fraction or 24 Gy/3 fractions). Using a two-tumor B16-F10 model, investigators found that the combination of CTLA4 blockade and radiotherapy was associated with the greatest delay in distant unirradiated tumor growth, compared to either treatment alone. Depletion of CD8 cells abrogated this effect. Among the 17 % treated with the combination and achieving a complete tumor response, tumor rechallenge demonstrated persistent immunity. Analysis of tumor-infiltrating lymphocytes demonstrated that resistance to therapy was associated with low numbers of infiltrating CD8 cells, and a low CD8/regulatory T cell ratio, and a higher number of "exhausted" CD8 cells. They also observed that upregulation of PD-L1 and interferon-stimulated genes in tumor cells was associated with resistance to combination treatment. The authors found that adding PD-L1 blockade to the combination of CTLA4 blockade and radiotherapy increased the response rate to 58 % and was associated with reinvigoration of the "exhausted" CD8 population infiltrating the tumor and in the periphery. They went on to characterize the effect of radiotherapy in the context of dual checkpoint blockade and found that radiotherapy was associated with diversification of the T cell receptor repertoire, while CTLA4 and PD-1 lowered the percent of Tregs and reversed T cell exhaustion in the tumor, respectively. Finally, the authors developed and tested the accuracy of a model to predict response to the combination of immunotherapy and radiotherapy which incorporated the proportion of "exhausted" CD8 cells, reinvigorated CD8 cells, and the ratio of CD8/regulatory T cells [37].

Combinations of Costimulatory and Inhibitory Receptor Modulators and Radiotherapy

Using a triple-negative (estrogen/progesterone/Her-2/neu receptor negative) breast cancer cell (AT-3) model, investigators explored the combination of PD-1 antagonism with a monoclonal antibody, with 4-1BB agonism alone immediately after radiotherapy (12 Gy/1 fraction or 16–20 Gy/4 fractions). The authors found that the combination of radiotherapy, 4-1BB agonism, and PD-1 antagonism was associated with a higher rate of response than the combination of radiotherapy and 4-1BB agonism or radiotherapy and PD-1 antagonism. In an orthotopic and subcutaneous model, this combination led to a 100 % and 40 % cure rate among the group treated with the triple combination of 4-1BB agonism, PD-1 blockade, and radiotherapy, respectively. A similar effect was noted when combining fractionated radiotherapy, PD-1 blockade, and 4-1BB agonism, with approximately 80 % achieving cure [24].

Investigators using a glioblastoma (GL261-luc) model examined the effect of focal radiotherapy (10 Gy/1 fraction) followed by CTLA4 (4F10) blockade and 4-1BB (2A) agonism. The combination of radiotherapy and CTLA4 blockade or radiotherapy and 4-1BB agonism was associated with longer survival than no treatment in their model; the CTLA4 combination with radiotherapy (but not the 4-1BB combination) was associated with significantly longer survival than radiotherapy alone. They found that delivering radiotherapy 2 days before, the day of, or 2 days after the first dose of CTLA4-blocking antibody was associated with similar survival benefits, compared to no treatment, although a lower proportion of long-term survivors and shortest median duration of survival was noted in the group treated with radiotherapy, followed 2 days later by CTLA4 blockade. The authors then went on to observe that the group treated with CTLA4 blockade, 4-1BB agonism, and radiotherapy had survival longer than any other combination treatment groups. They observed that CD4 and CD8 brain-infiltrating lymphocytes were more common in the groups treated with the combination of CTLA4 blockade and 4-1BB agonism, with or without radiotherapy, compared to non-tumor-bearing brains. The difference in infiltrating lymphocytes was not noted in draining cervical lymph nodes. Depletion of CD4 and CD8 abrogated the survival improvement with CTLA4 blockade and 4-1BB agonism, with the former being a more profound effect. Long-term survivors of the combination therapy underwent tumor rechallenge and were found to have long-term tumor-specific immunity [38].

An alternative strategy to tumor-specific irradiation is whole-body irradiation. Investigators used a combination of "lymphodepleting" whole-body irradiation (WBI) to 5 Gy in 1 dose 7 days after injection of multiple myeloma cell lines and found that this, in conjunction with a combination of checkpoint-blocking antibodies (against CTLA4, PD-1, PD-L1, TIM-3, or LAG3 or a combination thereof), improved the anti-myeloma immune response and survival. The authors could not elucidate the mechanism whereby WBI augmented immunotherapy other than to say it depleted lymphocytes with upregulated coinhibitory molecules, and this transient depletion facilitated effective immunotherapy. Notably, this strategy was only effective in hematopoietic cancer models, but not in solid tumor models [39].

Summary

Several noteworthy preclinical studies have examined the effect of combining lymphocyte costimulatory and inhibitor receptor modulators and radiotherapy. Most have demonstrated improvements in irradiated tumor control with the combination of receptor modulation and radiotherapy. In two-tumor models, this was associated with an improved control of unirradiated tumors, which translated into longer survival, cure, and immunologic memory. However, no improvement over radiotherapy alone was presented in some studies of CD40 and GITR. Moreover, some studies found that a combination of radiotherapy and more than one costimulatory or checkpoint modulator (CTLA4 and PD-1 or PD-L1, CD137/4-1BB and PD-L1, CD137/4-1BB and CTLA4) yielded the best outcomes. These effects have been observed in models of various cancers, including breast, lung, glioma, lymphoma, colon, mesothelioma, melanoma, kidney, pancreas, and multiple myeloma.

Variations in radiotherapeutic approach have been explored. The effect has been observed with single-dose and fractionated in vivo tumor radiotherapy, which most accurately recapitulates common clinical scenarios for patients with solid tumors. Importantly, some studies observed that a significant delay in checkpoint modulation after radiotherapy abrogated the therapeutic effects. In some models, a higher dose of tumor radiotherapy was associated with response, while lower doses were not. In some instances, irradiation of tumor cells demonstrated the effect, and in one study, two doses of radiotherapy appeared superior to a single dose. The target of radiotherapy was most often a tumor, but in the context of hematopoietic disease models, whole-body irradiation increased the response to checkpoint modulation and appeared to be dose dependent.

Immunologically, induction of the receptor ligands (PD-L1, 4-1BBL) by radiotherapy was associated with response to combination therapy in some studies. One study found that the T cell receptor diversification may be another important effect that radiotherapy has on the immune system. The infiltration of immune cells after combined checkpoint modulation and radiotherapy was greater than after either treatment alone; depletion of CD8 cells (and sometimes CD4, natural killer cells, or macrophages) typically abrogated therapeutic effects. In vitro assays typically demonstrated tumor-specific functionality of the infiltrating immune cells. Resistance to immune checkpoint modulation and radiotherapy was attributed to PD-L1 expression on tumor cells in two studies, and strategies to block this immunologic barrier appeared to overcome resistance. Finally, the use of immunocompromised model organisms demonstrated a lack of an antitumor effect after radiation demonstrating a critical role of the immune system in mediating the antitumor efficacy of radiation therapy.

The findings discussed herein clearly support future investigations combining lymphocyte costimulatory and inhibitory receptor modulation and radiotherapy. Preclinical evidence has suggested approaches that hold promise for cancer patients, but additional studies will be needed to clarify the optimal therapeutic approach. The design of rationale clinical trials will be imperative to validate the potential benefit for cancer patients.

References

1. Lee Y et al (2009) Therapeutic effects of ablative radiation on local tumor require CD8+ T cells: changing strategies for cancer treatment. Blood 114(3):589–595
2. Apetoh L et al (2007) Toll-like receptor 4-dependent contribution of the immune system to anticancer chemotherapy and radiotherapy. Nat Med 13(9):1050–1059
3. Reits EA et al (2006) Radiation modulates the peptide repertoire, enhances MHC class I expression, and induces successful antitumor immunotherapy. J Exp Med 203(5):1259–1271
4. Green DR et al (2009) Immunogenic and tolerogenic cell death. Nat Rev Immunol 9(5): 353–363
5. Golden EB, Apetoh L (2015) Radiotherapy and immunogenic cell death. Semin Radiat Oncol 25(1):11–17
6. Sharma A et al (2011) Gamma-Radiation promotes immunological recognition of cancer cells through increased expression of cancer-testis antigens in vitro and in vivo. PLoS One 6(11), e28217
7. Chakraborty M et al (2004) External beam radiation of tumors alters phenotype of tumor cells to render them susceptible to vaccine-mediated T-cell killing. Cancer Res 64(12):4328–4337
8. Matsumura S, Demaria S (2010) Up-regulation of the pro-inflammatory chemokine CXCL16 is a common response of tumor cells to ionizing radiation. Radiat Res 173(4):418–425
9. Formenti SC, Demaria S (2013) Combining radiotherapy and cancer immunotherapy: a paradigm shift. J Natl Cancer Inst 105(4):256–265

10. Sharma P, Allison JP (2015) The future of immune checkpoint therapy. Science 348(6230): 56–61
11. Golden EB et al (2012) The convergence of radiation and immunogenic cell death signaling pathways. Front Oncol 2:88
12. Burnette B, Weichselbaum RR (2013) Radiation as an immune modulator. Semin Radiat Oncol 23(4):273–280
13. Demaria S et al (2004) Ionizing radiation inhibition of distant untreated tumors (abscopal effect) is immune mediated. Int J Radiat Oncol Biol Phys 58(3):862–870
14. Vinay DS, Kwon BS (2012) Immunotherapy of cancer with 4-1BB. Mol Cancer Ther 11(5):1062–1070
15. Shi W, Siemann DW (2006) Augmented antitumor effects of radiation therapy by 4-1BB antibody (BMS-469492) treatment. Anticancer Res 26(5A):3445–3453
16. Newcomb EW et al (2010) Radiotherapy enhances antitumor effect of anti-CD137 therapy in a mouse Glioma model. Radiat Res 173(4):426–432
17. Weinberg AD et al (2011) Science gone translational: the OX40 agonist story. Immunol Rev 244(1):218–231
18. Yokouchi H et al (2008) Anti-OX40 monoclonal antibody therapy in combination with radiotherapy results in therapeutic antitumor immunity to murine lung cancer. Cancer Sci 99(2): 361–367
19. Gough MJ et al (2010) Adjuvant therapy with agonistic antibodies to CD134 (OX40) increases local control after surgical or radiation therapy of cancer in mice. J Immunother 33(8): 798–809
20. Schaer DA, Hirschhorn-Cymerman D, Wolchok JD (2014) Targeting tumor-necrosis factor receptor pathways for tumor immunotherapy. J Immunother Cancer 2:7
21. Yoshimoto Y et al (2014) Radiotherapy-induced anti-tumor immunity contributes to the therapeutic efficacy of irradiation and can be augmented by CTLA-4 blockade in a mouse model. PLoS One 9(3), e92572
22. Moran AE, Kovacsovics-Bankowski M, Weinberg AD (2013) The TNFRs OX40, 4-1BB, and CD40 as targets for cancer immunotherapy. Curr Opin Immunol 25(2):230–237
23. Honeychurch J et al (2003) Anti-CD40 monoclonal antibody therapy in combination with irradiation results in a CD8 T-cell-dependent immunity to B-cell lymphoma. Blood 102(4): 1449–1457
24. Verbrugge I et al (2012) Radiotherapy increases the permissiveness of established mammary tumors to rejection by immunomodulatory antibodies. Cancer Res 72(13):3163–3174
25. Leach DR, Krummel MF, Allison JP (1996) Enhancement of antitumor immunity by CTLA-4 blockade. Science 271(5256):1734–1736
26. Demaria S et al (2005) Immune-mediated inhibition of metastases after treatment with local radiation and CTLA-4 blockade in a mouse model of breast cancer. Clin Cancer Res 11(2 Pt 1):728–734
27. Dewan MZ et al (2009) Fractionated but not single-dose radiotherapy induces an immune-mediated abscopal effect when combined with anti-CTLA-4 antibody. Clin Cancer Res 15(17):5379–5388
28. Wu L et al (2015) Targeting the inhibitory receptor CTLA-4 on T cells increased abscopal effects in murine mesothelioma model. Oncotarget 6(14):12468–12480
29. Son CH et al (2014) CTLA-4 blockade enhances antitumor immunity of intratumoral injection of immature dendritic cells into irradiated tumor in a mouse colon cancer model. J Immunother 37(1):1–7
30. Nirschl CJ, Drake CG (2013) Molecular pathways: coexpression of immune checkpoint molecules: signaling pathways and implications for cancer immunotherapy. Clin Cancer Res 19(18):4917–4924
31. Topalian SL, Drake CG, Pardoll DM (2012) Targeting the PD-1/B7-H1(PD-L1) pathway to activate anti-tumor immunity. Curr Opin Immunol 24(2):207–212

32. Zeng J et al (2013) Anti-PD-1 blockade and stereotactic radiation produce long-term survival in mice with intracranial gliomas. Int J Radiat Oncol Biol Phys 86(2):343–349
33. Sharabi AB et al (2015) Stereotactic radiation therapy augments antigen-specific PD-1-mediated antitumor immune responses via cross-presentation of tumor antigen. Cancer Immunol Res 3(4):345–355
34. Park SS et al (2015) PD-1 restrains radiotherapy-induced abscopal effect. Cancer Immunol Res 3(6):610–619
35. Deng L et al (2014) Irradiation and anti-PD-L1 treatment synergistically promote antitumor immunity in mice. J Clin Invest 124(2):687–695
36. Dovedi SJ et al (2014) Acquired resistance to fractionated radiotherapy can be overcome by concurrent PD-L1 blockade. Cancer Res 74(19):5458–5468
37. Twyman-Saint Victor C et al (2015) Radiation and dual checkpoint blockade activate non-redundant immune mechanisms in cancer. Nature 520(7547):373–377
38. Belcaid Z et al (2014) Focal radiation therapy combined with 4-1BB activation and CTLA-4 blockade yields long-term survival and a protective antigen-specific memory response in a murine glioma model. PLoS One 9(7), e101764
39. Jing W et al (2015) Combined immune checkpoint protein blockade and low dose whole body irradiation as immunotherapy for myeloma. J Immunother Cancer 3(1):2

Chapter 8
Stereotactic Body Radiation Therapy (SBRT) or Alternative Fractionation Schedules

Aaron M. Laine, Zabi Wardak, Michael R. Folkert, and Robert D. Timmerman

Abstract The use of hypofractionated regimens for the treatment of tumors with radiation has come full circle. After the discovery of X-rays and their utilization for cancer treatment, the initial fractionation schemes were primarily hypofractionated in nature. However, due to technical limitations and associated toxicities, more protracted fractionated regimens eventually became the foundation for modern radiation therapy. With the advance of imaging and radiation delivery systems, interest in more hypofractionated approaches was revived. Stereotactic ablative radiation therapy (SABR; also referred as stereotactic body radiation therapy, SBRT) is the most abbreviated form of hypofractionation, typically utilizing 1–5 fractions for treatment. Its strengths include high rates of tumor control via a convenient, noninvasive outpatient procedure. Toxicities related to high, ablative radiation doses still are a potential concern; however, recent clinical trials for a variety of tumor sites have shown good outcomes in properly selected patients. This chapter will discuss the potential for SBRT/SABR to improve the therapeutic response. The use of SBRT/SABR regimens to treat lesions within the lung, liver, spine, and prostate will be reviewed. Due to more mature data in regard to the safety and efficacy, cost-effectiveness of the treatment, and potential for immunomodulatory effects, SBRT/SABR has become more wildly utilized in cancer treatment.

A.M. Laine • Z. Wardak • M.R. Folkert
Department of Radiation Oncology, Simmons Comprehensive Cancer Center,
UT Southwestern Medical Center, 5323 Harry Hines Blvd, Dallas, TX 75235, USA
e-mail: aaron.laine@utsouthwestern.edu; zabi.wardak@utsouthwestern.edu;
michael.folkert@utsouthwestern.edu

R.D. Timmerman (✉)
Department of Radiation Oncology, Simmons Comprehensive Cancer Center,
UT Southwestern Medical Center, 5323 Harry Hines Blvd, Dallas, TX 75235, USA

Departments of Radiation Oncology and Neurological Surgery, Simmons Comprehensive
Cancer Center, UT Southwestern Medical Center, 5323 Harry Hines Blvd, Dallas,
TX 75235, USA
e-mail: robert.timmerman@utsouthwestern.edu

© Springer International Publishing Switzerland 2017
P.J. Tofilon, K. Camphausen (eds.), *Increasing the Therapeutic
Ratio of Radiotherapy*, Cancer Drug Discovery and Development,
DOI 10.1007/978-3-319-40854-5_8

Keywords Stereotactic radiation • Stereotactic ablative therapy • SABR • SBRT • Therapeutic ratio • Lung radiation • Liver radiation • Spine radiation • Prostate radiation

Stereotactic Body Radiation Therapy (SBRT) or Stereotactic Ablative Body Radiosurgery (SABR)

Introduction

After the discovery of X-rays in 1895 and radioactivity in 1896, initial radiation cancer treatments were mostly hypofractionated. Treatments were limited in giving higher doses to the skin and superficial structures than to a deeper tumor target. Quality assurance measures were lacking to ensure accurate dose deposition. These approaches lead to tumor responses, however, with significant late tissue effects. Despite these limitations, hypofractionation remained the primary treatment schedule due to patient convenience and technical considerations with treatment delivery.

Early radiotherapy pioneers, including Friedrich Dessauer, identified the problems with the state of technology for delivering hypofractionated treatments. In 1905, Dessauer proposed that improvements could be achieved with the application of homogeneous dose to the tissue and eventually leading to the formulation of ideas of multibeam or multisource irradiation [1].

At the same time, Claudius Regaud was performing his seminal experiments relating to the irradiation of the testis. He observed that cells undergoing mitosis were more sensitive to radiation, whereas the more differentiated cells were less sensitive [2]. This work led to the "Law of Bergonie and Tribondeau" stating that the effects of irradiation on cells are more intense the greater their reproductive activity, the longer their mitotic phases, and the less differentiated, forming the biological basis for fractionation [3].

In 1932, Henri Coutard presented his groundbreaking findings at the American Congress of Roentgenology demonstrating that protracted fractionated radiotherapy had cured deep tumors with significantly less toxicity previously seen [4]. Afterward, radiation oncologists across the world mostly abandoned hypofractionated as a method for curative treatment. Interestingly, Coutard believed in both approaches stating that choice of fractionation should depend on the initial volume of the target (small targets warrant hypofractionation, whereas large should be more protracted) [5].

It took until the 1950s when Lars Leksell broke from the perceived rationale of conventionally fractionated radiotherapy (CFRT) by using large-dose single sessions of radiation delivery in the central nervous system [6]. Although a single large-dose radiation treatment was historically prohibitive, Leksell's approach defied conventional wisdom by its technology and administration. Unlike CFRT, which often irradiates much larger volumes of normal tissue to the prescription dose than the tumor itself, Leksell's stereotactic radiosurgery (SRS) went to great lengths to avoid delivering high dose to nontargeted normal tissues. Whatever normal tissue was included, either by being adjacent to the target or by inferior dosimetry, was likely damaged. However, if this damaged tissue was small in volume or noneloquent, the patient did not suffer clinically apparent toxicity, even as a late event.

Building upon these results, Lax and Blomgren at the Karolinska Institutet in Sweden separated from the established traditions of CFRT and began to explore the use of alternative hypofractionated radiation treatment regimens for lung, liver, and selected other malignant extracranial tumors. They constructed a stereotactic body frame that would simultaneously enable comfortable and reliable immobilization and dampening of respiratory motion treating patients with extracranial, localized tumors with ablative doses of radiation that ranged from 7.7 to 45 Gy in 1–4 fractions [7]. At the same time in Japan, Uematsu and colleagues developed technologies to deliver stereotactic radiation to lung tumors [8]. Initially the treatments were called extracranial stereotactic radioablation and later stereotactic body radiation therapy (SBRT) [9, 10]. More recently, the descriptive term stereotactic ablative radiotherapy (SABR) has been used [11].

Defining characteristics of SBRT/SABR include the following [12]: (1) secure immobilization avoiding patient movement for the typical long treatment sessions; (2) accurate repositioning from simulation to treatment; (3) minimization of normal tissue exposure attained by using multiple (e.g., 10 or more) or large-angle arcing small aperture fields; (4) rigorous accounting of organ motion; (5) stereotactic registration (i.e., via fiducial markers or surrogates) of tumor targets and normal tissue avoidance structures to the treatment delivery machine; and (6) ablative dose fractionation delivered to the patient with subcentimeter accuracy.

Radiobiological Modeling of SBRT/SABR

Classical understanding of the mechanisms of radiation-induced tumor cell killing centers on the hypothesis that DNA is the main target of ionizing radiation, leading to single- and double-strand breaks. Different mathematical models have been developed to compare tumor control and normal tissue toxicity profiles for various radiation schedules and fraction sizes. Since the development of the linear-quadratic (LQ) formalism by Lea and Catcheside to describe the relationship between radiation dose and the incidence of chromosomal translocations, it has served as the primary basis for modeling radiation dose effects [13]. The LQ model describes cell killing as a single-hit versus double-hit hypothesis, where the linear cell kill is expressed by the α component, while the quadratic cell kill is expressed by the β component [14]. The α/β ratio is obtained from isoeffect curves using the survival fractions of a cell line at different doses per fraction [15]. This ratio is primarily utilized to predict the clinical effects in response to changes in fraction size. With regard to tumors, a high α/β ratio predicts higher sensitivity to CFRT, while a lower α/β ratio predicts lower sensitivity to CFRT. Most tumors typically possess a high α/β ratio (approximately 8–10) relative to most normal tissues, which demonstrate lower α/β ratios (approximately 1–4).

Not all hypofractionated radiotherapy is ablative. In general, ablation occurs at dose levels that correspond to the exponential (linear region on a logarithmic scale) portion of the cell survival curve, which would generally involve daily dose levels of >8 Gy. Below this dose range, cells have more capacity to repair. The logarithm of cell survival as a function of dose in the lower-dose region exhibits a curviness called the shoulder. More conventional and nonablative hypofractionated radiotherapy is delivered on the shoulder. The range of 2.25–8 Gy per fraction, still considered hypofractionated, has mostly been used for palliation of metastatic disease. More recently, though, investigators treating common diseases like breast and prostate cancer have used nonablative hypofractionation in patients with curable tumors. This was partly for the cost savings associated with fewer overall fractions, but in some cases, such hypofractionation has a biological rationale for improving the therapeutic ratio.

Based on experimental and clinical data, the LQ model seems to predict biological effective dose (BED) accurately for fraction sizes less than 3.25 Gy [16]. Due to the fact that typical doses for SBRT/SABR fall outside of this range, the LQ model breaks down as does not accurately predict the BED for extremely hypofractionated regimens [16–19]. The development of more accurate models to predict the responses of tumors to hypofractionated radiotherapy has been attempted. The universal survival curve, modified linear-quadratic model (LQL), and the generalized linear-quadratic model all have shown better radiobiological modeling of high dose per fraction than the LQ model, with moderate success at maintaining accuracy within the conventionally fractionated range [16, 18, 20]. In an attempt to address this discrepancy, a universal survival curve was constructed which hybridized the LQ model and the multitarget model [20]. The multitarget model better describes the survival curve for ablative doses beyond the shoulder or the transition dose D_T. These models primarily predict the tumor control to hypofractionated radiotherapy; however, better estimation of normal tissue toxicity with larger doses per fraction is required.

Limitations to predict clinically relevant endpoints exist in simple radiobiological modeling due to the presence of additional factors, including dose rate, period of time over which treatment is delivered, tissue type irradiated, and competing cell death mechanisms besides DNA damage. These may include immunological activation mediated by the release of antigens, damage to cell membranes and organelles, and additional mechanisms related to ablative therapy [21].

Several groups have described tissues and their radiation response according to the organization of the smallest functional subunit [22, 23]. Structurally defined tissues can only repair radiation damage by recruiting their own stem cells and have a lower radiation tolerance per functional subunit. Generally, organs comprised of such structurally defined subunits, also called parallel functioning tissues, and are large organs like the peripheral lung and liver. Parallel organs display significant redundancy in the number of subunits performing the same function to overcome the poor tolerance to damage. In contrast, tissues made up predominately of structurally undefined subunits are much more tolerant of radiation damage per subunit because of their ability to recruit clonogenic cells from neighboring tissues for repair. Organs made up of structurally undefined subunits like the esophagus, major ducts and airways, and spinal cord are referred as serially functioning tissues and perform critical functions acting as a conduit. Despite possessing a higher radiation tolerance, if a section of a serially functioning tissue is damage anywhere along its length, all downstream function may be effected [12]. The potential to elicit such tissue injury when utilizing ablative doses is a major consideration needed to be taken into account when developing treatment plans.

The underpinning of radiobiological understanding of radiation therapy is based on the differences of chromosomal damage within tumor versus normal cells resulting from the relatively homogenous dose exposures of CFRT. It could then be expected that the large dose per fraction associated with SBRT/SABR would cause tremendous DNA damage within any tissue exposed to this dose. Therefore as mentioned above, it is critical to geometrically partition the dose levels received by the tumor and normal tissues. Additionally, SBRT/SABR dose distributions are typically engineered to be heterogeneous, allowing large variations of dose between tumor, adjacent normal tissue, and more removed normal tissues. Due to this dose variability, comparisons between SBRT/SABR and CFRT can become complicated [24].

Immunological Effects of Ablative Radiation

In addition to the DNA damage effects described above, a high intratumoral dose achieved with SBRT/SABR might optimize antitumor mechanisms by stimulating local and direct immune responses in the local microenvironment and antigen-presenting cells (APCs) [25]. High-dose-per-fraction radiation (>8 Gy per treatment fraction) may also generate stromal effects that are not accounted for in traditional radiobiological modeling [26, 27]. It has been suggested that higher doses per fraction result in increased tumor endothelial apoptosis and vascular damage, a phenomenon seen only in high-dose-per-fraction treatment schedules, may contribute significantly to cell kill [26, 28]. Relatively radiation-insensitive tumor stem cells may also compromise the ability of low-dose fractions to achieve durable tumor control; it has been hypothesized that higher doses per fraction can overcome these cells' ability to repair sublethal damage [29]. Higher doses per fraction, as opposed to conventional 2 Gy doses, can also prime T cells in lymphatic tissue, leading to more significant CD8+ T-cell-dependent eradication of disease, as well as the induction and expression of effector cytokines and other inflammatory mediators [30]. Such a pro-inflammatory environment laden with cytokine production can increase permeability of local vasculature and stimulate APCs to mature more effectively. More recently, increased interest in the potential ability of SBRT/SABR to promote an abscopal response in conjunction with immunomodulatory agents has been investigated. Two case reports of combination SBRT/SABR and ipilimumab (anti-CTLA-4) have shown abscopal effects in metastatic melanoma and non-small cell lung cancer [31, 32]. A Phase I trial of SBRT/SABR and high-dose interleukin-2 for patients with metastatic melanoma or renal cell carcinoma revealed abscopal responses in several patients [33]. The combination of greater degree and/or different modes of DNA damage as well as injury to the tumor microenvironment arising from the use of hypofractionated or single-fraction radiation therapy may work synergistically to cause irreparable and lethal injuries to the irradiated cells [28, 34, 35].

SBRT/SABR for Primary Management of NSCLC

Lung cancer is the second most diagnosed cancer and the leading cause of cancer-related mortality in the United States [36]. Of patients newly diagnosed with non-small cell lung cancer (NSCLC), 15–20 % are found to have stage I disease [37]. Surgical resection is the treatment of choice for these patients. However, up to 30 % are deemed inoperable because of comorbidities [38]. SBRT/SABR has proven efficacy in the treatment of patients with early-stage, medically inoperable NSCLC [39, 40] with an emerging indication in the setting of limited metastatic disease [41–52].

For patients with medically inoperable NSCLC, dose escalation using conventional fractionation was initially explored to improve the probability of local control. Radiation Therapy Oncology Group (RTOG) Protocol 7301 investigated multiple dosing regimens for patients with T1-3 N0-2 disease, including 40 Gy delivered in a split regimen of two courses of 20 Gy delivered in 5 fractions (40 Gy total in 10 fractions) with a 2-week break between courses, and continuous regiments escalating the dose from 40 to 60 Gy. The failure rate within the irradiated volume was 48 % in the 40 Gy continuous regimen, 38 % for the 40 Gy split course and 50 Gy regimen, and 27 % in the 60 Gy continuous regimen [53]. RTOG Protocol 9311 then escalated doses from 65 to 90.3 Gy using 3D conformal radiation therapy in inoperable patients and found that treatment could safely be delivered in daily fraction sizes of 2.15 Gy to a total dose of 77.4 Gy or 83.8 Gy provided that the volume of the lung receiving 20 Gy could be constrained to less than 25 % of the total lung volume. The study attained locoregional control rates at 2 years of 55–78 % at the MTD [54].

A later dose-escalation study conducted by Rosenzweig et al. treated patients with inoperable NSCLC using 3D conformal radiation therapy, with fraction sizes of 1.8 Gy for doses ≤81 Gy and 2 Gy for doses >81 Gy. Dose-escalation levels included 70.2, 75.6, 81.0, 84.0, and 90 Gy; unacceptable pulmonary toxicity occurred at 90 Gy, and the maximum tolerated dose (MTD) was established at 84 Gy [55]. Long-term results of this study were reported by Sura et al. and included 55 patients with stage I/II disease. They demonstrated that treating the primary lesion with escalated doses >80 Gy in 2 Gy fractions resulted in 5-year local control (LC) and overall survival (OS) outcomes of 67 % and 36 %, respectively [56].

In order to continue to improve LC and OS in this patient population, protocols have sought to improve the therapeutic ratio with the addition of chemotherapy or by changing the dose per fraction. Researchers at Indiana University reported a

Phase I study in which patients with T1–T2 N0 NSCLC were treated with escalating doses of SBRT/SABR, starting at 24 Gy in 3 fractions and increasing to 60 Gy (for T1 lesions) or 72 Gy (for T2 lesions) in 3 fractions to determine the maximum tolerated dose (MTD). The MTD was not reached for T1 lesions at 60 Gy, and for T2 lesions an MTD of 66 Gy was established based on bronchitis, pericardial effusion, hypoxia, and pneumonitis. Crude rates of local failure were 21 % in both the T1 and T2 cohorts, and a dose response was noted with only one local failure observed with fraction sizes of >16 Gy per fraction [10, 39]. These doses were calculated without correction for tissue inhomogeneity; subsequent doses used inhomogeneity correction and as a result appear slightly lower.

A subsequent Phase II multicenter trial (RTOG 0236) further evaluated the toxicity and efficacy of stereotactic body radiation therapy in a high-risk population of patients with T1-2aN0 (lesions <5 cm in size) early-stage, medically inoperable NSCLC. Doses of 54 Gy in 3 fractions were delivered, and an estimated 3-year local control rate of 97.6 % was observed, with an overall survival rate of 55.8 % at 3 years [40]. Based on this study, stereotactic body radiotherapy (SBRT) is now the standard of care for medically inoperable early-stage non-small cell lung cancer (NSCLC) or those patients who refuse surgery. Further work is being done to optimize dose delivery for early-stage NSCLC; the RTOG conducted RTOG Protocol 0915, a randomized Phase II study that compared two different SBRT/SABR treatment schedules for medically inoperable patients with stage I peripheral NSCLC, in which patients were randomized to receive 34 Gy in a single fraction or 48 Gy in four daily consecutive fractions of 12 Gy per fraction. This protocol is now closed to accrual, and final results are pending; preliminary data suggest that 34 Gy may be more efficacious with respect to local control and equivalent in toxicity profile, and a comparison of 34 Gy in one fraction to 54 Gy in 3 fractions is planned.

Continued evaluation of dose response outside of trials has been performed. In a review of the National Cancer Data Base (NCDB), 498 patients were identified and evaluated for response to SBRT/SABR. These patients were treated with a range of dosing regimens, with the most common being 60 Gy in 3 fractions, 48 Gy in 4 fractions, 54 Gy in 3 fractions, 45 Gy in 3 fractions, and 48 Gy in 3 fractions. Outcomes were evaluated with respect to biologically effective dose (BED) [57], which is calculated according to the simplified formula:

$$BED = nd\left(1 + d/\left(\alpha/\beta\right)\right)$$

where n = number of treatment fractions, d = dose per fraction, and α/β is the ratio of the linear and quadratic components of the cell survival curve; for the purposes of their study, an α/β ratio of 10 was assumed. For example, a regimen of 54 Gy in 3 fractions would have a BED of $18 \times 3 \times \left(1 + 18/10\right)$ or 151.2. They found that increasing BED to doses >150 Gy equivalent was associated with improved survival in patients undergoing SBRT/SABR for larger (T2) tumors [58].

While local control rates with SBRT/SABR in early-stage NSCLC are excellent [40, 59], distant failure is common, occurring in 20–30 % of patients in 3–5 years [40, 60–62]. Future efforts in the treatment of early-stage NSCLC will naturally include optimization of treatment delivery to safely and accurately deliver ablative doses to tumor while limiting normal tissue toxicity, but it is likely that incorporation of appropriately timed and administered cytotoxic, targeted, and immunotherapy-based treatments will be required to optimize outcomes in terms of out-of-field tumor recurrence and overall patient survival after SBRT/SABR.

Specific Issues Associated with SBRT/SABR for Targets in the Lung

Escalating the dose to the target in the lung has been shown to be effective in terms of killing the tumor cells, but the normal nearby tissues must be taken into account; tumor control does come at a price. The lung may be considered both a parallel and serial organ, in that there is some redundancy due to its paired nature and parenchymal reserve, but injury to a central structure may impair function of a large downstream volume; one aspect of this is the proximal bronchial tree. Ablative doses given to a very proximal branch of the airway could cause injury that impairs downstream function and lead to significant patient pulmonary toxicity; additionally, large vessels run in close approximation to these large branches and could also potentially be a target for injury. In a study by Timmerman et al., building on an earlier dose-escalation study [10], 70 patients with T1-2 N0 medical inoperable NSCLC were treated with either 60 Gy in 3 fractions (for T1 disease) or 66 Gy in 3 fractions (for T2 disease); these doses were also calculated without correction for tissue inhomogeneity, and there was no restriction on tumor location. Local tumor control remained very high, 95 % at 2 years; however, on follow-up, eight patients had serious grade 3 or 4 toxicities (declining pulmonary function, pneumonia, effusion, apnea), and six patients died of possible grade 5 toxicities, including one fatal hemoptysis four infectious pneumonias, and one pericardial effusion. Tumor location was associated with severe toxicity, and this study identified that dose delivery to targets overlapping the proximal bronchial tree with a 2 cm expansion (consisting of the carina, the right and left main bronchi, the right and left upper lobe bronchi, the bronchus intermedius, the right middle lobe bronchus the lingular bronchus;, and the right and left lower lobe bronchi) was most predictive of serious adverse effects. This area was defined as a "no-fly zone" for SBRT/SABR in the lung of very high fraction sizes (>10 Gy per fraction) [63].

Effective dose delivery for patients with "central tumors" is an area of active investigation. The RTOG recently closed RTOG Protocol 0813, which was a Phase I/II study of SBRT/SABR for the treatment of early-stage, centrally located NSCLC in medically inoperable patients. They defined central tumors as those with any overlap with a 2 cm expansion from the previously defined proximal bronchial tree, as well as any lesions adjacent to the mediastinal or pericardial pleura. Dose was delivered in 5 fractions every other day, starting at 50 Gy in 5 fractions and escalating to 60 Gy in 5 fractions.

SBRT/SABR for Metastases to the Spine

Radiation therapy has a role in the management of both primary and metastatic lesions of the spine, although the vast preponderance of metastatic disease has led to more extensive research and clinical evaluation of treatment techniques. Metastatic disease in the spine is common, accounting for up to 70% of all metastases to the bone and affecting up to 10% of all cancer patients [35, 64]. Spine involvement can result in back pain (the most common presenting symptom) and deterioration in functional status and quality of life [65]. Compression or invasion of the spinal cord, cauda equina, or exiting nerve roots can lead to disabling or even life-threatening neurological symptoms [66].

Conventionally fractionated radiation therapy for spine metastases is generally a palliative therapy and may not be sufficient alone to restore and maintain neurological function; in a study by Patchell et al., patients with epidural spinal cord compression were randomized to conventional external beam radiation therapy (30 Gy in 10 fractions) alone or direct decompressive surgery followed by radiation therapy. Patients who underwent combined modality treatment had significantly improved neurological outcomes, with more patients able to ambulate after treatment (84% vs 57%, $P=0.001$) and longer sustained ambulatory status (122 days vs 13 days, $P=0.003$). A small survival benefit was also noted (126 days vs 100 days, $P=0.033$) [67]. Conventional external beam therapy has been shown to achieve local control rates range less than 50% [68–71]. Even in the postoperative setting, in a large retrospective study by Klekamp and Samii, patients receiving low-dose conventional external beam radiation therapy following surgery for spinal lesions had documented local failure as high as 58% at 6 months, and these local failures led to neurologic deterioration in 69% of the patients within 1 year and in 96% of patients within 4 years [69].

Multiple studies support the hypothesis that dose escalation, particularly in terms of dose per fraction, improves the likelihood of local control in lesions metastatic to the spine [72–75]. Hartsell et al. conducted a randomized trial in which 898 patients with painful bone lesions (patients with spinal cord or cauda equina compression were excluded) were treated with either 8 Gy in 1 fraction or 30 Gy in 10 fractions. The two regimens were equivalent in terms of pain and narcotic relief at 3 months, with less acute grade 2–4 toxicity in the 8 Gy arm (10% vs 17%); retreatment rates were doubled in the 8 Gy arm (18% vs 9%), suggesting that a single high-dose fraction could provide comparable benefit to a more protracted course [76]. With advances in radiation therapy delivery, fraction sizes above 8 Gy could be delivered to spinal targets while constraining dose to the spinal cord and/or cauda equina [77]. The use of SBRT/SABR techniques with precise target delineation allows for safe delivery of radiation while limiting dose to the nearby spinal cord; techniques for defining the spinal cord vary, with some institutions preferring a CT-myelogram-defined cord immediately prior to simulation [78, 79], while other institutions define the cord on the basis of a registered and fused T1- and T2-weighted MRI, which is the method used in the current RTOG (now NRG Oncology) 0631 protocol.

A more conservative approach pursued at some institutions defines the organ at risk as the entire thecal sac or canal [80]; this approach is often used at the level of the cauda equina [74].

A Phase I/II non-dose-escalating study was performed by Chang et al. using SBRT/SABR for spinal metastasis, pattern of failure analysis. In their initial Phase I report [81], they treated 15 patients with SBRT/SABR to a goal dose of 30 Gy in 5 fractions, constraining the spinal cord to a maximum dose of 10 Gy. Five of the patients treated on the study had been previously irradiated. No neurotoxicity or grade 3–4 toxicities were observed. In the subsequent failure analysis report [82], a total of 63 patients with 74 tumors had been treated to doses of 30 Gy in 5 fractions or 27 Gy in 3 fractions; 1-year freedom from tumor progression was 84%. Of the local recurrences, 47% were located in the epidural space, where effective dose delivery was most constrained by the proximity of the spinal cord [81, 82]. The correlation between failure to deliver maximal dose and increased risk of failure has received attention from multiple investigators. Lovelock et al. [83] reported a study of dosimetric coverage of target lesions and found that portions of gross tumor volumes (GTV) receiving less than 15 Gy were at highest risk of failure. These deficits in GTV dosimetry were often due to constraints placed on the radiation treatment planning process in terms of the maximum dose (D_{max}) permitted to the spinal cord.

A dose-escalation protocol initiated at Memorial Sloan Kettering Cancer Center (MSKCC) using image-guided single-fraction high-dose radiotherapy for metastatic disease established 24 Gy to the planning target volume (PTV) as an effective dose to achieve 85–95% tumor control for spine lesions, osseous metastases, and soft-tissue/lymph node metastatic deposits (MSKCC Protocol 06-101) [77, 84]. Yamada et al. reported on 93 patients with 103 spinal metastases treated with 18–24 Gy in a single fraction. Using this regimen, 90% overall actuarial local control was achieved at a median follow-up of 15 months; patients treated with the highest dose level of 24 Gy had superior local control (95% vs 80% for single-fraction treatments <24 Gy) [77].

Some tumors, such as renal carcinoma and sarcoma, have been shown to be less sensitive to fractionated radiation than other histologies and also have limited systemic treatment options. These tumor histologies provide a particularly useful model for testing the efficacy of SBRT/SABR, as local control outcomes are not confounded by competing therapies [85]. Zelefsky et al. reported on tumor control outcomes after hypofractionated and single-dose SBRT/SABR for extracranial metastases from renal cell carcinoma; of the 105 lesions treated on the study, 59 (56%) were located in the spine. For patients who received 24 Gy in a single fraction, 3-year local progression free survival was 88%; for patients receiving single fractions of less than 24 Gy or hypofractionated regimens of 24–30 Gy in 3–5 fractions, 3-year local progression free survival was 21% and 17%, respectively [75]. Folkert et al. reported on 88 patients with 120 discrete metastases from high-grade sarcoma to the spine, treated with hypofractionated or single-fraction SBRT/SABR. Local control at 12 months was 88%, with single-fraction treatments of 24 Gy having superior outcomes (1-year local control of 91%, compared to 84% for hypofractionated courses of 24–26 Gy in 3–6 fractions) [73].

A currently open RTOG trial, RTOG 0631 (NCI designation NCT00922974), is comparing the relative benefit of 2 single-fraction regimens: 8 Gy in 1 fraction delivered with conventional techniques and 16–18 Gy delivered in 1 fraction using SBRT/SABR techniques. Clinical response, in terms of pain reduction at 3 months, is the primary objective of the Phase III portion of the study. Initial Phase II results have been published demonstrating the feasibility and reproducibility of the technique [86]; while local control outcomes are not a specific objective of the study, the potential exists to provide a direct comparison of objective radiographic response to low- and high-dose single-fraction regimens.

Specific Issues Associated with SBRT/SABR for Targets in the Spine

Treatment of targets in the spine can be particularly complex as the spine circumferentially encloses critical neural structures. A critical toxicity that must be taken into account with treatments affecting the spinal cord is radiation myelitis. Radiation myelopathy is defined as clinical signs and/or symptoms of sensory or motor deficits, with progressive loss of function or neuropathic pain, referable to a level of the spinal cord treated by radiation therapy and confirmed by radiographic means [87–89].

The generally accepted dose limit for the spinal cord is 45 Gy at 1.8–2.0 Gy/fraction [89]; 50 Gy is observed in otherwise healthy patients treated with curative intent where the tumor location prohibits limiting the cord to a lower dose, with an attendant 5 % risk of myelopathy at 5 years [87, 89]. For patients undergoing high-dose spinal cord radiosurgical procedures, spinal cord tolerance is defined as a cord maximal dose of 14 Gy or less than 10 Gy to 10 % volume of the spinal cord per level [77, 90]. In the event of failure, these limitations may preclude or impair the ability of radiation oncologists to offer effective salvage therapy with external beam techniques. Toxicity resulting from repeat irradiation is a subject of open investigation, with thresholds of 100–135 Gy in biologically effective dose (BED) proposed for late complications due to repeat irradiation of the spinal cord [91–93]. Outcomes were evaluated with respect to biologically effective dose (BED) [57], which is calculated according to the simplified formula:

$$ BED = nd\left(1 + d/\left(\alpha/\beta\right)\right) $$

where n = number of treatment fractions, d = dose per fraction, and α/β is the ratio of the linear and quadratic components of the cell survival curve; for the purposes of spine irradiation, an α/β ratio of 2 may be assumed. For example, a tolerance dose of 14 Gy in 1 fraction would have a BED of $14 * 1 * \left(1 + 14/2\right)$ or 112 Gy.

Preclinical data exists in swine models, as well as several published institutional experiences with multiply irradiated patients, that suggests that the tolerance of the human spinal cord to re-irradiation may be greater than currently assumed and practiced. A study by Medin et al. [94] used a swine model in which two sets of pigs underwent single-fraction SRS at a series of increasing spinal cord D_{max} (approximately 15, 17, 19, 21, 23, and 25 Gy); one set had previously undergone irradiation of the spinal cord 1 year prior to SBRT/SABR, receiving 30 Gy in 10 fractions (BED = 75 Gy). No differences in the rates of spinal cord injury were noted in the previously irradiated swine cohort compared to the unirradiated cohort, and no neurologic injuries were noted at spinal cord D_{max} <18.8 Gy. In humans, Katsoulakis et al. [95] studied a cohort of ten patients treated with three courses of radiation to the same site in the spine; the median spinal cord total D_{max} BED for the cohort was 141.5 Gy BED (range 103.8–203.4 Gy BED). In this cohort, no cases of clinical radiation myelopathy were observed with a median total follow-up of 40 months from the first course of radiation and 12 months from the third course of radiation. Additionally, no MRI spinal cord signal changes were noted.

Determining the re-irradiation tolerance of the spinal cord is the objective of a prospective Phase I clinical trial investigating the use of single-fraction re-irradiation following local progression of mobile spine and sacral lesions that have previously received radiation therapy. Patients on this trial will be treated with single-fraction SBRT/SABR at three cord tolerance levels, starting with a spinal cord/cauda D_{max} of 14 Gy, escalating to 16 and then 18 Gy (NCI designation NCT02278744).

SBRT/SABR for Primary Liver Cancer

Hepatocellular carcinoma (HCC) is the sixth most common cancer worldwide and the third most common cause of cancer death [96]. Hepatocellular carcinoma most commonly arises within a background of chronic liver disease [97], and the most common risk factors for the development of HCC are alcohol use and viral infection with hepatitis B and/or hepatitis C [98]. In the United States, the incidence will continue to rise dramatically necessitating early diagnosis and definitive therapy [99]. Due to the increasing incidence of HCC, routine surveillance strategies are in place which allow for earlier detection of disease in patients at high risk [100].

The current treatment schema for patients with HCC is defined by the Barcelona Clinic Liver Cancer (BCLC) strategy. This takes into account the quantity of tumors, the size of tumors, Child-Pugh's score, and extent of invasion [101]. Potentially curative treatment for patients with HCC can be performed with orthotopic liver transplantation (OLT), which treats both the underlying cirrhosis as well as the malignancy. Candidacy for liver transplantation is based on patients with early-stage disease, consisting of Child-Pugh score A–B, a single nodule <5 cm or 3 nodules <3 cm, and candidacy for transplantation.

Aside from OLT, surgical resection and percutaneous ablation are the treatments which provided the highest potential of cure [100]. Percutaneous radiofrequency ablation is the treatment of choice for patients not candidates for surgical resection. During treatment, the tumor and a margin of adjacent hepatic tissue are treated with results as effective as resection for small, solitary nodules of HCC [102]. Transarterial chemoembolization is a procedure which takes advantage of the dual blood supply of the liver to deliver antineoplastics plus a gelatin sponge to arterial vasculature supplying the tumor [103]. The seminal meta-analysis of TACE versus systemic therapy found an improvement in the 2-year survival rate [104], and it is recommended for patients with BCLC intermediate-stage disease.

For patients with BCLC early-stage disease, SBRT/SABR can be considered as an alternative for patients not amenable to RFA due to tumor size or proximity to vessels. A substantial proportion of patients present with disease outside of transplant criteria or will progress outside of transplant criteria while on the waiting list, which necessitates the need for "bridging" therapies. It is here where modalities for downstaging or bridging can be aided by the utilization of SBRT/SABR. Furthermore, among patients with BCLC intermediate-stage disease, SBRT/SABR can be used following failure of TACE or as an alternative for TACE in patients who are not candidates for therapy. Follow-up of patients treated with SBRT/SABR with HCC includes dedicated liver imaging, ideally with MRI. There is considerable work being performed on characterizing imaging features in the cirrhotic liver post-SBRT/SABR, with Fig. 8.1 showing features of a treated lesion.

Our commonly utilized dose regimen for patients with HCC is based on the Indiana University experience. In a Phase I feasibility trial, patients with HCC were treated with dose escalation from 36 Gy in 3 fractions to a total dose of 48 Gy in 3 fractions if dose-limiting toxicities were not suffered [105]. Patients were eligible for this trial if they had Child-Pugh score A or B, a solitary tumor less than 6 cm in size or three lesions with total diameter less than 6 cm, and adequate liver function. In this trial, patients were treated in the Elekta Stereotactic Body Frame with abdominal compression to minimize diaphragmatic motion to less than 0.5 cm.

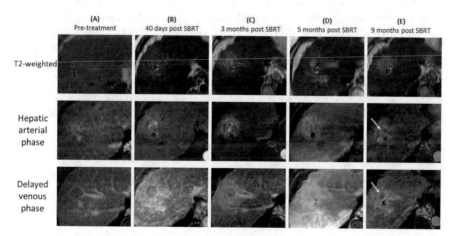

Fig. 8.1 HCC treated with SBRT. Pathognomonic arterial enhancement and venous washout seen pretreatment, which gradually resolved representing tumor response. T2-weighted imaging shows progressive evolution of edema within irradiated volume (**a–e**) [145]

Patients had daily image guidance with cone-beam CT scans prior to the delivery of each fraction. The target volume was delineated based on CT-based imaging, with no clinical target volume expansion and a minimum of 5 mm axial and 10 mm craniocaudal planning target volume expansion. Patients with portal vein thrombosis were allowed on the protocol, and the entire length of the thrombus was treated with a 1 cm margin. Key normal tissue constraints were that 1/3 of the uninvolved liver received less than or equal to 10 Gy for Child-Pugh class A patients and that 1/3 of the uninvolved liver received less than or equal to 15 Gy for Child-Pugh class B patients. Renal constraints included less than 2/3 of the right kidney receiving greater than 15 Gy and 1/3 of the left kidney receiving greater than 15 Gy. The maximum bowel and stomach dose were 12 Gy. In this study, the dose was successfully escalated to patients with Child-Pugh class A to 48 Gy in 3 fractions without reaching dose-limiting toxicity. However, in patients with Child-Pugh class B cirrhosis, the maximum tolerated dose was 40 Gy in 5 fractions due to two patients suffering grade 3 liver toxicity. With long-term follow-up, the Indiana experience found positive rates of 2-year local control of 90 % among the treated population. There were no long-term grade 3 or higher non-hematologic toxicities, and 20 % of patients were found to experience progression in the Child-Pugh score at 3 months [106].

A second key Phase I/II trial was performed by Princess Margaret University and the University of Toronto [107]. In this trial, patients with Child-Pugh score A with no more than five liver tumors with a maximal dimension of 15 cm were enrolled. Patients in this trial were treated to a dose of 30–54 Gy in six fractions, with the maximum effective irradiated liver volume of 60 %. No patients in this trial suffered classic RILD or dose-limiting toxicity, with a decline in Child-Pugh score at 3 months occurring in 29 % of the cohort. Like the Indiana experience, the local tumor control was excellent at 87 % at 1 year. These two trials provide data for the efficacy for SBRT in the setting of well-controlled and designed clinical trials.

While these studies were limited to patients with preserved to mildly elevated liver function, there is evidence for the treatment of patients with Child-Pugh B7 or B8 with SBRT/SABR as well. The Princess Margaret group performed a prospective study with patients with Child-Pugh B7 or 8 with less than 10 cm of HCC tumor [108]. Patients received a median dose of 30 Gy in 5 fractions; however, as expected with their more fragile liver function, 63 % of the cohort had a decline in their Child-Pugh score at 3 months. Sorafenib is a tyrosine kinase inhibitor which is used in patients with advanced HCC, showing an improvement in overall survival compared to placebo. Currently an RTOG trial (RTOG 1112) is enrolling patients with advanced-stage HCC to daily sorafenib versus SBRT/SABR alone followed by daily sorafenib. The primary endpoint of the trial is overall survival with secondary endpoints evaluating the safety profile of SBRT/SABR plus sorafenib. This trial will potentially further expand the utilization of SBRT/SABR patients with advanced HCC.

SBRT/SABR for the Treatment of Liver Metastases

Because of its rich blood supply, hematogenous metastases to the liver are common among patients with solid organ malignancies [109]. Colorectal cancers are the most common primary malignancy to metastasize to the liver due to drainage via the portal circulation, with up to 50 % of patients suffering hepatic metastases within 5 years [110]. A subset of patients with metastatic disease present with oligometastases, a hypothesis popularized in 1995 by Hellman and Weichselbaum. It states that metastatic disease occurs in a stepwise manner, with limited metastases initially followed by progression to widespread disease [111]. Early in the spectrum, metastases may be limited in number and location [112]. Improvements in imaging including PET/CT and MRI have allowed for identification of isolated metastatic deposits with higher sensitivity and specificity than ever before. A significantly greater proportion of patients may be identified early in the metastatic spectrum and offered potentially curative local treatment with liver metastases.

Treatment of oligometastases was first performed via surgical metastasectomy with surgical resection of hepatic, pulmonary, or adrenal metastases having improved rates of survival with resection [113–115]. Furthermore, systemic therapy may convert patients with widely metastatic disease to a limited volume metastatic state, increasing the proportion of patients who may be candidates for early treatment of oligometastatic disease. Surgical metastasectomy is the standard of care in patients who are candidates; however, this is available only to approximately a quarter of patients with hepatic metastases due to the extent of disease or comorbidities [116]. RFA and TACE, much like utilized in hepatocellular carcinoma, are treatment options for patients with hepatic metastases as well.

Noninvasive treatment of hepatic metastases is also possible with external beam radiotherapy. Stereotactic body radiotherapy has allowed the delivery of high doses of therapy in single and multiple fractions with excellent rates of local control. A multi-institutional Phase I/II trial from the University of Colorado enrolled patients with 1–3 liver metastases from any solid tumor, cumulative maximum tumor diameter <6 cm, adequate liver and kidney function, and no chemotherapy 14 days before or after SBRT [47]. In the Phase I portion, the SBRT/SABR dose was escalated from 36 to 60 Gy in 3 fractions. Thirteen patients were treated with a dose of less than 60 Gy and 36 patients treated at 60 Gy, for a total of 63 hepatic lesions. Volume delineation was similar to that in the lung oligometastases trial, with the PTV defined as GTV expanded by 5 mm radially and 10 mm craniocaudally and 7 mm radially and 15 mm craniocaudally, with active breathing control and abdominal compression, respectively. At least 700 cc of normal liver had to receive a total dose <15 Gy, and the sum of the left and right kidney volume receiving 15 Gy had to be less than 35 %. With a median follow-up of 16 months, the 2-year actuarial in-field local control was 92 % with a median overall survival of 20.5 months. Treatment was well tolerated with one patient suffering grade 3 soft-tissue toxicity, no grade 4 or 5 toxicity, and no instances of radiation-induced liver dysfunction (RILD).

Fig. 8.2 Stereotactic body
radiation therapy (SBRT)
of a colorectal liver
metastasis. (**a**) Beam
arrangements for treatment
of liver dome lesion.
Diaphragmatic motion was
limited by the use of a
compression plate on the
abdomen. (**b**) Dose
distributions for treatment
of large lesion in liver
dome in axial, sagittal, and
coronal planes, receiving
35 Gy in a single fraction

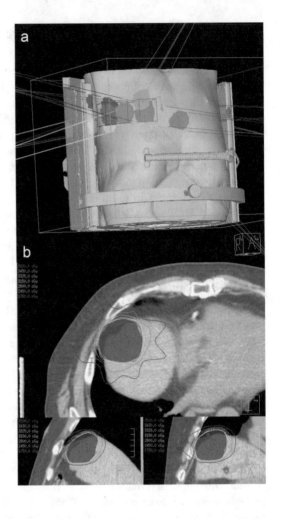

Recently, interest has been increased in the delivery of single-fraction liver
SBRT/SABR. Wulf et al. demonstrated that single-fraction doses of 26 Gy improved
local control at 12 months to approximately 100 % with no grade 3 or higher toxicity [117]. More recently, SBRT/SABR was successfully escalated to 40 Gy in a
single fraction with no grade 3 or higher toxicities related to treatment observed
[118]. Furthermore, the 36-month rate of local control was 100 % showing an excellent opportunity to control liver metastases. Figure 8.2 shows dosimetry and beam
geometry for single-fraction liver SBRT/SABR.

Specific Issues Associated with SBRT/SABR for Targets in the Liver

Liver SBRT/SABR for metastatic disease is often performed in patients without concomitant cirrhosis. Nonetheless, normal liver reserve, much like surgical resection, is a key consideration with treatment planning, with a minimal residual functional volume of approximately 700 cc desired. In patients with HCC, the doses delivered, as seen above, are lower than for metastatic disease due to the sensitive, cirrhotic liver.

Traditional SBRT/SABR is delivered via photon beams with energies between 6 and 18 MV. Patient immobilization is a key factor in the delivery of stereotactic treatment, with stereotactic frames with reference to the stereotactic coordinate system, a commonly utilized system. Motion management for treatment of the liver is essential, given the considerable motion of the organ and diaphragm. During CT simulation, the movement of the dome of the diaphragm should be visualized via fluoroscopy or alternative means with techniques to limit motion including breath-hold and abdominal compression. Target volume delineation of liver lesions is ideally done with registration of an abdominal MRI, done in the treatment planning position with motion management, if possible. Planning can be performed with noncoplanar 3D-conformal techniques, intensity-modulated radiation therapy, or volumetric-modulated arc therapy. Prescription isodose lines covering the PTV are between 60 and 90 %, and suggested dose constraints for adjacent normal structures for 1, 3, and 5 fractions are shown below in Table 8.1.

SBRT/SABR for the Treatment of Prostate Cancer

Prostate cancer is the most common cancer in Western males after non-melanomatous skin cancer [36]. Among males, prostate carcinoma was the second leading cause of cancer mortality behind lung cancer. About 60 % of prostate cancer is diagnosed in men age 65 or older which impacts therapy options as a result of competing comorbidities. With introduction of PSA screening, the majority of prostate cancer is diagnosed in organ-confined disease, which is typically treated with radical prostatectomy or radiotherapy [119]. Dose escalation of conventionally fractionated external beam radiation therapy (CF-EBRT) has demonstrated improved biochemical control and even a survival advantage for patients with intermediate and high-risk disease [120–122]. These results can be achieved with acceptably low toxicity using modern conformal techniques, however, at the increased cost and inconvenience of delivering a large number of fractions, 5 days a week over 8–9 weeks. Additionally, the potential unusual radiobiological characteristics of prostate cancer suggest that it may be more sensitive to larger fractions of radiation. More hypofractionated regimens have been proposed to improve the efficacy and convenience of treatment for prostate cancer.

Table 8.1 Proposed dose constraints for SBRT/SABR treatments of 1, 3, and 5 fractions

Serial tissue	Volume (cc)	Volume max (Gy)	Max point dose (Gy)[a]	Endpoint (≥grade 3)
One fraction				
Spinal cord and medulla	<0.35	10	14	Myelitis
Esophagus[b]	<5	11.9	15.4	Stenosis/fistula
Heart/Pericardium	<15	16	22	Pericarditis
Rib	<5	28	33	Pain or fracture
Skin	<10	25.5	27.5	Ulceration
Stomach	<5	17.4	22	Ulceration/fistula
Bile duct			30	Stenosis
Duodenum[b]	<5	11.2	17	Ulceration
	<10	9		
Jejunum/ileum[b]	<30	12.5	22	Enteritis/obstruction
Colon[b]	<20	18	29.2	Colitis/fistula
Parallel tissue	**Critical volume (cc)**	**Critical volume dose max (Gy)**		
Liver	700	11		Basic liver function
Renal cortex (right and left)	200	9.5		Basic renal function
Serial tissue	**Volume (cc)**	**Volume max (Gy)**		
Three fractions				
Spinal cord and medulla	<0.35	15.9	22.5	Myelitis
Esophagus[b]	<5	17.7	25.2	Stenosis/fistula
Heart/pericardium	<15	24	30	Pericarditis
Rib	<5	40	50	Pain or fracture
Skin	<10	31	33	Ulceration
Stomach	<5	22.5	30	Ulceration/fistula
Bile duct			36	Stenosis
Duodenum[b]	<5	15.6	22.2	Ulceration
	<10	12.9		
Jejunum/ileum[b]	<30	17.4	27	Enteritis/obstruction
Colon[b]	<20	24	34.5	Colitis/fistula
Parallel tissue	**Critical volume (cc)**	**Critical volume dose max (Gy)**		
Liver	700	17.1		Basic liver function
Renal cortex (right and left)	200	15		Basic renal function
Serial tissue	**Volume (cc)**	**Volume max (Gy)**		

(continued)

Table 8.1 (continued)

Serial tissue	Volume (cc)	Volume max (Gy)	Max point dose (Gy)[a]	Endpoint (≥grade 3)
Five fractions				
Spinal cord and medulla	<0.35	22	28	Myelitis
Esophagus[b]	<5	19.5	35	Stenosis/fistula
Heart/pericardium	<15	32	38	Pericarditis
Rib	<5	45	57	Pain or fracture
Skin	<10	36.5	38.5	Ulceration
Stomach	<5	26.5	35	Ulceration/fistula
Bile duct			41	Stenosis
Duodenum[b]	<5	18.5	26	Ulceration
	<10	14.5		
Jejunum/ileum[b]	<30	20	32	Enteritis/obstruction
Colon[b]	<20	28.5	40	Colitis/fistula
Parallel tissue	**Critical volume (cc)**	**Critical volume dose max (Gy)**		
Liver	700	21		Basic liver function
Renal cortex (right and left)	200	18		Basic renal function

[a]"Point" defined as 0.035 cc or less
[b]Avoid circumferential irradiation

CF-EBRT schemes employing fraction sizes of 1.8–2.0 Gy are based on the premise that tumors are less responsive to faction size than are late-responding normal tissues. The α/β ratio is a measure of fractionation response with low ratio typically associated with late-responding tissues (normal tissues) and higher ratios associated with acute-responding tissues (tumors). Convention states that a low α/β ratio is consistent with a higher capacity for repair between fractions with an accompanying greater relative sparing with smaller fraction sizes. Therefore under these conditions, an improved therapeutic ratio would be achieved with multiple small fractions for most tumor types. However, if a tumor has a lower α/β ratio than surrounding organs, decreasing dose per fraction preferentially spares the tumor, suggestion that for tumors with a low α/β, hypofractionation may be more effective [57].

Recent analysis and review of clinical outcomes, primarily after treatment with brachytherapy, argue for a low α/β for prostate cancer of approximately 1.5 [123–127]. Several recent clinical trials were designed with the explicit assumption of this low α/β ratio by utilizing more hypofractionated regimens in comparison with conventional schedules [128–133]. Altogether, these trials show that the treatment can be delivered much more quickly and conveniently using equivalent effective doses with hypofractionation without compromising PSA control or significant toxicity so long as careful technique and normal tissue dose tolerance are respected. Building upon this premise, even more extreme hypofractionated approaches (6.5–10 Gy per fraction) have been investigated.

Madsen et al. published one of the first experiences with prostate SABR describing their results from a Phase I/II trial at the Virginia Mason Medical Center [134]. Forty men with low-risk disease (Gleason score ≤6, PSA <10 ng/mL, and clinical stage ≤T2a) were treated with 5 fractions of 6.7 Gy per fraction for a total dose of 33.5 Gy. The target was the prostate plus a 4–5 mm margin. Daily image guidance was used using implanted fiducial markers. Median follow-up was 41 months. There was one acute grade 3 urinary toxicity (urinary retention requiring catheterization) and no acute grade 4–5 toxicities. Late grade 2 GU and GI toxicity rates were 20 % and 7.5 %, respectively, with no grade 3 or higher toxicities. Four-year actuarial freedom from biochemical recurrence (FFBR) was 90 %.

The feasibility of increasing SBRT/SABR dose was investigated by King et al. at Stanford University in a Phase II trial [135]. 36.25 Gy in 5 fractions of 7.25 Gy was delivered to the prostate plus a 3–5 mm margin. In 67 patients with low- to intermediate-risk features (Gleason score 3+3 or 3+4, PSA ≤10 ng/mL, and clinical stage ≤T2b), there were no grade 4 or higher toxicities. Late grade 2 and 3 GU toxicity rates were 5 % and 3.5 %, respectively. Late grade 2 GI toxicity was 2 % with no grade 3 or higher toxicities seen. Patients who received QOD treatments were less likely to experience grade 1–2 GI and GU toxicities than those who received QD treatments. Four-year PSA relapse-free su rvival was 94 %.

The largest prospective study of prostate SBRT/SABR is from Katz et al. at the Winthrop University Hospital [136]. Three hundred four patients (69 % low-risk, 27 % intermediate-risk, 4 % high-risk) were treated. The first 50 patients received 35 Gy in 5 fractions of 7 Gy with the subsequent 254 patients receiving 36.25 Gy in 5 fractions of 7.25 Gy. Lower-dose patients had a median follow-up of 30 months and the higher-dose patients a median follow-up of 17 months. There were no grade 3–4 acute complications. Late grade 2 GU and GI toxicities were 14 % and 7 %, respectively. Five patients had late grade 3 GU toxicity with no late grade 4–5 toxicities. For patients that were potent prior to treatment, 75 % stated that they remained sexually potent. Actuarial 5-year biochemical recurrence-free survival was 97 % for low-risk, 90.7 % for intermediate-risk, and 74.1 % for high-risk patients.

A recent pooled analysis of 1100 patients from prospective Phase II trials using SBRT/SABR for the treatment of prostate cancer in which a median dose of 36.25 Gy was delivered in 4–5 fractions demonstrated a 93 % 5-year biochemical relapse-free survival rate for all patients (95 % for low-risk, 84 % for intermediate-risk, and 81 % for high-risk) with favorable long-term patient-reported outcomes with respect to urinary and bowel functions [137, 138].

Compared to the prior studies using similar dose fractionation regimens, we commenced a multicenter Phase I/II trial investigating using significantly higher doses [139]. We chose to start at a dose similar to the biologic equivalent margin dose of the HDR brachytherapy experience (i.e., 45 Gy in 5 fractions) and escalate to 50 Gy in 5 fractions. In the Phase I portion, 45 patients, in 3 cohorts of 15, were treated with 45, 47.5, and 50 Gy in 5 equal fractions, respectively. Forty percent had low-risk disease (Gleason score ≤6, PSA <10 ng/mL, and clinical stage ≤T2a) and 60 % with intermediate-risk (Gleason score=7 or PSA >10 ng/mL, <15 ng/mL, or clinical stage T2b). No dose-limiting toxicities (grade 3–5) occurred within the first 90 days posttreatment. GI grade $\geq$2 and grade $\geq$3 toxicity occurred in 18 % and 2 %, respectively, and GU grade $\geq$2 and grade $\geq$3 toxicity occurred in 31 % and 4 %, respectively. Initial PSA control was 100 %. These encouraging results led to the further enrollment on the Phase II trial at the 50 Gy dose level studying late toxicity. An additional 46 patients were enrolled for a total of 91 (64 % intermediate-risk and 36 % low-risk). With a median follow-up of 42 months, PSA control remained at 99 % [140]. One patient with unfavorable intermediate-risk disease, who was treated on the 45 Gy arm, demonstrated failure to therapy.

Specific Issues Associated with SBRT/SABR for Targets in the Prostate

Ultimately, dose escalation to treat prostate cancer is limited by toxicity to the bladder or rectum. As reported in an update by Kim et al., the toxicity profile was favorable in the initial Phase I results; however, in the Phase II portion, the profile changed and five patients (10.6 %) developed high-grade rectal toxicity [141]. Injury was primarily to the anterior rectal wall and required a diverting colostomy for resolution.

Dosimetric analysis was performed on treatment planning data to determine predictors for rectal tolerance when using SBRT/SABR [141]. We predicted that the key to tolerance for SBRT/SABR would relate to the degree of damage inflicted and the success of normal tissue injury repair permitted. The most successful surgical repair of radiation-induced rectal injury with deep ulceration and/or fistula is by inserting a myocutaneous graft. A myocutaneous graft provides both a blood supply to devascularized areas via transferred muscle (i.e., the myo-component) as well as epithelial stem cells via skin and mucosal grafting (i.e., the cutaneous component) capable of proliferation over the denuded areas. We hypothesized that the two primary physiological requirements learned from surgical repair studies, a robust blood supply and adequate stem cells capable of repairing mucosal injury, are impaired by high dose of radiation therapy, and therefore, injuries would primarily fall into two categories: (1) mucosal damage including injury to stem cells and/or (2) vascular/stromal damage leading to devitalization of tissues. In turn, the inability to heal may be due to (1) stem cell (crypt cell) depletion at the site of injury and inability to efficiently recruit neighboring viable stem cells, due to excessive distance required to migrate to the site of injury, and/or (2) significant destruction of stroma and vasculature by excess volume of rectal wall being irradiated to an ablative dose of radiation. In line with this hypothesis, high-grade rectal events were correlated with the volume of rectal wall receiving 50 Gy >3 cm^3 and treatment of >35 % of rectal wall to 39 Gy (Fig. 8.3a, b). Additionally, a high rate of acute grade $\geq$2 rectal injury occurred if more than 50 % of the rectal mucosa was irradiated beyond 24 Gy. Therefore, strategies of limiting percent rectal circumference (PRC)

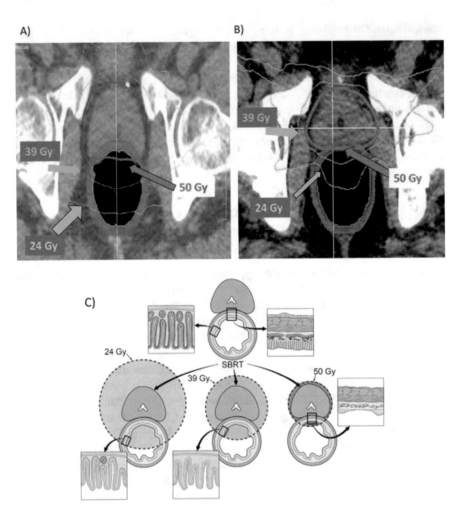

Fig. 8.3 Determination of rectal toxicity when treating the prostate with ablative doses. Representative treatment plans of patients treated with 50 Gy in 5 fractions. (**a**) Experienced grade 2 acute and grade 3 late rectal toxicity. (**b**) Only experienced grade 1 acute/late rectal toxicity. (**c**) Potential biological consequence of rectal wall irradiation. (Reprinted with permission from [141])

treated to 24 Gy may reduce risk of acute grade ≥2 rectal events, whereas reducing PRC treated to 39 Gy may reduce the risk of high-grade late rectal toxicity (Fig. 8.3c).

In an attempt to optimize treatment planning and reduce rectal toxicity, we are currently investigating the use of a biodegradable spacer to increase the distance between the target organ (prostate) and the tissue at risk (rectum). This spacer has been shown to be well tolerated and able to reduce patients experiencing declines in bowel and urinary quality of life when used with conventionally fractionated image-guided radiation therapy [142–144]. These spacers would likely be particularly

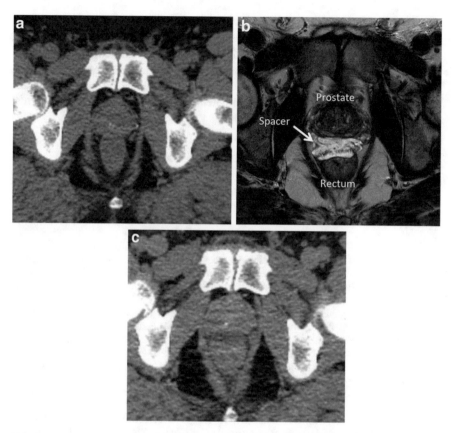

Fig. 8.4 Increased separation with the use of a biodegradable spacer (SpaceOAR system; Augmenix, Waltham, MA). (**a**) Planning computer tomography (CT) axial imaging prior to spacer placement. (**b**) T2-weighted axial magnetic resonance images and (**c**) planning CT axial imaging post spacer placement

effective at reducing the high dose associated with vascular/stromal injury and will likely lead to significant reduction of high-grade rectal toxicity events while allowing the highly effective tumor ablative dose to be delivered, thereby increasing the therapeutic ratio (Fig. 8.4).

Conclusions

Through advances in imaging and radiation delivery techniques, the use of stereotactic radiation in the body has become a common treatment approach in a relatively quick fashion. Well-conducted clinical studies have shown that SBRT/SABR can be utilized for a broad scope of indications, especially for the eradication for gross primary disease. In addition, due to its oligofractionation approach, SBRT/SABR can easily integrate into systemic therapeutic regimens without causing significant delays or disruptions. Further investigation of the potential immunological stimulation of ablative radiation could lead to more efficacious therapies, especially for the treatment of metastatic disease. Going forward, ablative therapies utilizing particles will be of increased interest due to the potential for increased sparing of normal tissue dose and higher radiobiological potency.

Disclosures

The authors have reported no relevant financial disclosures.

References

1. Dessauer F (1905) Beiträge zur Bestrahlung tiefliegender Prozesse. Med Klin 1:526–529
2. Regaud C, Blanc J (1906) Actions des rayons X sur les diverses generations de la lignée spermatique: Extrème sensibilié des spermatogonies à ces rayons. Compt Rend Soc Biol 61:163–165
3. Bergonie J, Tribondeau L (1906) Interpretation de quelques resultats de la radiotherapie et essai de fixaation d'une technique rationelle. CR Acad Sci Paris 143:983–985
4. Coutard H (1932) Roentgen therapy of epitheliomas of the tonsillar region, hypopharynx and larynx from 1920 to 1926. AJR Am J Roentgenol 28:313–331
5. Coutard H (1924) Note preliminaire sur la radiographic du larynx normal et du larynx cancereux. J Belge Radiol 13:487–490
6. Leksell L (1951) The stereotaxic method and radiosurgery of the brain. Acta Chir Scand 102:316–319
7. Blomgren H, Lax I, Naslund I, Svanstrom R (1995) Stereotactic high dose fraction radiation therapy of extracranial tumors using an accelerator. Clinical experience of the first thirty-one patients. Acta Oncol 34:861–870
8. Uematsu M, Shioda A, Tahara K, Fukui T, Yamamoto F, Tsumatori G, Ozeki Y, Aoki T, Watanabe M, Kusano S (1998) Focal, high dose, and fractionated modified stereotactic radiation therapy for lung carcinoma patients: a preliminary experience. Cancer 82:1062–1070
9. Potters l, Steinberg M, Rose C, Timmerman R, Ryu S, Hevezi JM, Welsh J, Mehta M, Larson DA, Janjan NA, American Society for Therapeutic Radiology and Oncology, American College of Radiology (2004) American Society for Therapeutic Radiology and Oncology and American College of Radiology practice guideline for the performance of stereotactic body radiation therapy. Int J Radiat Oncol Biol Phys 60:1026–1032
10. Timmerman R, Papiez L, Mcgarry R, Likes L, Desrosiers C, Frost S, Williams M (2003) Extracranial stereotactic radioablation: results of a phase I study in medically inoperable stage I non-small cell lung cancer. Chest 124:1946–1955
11. Loo BW Jr, Chang JY, Dawson LA, Kavanagh BD, Koong AC, Senan S, Timmerman RD (2011) Stereotactic ablative radiotherapy: what's in a name? Pract Radiat Oncol 1:38–39
12. Timmerman RD, Kavanagh BD, Cho LC, Papiez L, Xing L (2007) Stereotactic body radiation therapy in multiple organ sites. J Clin Oncol 25:947–952
13. Lea DE, Catcheside DG (1942) The mechanism of the induction by radiation of chromosome aberrations in Tradescantia. J Genet 44:216–245
14. Joiner M, Kogel AVD (2009) Basic clinical radiobiology, 4th edn. Hodder Arnold, London
15. Lee SP, Leu MY, Smathers JB, McBride WH, Parker RG, Withers HR (1995) Biologically effective dose distribution based on the linear quadratic model and its clinical relevance. Int J Radiat Oncol Biol Phys 33:375–389

16. Wang JZ, Huang Z, Lo SS, Yuh WT, Mayr NA (2010) A generalized linear-quadratic model for radiosurgery, stereotactic body radiation therapy, and high-dose rate brachytherapy. Sci Transl Med 2:39–48

17. Astrahan M (2008) Some implications of linear-quadratic-linear radiation dose-response with regard to hypofractionation. Med Phys 35:4161–4172

18. Guerrero M, LI XA (2004) Extending the linear-quadratic model for large fraction doses pertinent to stereotactic radiotherapy. Phys Med Biol 49:4825–4835

19. Kirkpatrick JP, Meyer JJ, Marks LB (2008) The linear-quadratic model is inappropriate to model high dose per fraction effects in radiosurgery. Semin Radiat Oncol 18:240–243

20. Park C, Papiez L, Zhang S, Story M, Timmerman RD (2008) Universal survival curve and single fraction equivalent dose: useful tools in understanding potency of ablative radiotherapy. Int J Radiat Oncol Biol Phys 70:847–852

21. Story M, Kodym R, Saha D (2008) Exploring the possibility of unique molecular, biological, and tissue effects with hypofractionated radiotherapy. Semin Radiat Oncol 18:244–248

22. Wolbarst AB, Chin LM, Svensson GK (1982) Optimization of radiation therapy: integral-response of a model biological system. Int J Radiat Oncol Biol Phys 8:1761–1769

23. Yaes RJ, Kalend A (1988) Local stem cell depletion model for radiation myelitis. Int J Radiat Oncol Biol Phys 14:1247–1259

24. Kavanagh BD, Timmerman R, Meyer JL (2011) The expanding roles of stereotactic body radiation therapy and oligofractionation: toward a new practice of radiotherapy. Front Radiat Ther Oncol 43:370–381

25. Finkelstein SE, Timmerman R, McBride WH, Schaue D, Hoffe SE, Mantz CA, Wilson GD (2011) The confluence of stereotactic ablative radiotherapy and tumor immunology. Clin Dev Immunol 2011:439752

26. Garcia-Barros M, Paris F, Cordon-Cardo C, Lyden D, Rafii S, Haimovitz-Friedman A, Fuks Z, Kolesnick R (2003) Tumor response to radiotherapy regulated by endothelial cell apoptosis. Science 300:1155–1159

27. Lee Y, Auh SL, Wang Y, Burnette B, Wang Y, Meng Y, Beckett M, Sharma R, Chin R, Tu T, Weichselbaum RR, Fu YX (2009) Therapeutic effects of ablative radiation on local tumor require CD8+ T cells: changing strategies for cancer treatment. Blood 114:589–595

28. Fuks Z, Kolesnick R (2005) Engaging the vascular component of the tumor response. Cancer Cell 8:89–91

29. Hill RP, Marie-Egyptienne DT, Hedley DW (2009) Cancer stem cells, hypoxia and metastasis. Semin Radiat Oncol 19:106–111

30. Burnette B, Weichselbaum RR (2015) The immunology of ablative radiation. Semin Radiat Oncol 25:40–45

31. Golden EB, Demaria S, Schiff PB, Chachoua A, Formenti SC (2013) An abscopal response to radiation and ipilimumab in a patient with metastatic non-small cell lung cancer. Cancer Immunol Res 1:365–372

32. Postow MA, Callahan MK, Barker CA, Yamada Y, Yuan J, Kitano S, Mu Z, Rasalan T, Adamow M, Ritter E, Sedrak C, Jungbluth AA, Chua R, Yang AS, Roman RA, Rosner S, Benson B, Allison JP, Lesokhin AM, Gnjatic S, Wolchok JD (2012) Immunologic correlates of the abscopal effect in a patient with melanoma. N Engl J Med 366:925–931

33. Seung SK, Curti BD, Crittenden M, Walker E, Coffey T, Siebert JC, Miller W, Payne R, Glenn L, Bageac A, Urba WJ (2012) Phase 1 study of stereotactic body radiotherapy and interleukin-2—tumor and immunological responses. Sci Transl Med 4:137–174

34. Brown JM, Koong AC (2008) High-dose single-fraction radiotherapy: exploiting a new biology? Int J Radiat Oncol Biol Phys 71:324–325

35. Gerszten PC, Mendel E, Yamada Y (2009) Radiotherapy and radiosurgery for metastatic spine disease: what are the options, indications, and outcomes? Spine (Phila Pa 1976) 34:S78–S92

36. Siegel RL, Miller KD, Jemal A (2015) Cancer statistics, 2015. CA Cancer J Clin 65:5–29

37. Midthun DE, Jett JR (2008) Update on screening for lung cancer. Semin Respir Crit Care Med 29:233–240

38. Iyengar P, Timmerman RD (2012) Stereotactic ablative radiotherapy for non-small cell lung cancer: rationale and outcomes. J Natl Compr Canc Netw 10:1514–1520

39. Mcgarry RC, Papiez L, Williams M, Whitford T, Timmerman RD (2005) Stereotactic body radiation therapy of early-stage non-small-cell lung carcinoma: phase I study. Int J Radiat Oncol Biol Phys 63:1010–1015

40. Timmerman R, Paulus R, Galvin J, Michalski J, Straube W, Bradley J, Fakiris A, Bezjak A, Videtic G, Johnstone D, Fowler J, Gore E, Choy H (2010) Stereotactic body radiation therapy for inoperable early stage lung cancer. JAMA 303:1070–1076

41. Gan GN, Weickhardt AJ, Scheier B, Doebele RC, Gaspar LE, Kavanagh BD, Camidge DR (2014) Stereotactic radiation therapy can safely and durably control sites of extra-central nervous system oligoprogressive disease in anaplastic lymphoma kinase-positive lung cancer patients receiving crizotinib. Int J Radiat Oncol Biol Phys 88:892–898

42. Hasselle MD, Haraf DJ, Rusthoven KE, Golden DW, Salgia R, Villaflor VM, Shah N, Hoffman PC, Chmura SJ, Connell PP, Vokes EE, Weichselbaum RR, Salama JK (2012) Hypofractionated image-guided radiation therapy for patients with limited volume metastatic non-small cell lung cancer. J Thorac Oncol 7:376–381

43. Kelsey CR, Salama JK (2013) Stereotactic body radiation therapy for treatment of primary and metastatic pulmonary malignancies. Surg Oncol Clin N Am 22:463–481

44. Milano MT, Katz AW, Zhang H, Okunieff P (2012) Oligometastases treated with stereotactic body radiotherapy: long-term follow-up of prospective study. Int J Radiat Oncol Biol Phys 83:878–886

45. Milano MT, Philip A, Okunieff P (2009) Analysis of patients with oligometastases undergoing two or more curative-intent stereotactic radiotherapy courses. Int J Radiat Oncol Biol Phys 73:832–837

46. Rusthoven KE, Kavanagh BD, Burri SH, Chen C, Cardenes H, Chidel MA, Pugh TJ, Kane M, Gaspar LE, Schefter TE (2009) Multi-institutional phase I/II trial of stereotactic body radiation therapy for lung metastases. J Clin Oncol 27:1579–1584

47. Rusthoven KE, Kavanagh BD, Cardenes H, Stieber VW, Burri SH, Feigenberg SJ, Chidel MA, Pugh TJ, Franklin W, Kane M, Gaspar LE, Schefter TE (2009) Multi-institutional phase I/II trial of stereotactic body radiation therapy for liver metastases. J Clin Oncol 27:1572–1578

48. Salama JK, Hasselle MD, Chmura SJ, Malik R, Mehta N, Yenice KM, Villaflor VM, Stadler WM, Hoffman PC, Cohen EE, Connell PP, Haraf DJ, Vokes EE, Hellman S, Weichselbaum RR (2012) Stereotactic body radiotherapy for multisite extracranial oligometastases: final report of a dose escalation trial in patients with 1 to 5 sites of metastatic disease. Cancer 118:2962–2970

49. Salama JK, Kirkpatrick JP, Yin FF (2012) Stereotactic body radiotherapy treatment of extracranial metastases. Nat Rev Clin Oncol 9:654–665

50. Tree AC, Khoo VS, Eeles RA, Ahmed M, Dearnaley DP, Hawkins MA, Huddart RA, Nutting CM, Ostler PJ, van As NJ (2013) Stereotactic body radiotherapy for oligometastases. Lancet Oncol 14:e28–e37

51. Villaruz LC, Kubicek GJ, Socinski MA (2012) Management of non-small cell lung cancer with oligometastasis. Curr Oncol Rep 14:333–341

52. Weickhardt AJ, Scheier B, Burke JM, Gan G, Lu X, Jr BUNNPA, Aisner DL, Gaspar LE, Kavanagh BD, Doebele RC, Camidge DR (2012) Local ablative therapy of oligoprogressive disease prolongs disease control by tyrosine kinase inhibitors in oncogene-addicted non-small-cell lung cancer. J Thorac Oncol 7:1807–1814

53. Perez CA, Pajak TF, Rubin P, Simpson JR, Mohiuddin M, Brady LW, Perez-Tamayo R, Rotman M (1987) Long-term observations of the patterns of failure in patients with unresectable non-oat cell carcinoma of the lung treated with definitive radiotherapy. Report by the Radiation Therapy Oncology Group. Cancer 59:1874–1881

54. Bradley J, Graham MV, Winter K, Purdy JA, Komaki R, Roa WH, Ryu JK, Bosch W, Emami B (2005) Toxicity and outcome results of RTOG 9311: a phase I-II dose-escalation study using three-dimensional conformal radiotherapy in patients with inoperable non-small-cell lung carcinoma. Int J Radiat Oncol Biol Phys 61:318–328

55. Rosenzweig KE, Fox JL, Yorke E, Amols H, Jackson A, Rusch V, Kris MG, Ling CC, Leibel SA (2005) Results of a phase I dose-escalation study using three-dimensional conformal radiotherapy in the treatment of inoperable nonsmall cell lung carcinoma. Cancer 103: 2118–2127

56. Sura S, Yorke E, Jackson A, Rosenzweig KE (2007) High-dose radiotherapy for the treatment of inoperable non-small cell lung cancer. Cancer J 13:238–242

57. Fowler JF (1989) The linear-quadratic formula and progress in fractionated radiotherapy. Br J Radiol 62:679–694

58. Koshy M, Malik R, Weichselbaum RR, Sher DJ (2015) Increasing radiation therapy dose is associated with improved survival in patients undergoing stereotactic body radiation therapy for stage I non-small-cell lung cancer. Int J Radiat Oncol Biol Phys 91:344–350

59. Mehta N, King CR, Agazaryan N, Steinberg M, Hua A, Lee P (2012) Stereotactic body radiation therapy and 3-dimensional conformal radiotherapy for stage I non-small cell lung cancer: a pooled analysis of biological equivalent dose and local control. Pract Radiat Oncol 2:288–295

60. Bradley JD, El Naqa I, Drzymala RE, Trovo M, Jones G, Denning MD (2010) Stereotactic body radiation therapy for early-stage non-small-cell lung cancer: the pattern of failure is distant. Int J Radiat Oncol Biol Phys 77:1146–1150

61. Grills IS, Mangona VS, Welsh R, Chmielewski G, McInerney E, Martin S, Wloch J, Ye H, Kestin LL (2010) Outcomes after stereotactic lung radiotherapy or wedge resection for stage I non-small-cell lung cancer. J Clin Oncol 28:928–935

62. Senthi S, Lagerwaard FJ, Haasbeek CJ, Slotman BJ, Senan S (2012) Patterns of disease recurrence after stereotactic ablative radiotherapy for early stage non-small-cell lung cancer: a retrospective analysis. Lancet Oncol 13:802–809

63. Timmerman R, Mcgarry R, Yiannoutsos C, Papiez L, Tudor K, Deluca J, Ewing M, Abdulrahman R, Desrosiers C, Williams M, Fletcher J (2006) Excessive toxicity when treating central tumors in a phase II study of stereotactic body radiation therapy for medically inoperable early-stage lung cancer. J Clin Oncol 24:4833–4839

64. Chao ST, Koyfman SA, Woody N, Angelov L, Soeder SL, Reddy CA, Rybicki LA, Djemil T, Suh JH (2012) Recursive partitioning analysis index is predictive for overall survival in patients undergoing spine stereotactic body radiation therapy for spinal metastases. Int J Radiat Oncol Biol Phys 82:1738–1743

65. Sze WM, Shelley M, Held I, Wilt T, Mason M (2003) Palliation of metastatic bone pain: single fraction versus multifraction radiotherapy—a systematic review of randomised trials. Clin Oncol 15:345–352

66. Desforges JF, Byrne TN (1992) Spinal cord compression from epidural metastases. N Engl J Med 327:614–619

67. Patchell RA, Tibbs PA, Regine WF, Payne R, Saris S, Kryscio RJ, Mohiuddin M, Young B (2005) Direct decompressive surgical resection in the treatment of spinal cord compression caused by metastatic cancer: a randomised trial. Lancet 366:643–648

68. Greenberg HS, Kim JH, Posner JB (1980) Epidural spinal cord compression from metastatic tumor: results with a new treatment protocol. Ann Neurol 8:361–366

69. Klekamp J, Samii H (1998) Surgical results for spinal metastases. Acta Neurochir (Wien) 140:957–967

70. Maranzano E, Latini P, Beneventi S, Marafioti L, Piro F, Perrucci E, Lupattelli M (1998) Comparison of two different radiotherapy schedules for spinal cord compression in prostate cancer. Tumori 84:472–477

71. Young RF, Post EM, King GA (1980) Treatment of spinal epidural metastases. Randomized prospective comparison of laminectomy and radiotherapy. J Neurosurg 53:741–748

72. Damast S, Wright J, Bilsky M, Hsu M, Zhang Z, Lovelock M, Cox B, Zatcky J, Yamada Y (2011) Impact of dose on local failure rates after image-guided reirradiation of recurrent paraspinal metastases. Int J Radiat Oncol Biol Phys 81:819–826

73. Folkert MR, Bilsky MH, Tom AK, Oh JH, Alektiar KM, Laufer I, Tap WD, Yamada Y (2014) Outcomes and toxicity for hypofractionated and single-fraction image-guided stereotactic radiosurgery for sarcomas metastasizing to the spine. Int J Radiat Oncol Biol Phys 88: 1085–1091

74. Gerszten PC, Burton SA, Ozhasoglu C, Welch WC (2007) Radiosurgery for spinal metastases: clinical experience in 500 cases from a single institution. Spine (Phila Pa 1976) 32:193–199

75. Zelefsky MJ, Greco C, Motzer R, Magsanoc JM, Pei X, Lovelock M, Mechalakos J, Zatcky J, Fuks Z, Yamada Y (2012) Tumor control outcomes after hypofractionated and single-dose stereotactic image-guided intensity-modulated radiotherapy for extracranial metastases from renal cell carcinoma. Int J Radiat Oncol Biol Phys 82:1744–1748

76. Hartsell WF, Scott CB, Bruner DW, Scarantino CW, Ivker RA, Roach M 3rd, Suh JH, Demas WF, Movsas B, Petersen IA, Konski AA, Cleeland CS, Janjan NA, Desilvio M (2005) Randomized trial of short- versus long-course radiotherapy for palliation of painful bone metastases. J Natl Cancer Inst 97:798–804

77. Yamada Y, Bilsky MH, Lovelock DM, Venkatraman ES, Toner S, Johnson J, Zatcky J, Zelefsky MJ, Fuks Z (2008) High-dose, single-fraction image-guided intensity-modulated radiotherapy for metastatic spinal lesions. Int J Radiat Oncol Biol Phys 71:484–490

78. Lovelock DM, Hua C, Wang P, Hunt M, Fournier-Bidoz N, Yenice K, Toner S, Lutz W, Amols H, Bilsky M, Fuks Z, Yamada Y (2005) Accurate setup of paraspinal patients using a noninvasive patient immobilization cradle and portal imaging. Med Phys 32:2606–2614

79. Yamada Y, Lovelock DM, Yenice KM, Bilsky MH, Hunt MA, Zatcky J, Leibel SA (2005) Multifractionated image-guided and stereotactic intensity-modulated radiotherapy of para-spinal tumors: a preliminary report. Int J Radiat Oncol Biol Phys 62:53–61

80. Sahgal A, Bilsky M, Chang EL, Ma L, Yamada Y, Rhines LD, Letourneau D, Foote M, Yu E, Larson DA, Fehlings MG (2011) Stereotactic body radiotherapy for spinal metastases: current status, with a focus on its application in the postoperative patient. J Neurosurg Spine 14:151–166

81. Chang EL, Shiu AS, Lii MF, Rhines LD, Mendel E, Mahajan A, Weinberg JS, Mathews LA, Brown BW, Maor MH, Cox JD (2004) Phase I clinical evaluation of near-simultaneous computed tomographic image-guided stereotactic body radiotherapy for spinal metastases. Int J Radiat Oncol Biol Phys 59:1288–1294

82. Chang EL, Shiu AS, Mendel E, Mathews LA, Mahajan A, Allen PK, Weinberg JS, Brown BW, Wang XS, Woo SY, Cleeland C, Maor MH, Rhines LD (2007) Phase I/II study of stereotactic body radiotherapy for spinal metastasis and its pattern of failure. J Neurosurg Spine 7:151–160

83. Lovelock DM, Zhang Z, Jackson A, Keam J, Bekelman J, Bilsky M, Lis E, Yamada Y (2010) Correlation of local failure with measures of dose insufficiency in the high-dose single-fraction treatment of bony metastases. Int J Radiat Oncol Biol Phys 77:1282–1287

84. Moulding HD, Elder JB, Lis E, Lovelock DM, Zhang Z, Yamada Y, Bilsky MH (2010) Local disease control after decompressive surgery and adjuvant high-dose single-fraction radiosurgery for spine metastases. J Neurosurg Spine 13:87–93

85. Rades D, Freundt K, Meyners T, Bajrovic A, Basic H, Karstens JH, Adamietz IA, Wildfang I, Rudat V, Schild SE, Dunst J (2011) Dose escalation for metastatic spinal cord compression in patients with relatively radioresistant tumors. Int J Radiat Oncol Biol Phys 80:1492–1497

86. Ryu S, Pugh SL, Gerszten PC, Yin FF, Timmerman RD, Hitchcock YJ, Movsas B, Kanner AA, Berk LB, Followill DS, Kachnic LA (2011) RTOG 0631 phase II/III study of image-guided stereotactic radiosurgery for localized (1-3) spine metastases: phase II results. Int J Radiat Oncol Biol Phys 81:S131–S132

87. Emami B, Lyman J, Brown A, Coia L, Goitein M, Munzenrider JE, Shank B, Solin LJ, Wesson M (1991) Tolerance of normal tissue to therapeutic irradiation. Int J Radiat Oncol Biol Phys 21:109–122

88. Kirkpatrick JP, van der Kogel AJ, Schultheiss TE (2010) Radiation dose-volume effects in the spinal cord. Int J Radiat Oncol Biol Phys 76:S42–S49

89. Schultheiss TE, Kun LE, Ang KK, Stephens LC (1995) Radiation response of the central nervous system. Int J Radiat Oncol Biol Phys 31:1093–1112

90. Ryu S, Jin JY, Jin R, Rock J, Ajlouni M, Movsas B, Rosenblum M, Kim JH (2007) Partial volume tolerance of the spinal cord and complications of single-dose radiosurgery. Cancer 109:628–636

91. Nieder C, Grosu AL, Andratschke NH, Molls M (2005) Proposal of human spinal cord reirradiation dose based on collection of data from 40 patients. Int J Radiat Oncol Biol Phys 61:851–855
92. Rades D, Stalpers LJ, Veninga T, Hoskin PJ (2005) Spinal reirradiation after short-course RT for metastatic spinal cord compression. Int J Radiat Oncol Biol Phys 63:872–875
93. Sahgal A, Ma L, Weinberg V, Gibbs IC, Chao S, Chang UK, Werner-Wasik M, Angelov L, Chang EL, Sohn MJ, Soltys SG, Letourneau D, Ryu S, Gerszten PC, Fowler J, Wong CS, Larson DA (2012) Reirradiation human spinal cord tolerance for stereotactic body radiotherapy. Int J Radiat Oncol Biol Phys 82:107–116
94. Medin PM, Foster RD, van der Kogel AJ, Sayre JW, McBride WH, Solberg TD (2012) Spinal cord tolerance to reirradiation with single-fraction radiosurgery: a swine model. Int J Radiat Oncol Biol Phys 83:1031–1037
95. Katsoulakis E, Riaz N, Cox B, Mechalakos J, Zatcky J, Bilsky M, Yamada Y (2013) Delivering a third course of radiation to spine metastases using image-guided, intensity-modulated radiation therapy. J Neurosurg Spine 18:63–68
96. Ferlay J, Shin HR, Bray F, Forman D, Mathers C, Parkin DM (2010) Estimates of worldwide burden of cancer in 2008: GLOBOCAN 2008. Int J Cancer 127:2893–2917
97. Sherman M (2010) Hepatocellular carcinoma: epidemiology, surveillance, and diagnosis. Semin Liver Dis 30:3–16
98. El-Serag HB (2012) Epidemiology of viral hepatitis and hepatocellular carcinoma. Gastroenterology 142:1264–1273e1
99. Davis GL, Alter MJ, El-Serag H, Poynard T, Jennings LW (2010) Aging of hepatitis C virus (HCV)-infected persons in the United States: a multiple cohort model of HCV prevalence and disease progression. Gastroenterology 138:513–521, 521 e1–6
100. Bruix J, Sherman M, American Association for the Study of Liver D (2011) Management of hepatocellular carcinoma: an update. *Hepatology* 53:1020–1022
101. Llovet JM, Bru C, Bruix J (1999) Prognosis of hepatocellular carcinoma: the BCLC staging classification. Semin Liver Dis 19:329–338
102. Chen MS, LI JQ, Zheng Y, Guo RP, Liang HH, Zhang YQ, Lin XJ, Lau WY (2006) A prospective randomized trial comparing percutaneous local ablative therapy and partial hepatectomy for small hepatocellular carcinoma. Ann Surg 243:321–328
103. Wang YX, de Baere T, Idee JM, Ballet S (2015) Transcatheter embolization therapy in liver cancer: an update of clinical evidences. Chin J Cancer Res 27:96–121
104. Llovet JM, Bruix J (2003) Systematic review of randomized trials for unresectable hepatocellular carcinoma: chemoembolization improves survival. Hepatology 37:429–442
105. Cardenes HR, Price TR, Perkins SM, Maluccio M, Kwo P, Breen TE, Henderson MA, Schefter TE, Tudor K, Deluca J, Johnstone PA (2010) Phase I feasibility trial of stereotactic body radiation therapy for primary hepatocellular carcinoma. Clin Transl Oncol 12:218–225
106. Andolino DL, Johnson CS, Maluccio M, Kwo P, Tector AJ, Zook J, Johnstone PA, Cardenes HR (2011) Stereotactic body radiotherapy for primary hepatocellular carcinoma. Int J Radiat Oncol Biol Phys 81:e447–e453
107. Bujold A, Massey CA, Kim JJ, Brierley J, Cho C, Wong RK, Dinniwell RE, Kassam Z, Ringash J, Cummings B, Sykes J, Sherman M, Knox JJ, Dawson LA (2013) Sequential phase I and II trials of stereotactic body radiotherapy for locally advanced hepatocellular carcinoma. J Clin Oncol 31:1631–1639
108. Culleton S, Jiang H, Haddad CR, Kim J, Brierley J, Brade A, Ringash J, Dawson LA (2014) Outcomes following definitive stereotactic body radiotherapy for patients with Child-Pugh B or C hepatocellular carcinoma. Radiother Oncol 111:412–417
109. Aitken KL, Hawkins MA (2015) Stereotactic body radiotherapy for liver metastases. Clin Oncol (R Coll Radiol) 27:307–315
110. Bengmark S, Hafstrom L (1969) The natural history of primary and secondary malignant tumors of the liver. I The prognosis for patients with hepatic metastases from colonic and rectal carcinoma by laparotomy. Cancer 23:198–202

111. Hellman S, Weichselbaum RR (1995) Oligometastases. J Clin Oncol 13:8–10
112. Weichselbaum RR, Hellman S (2011) Oligometastases revisited. Nat Rev Clin Oncol 8:378–382
113. Fong Y, Fortner J, Sun RL, Brennan MF, Blumgart LH (1999) Clinical score for predicting recurrence after hepatic resection for metastatic colorectal cancer: analysis of 1001 consecutive cases. Ann Surg 230:309–318, Discussion 318–321
114. Pastorino U, Buyse M, Friedel G, Ginsberg RJ, Girard P, Goldstraw P, Johnston M, McCormack P, Pass H, Putnam JB Jr, International Registry of Lung M (1997) Long-term results of lung metastasectomy: prognostic analyses based on 5206 cases. J Thorac Cardiovasc Surg 113, 37–49
115. Strong VE, D'Angelica M, Tang L, Prete F, Gonen M, Coit D, Touijer KA, Fong Y, Brennan MF (2007) Laparoscopic adrenalectomy for isolated adrenal metastasis. Ann Surg Oncol 14:3392–3400
116. Hewish M, Cunningham D (2011) First-line treatment of advanced colorectal cancer. Lancet 377:2060–2062
117. Wulf J, Guckenberger M, Haedinger U, Oppitz U, Mueller G, Baier K, Flentje M (2006) Stereotactic radiotherapy of primary liver cancer and hepatic metastases. Acta Oncol 45:838–847
118. Meyer JJ, Foster RD, Lev-Cohain N, Yokoo T, Dong Y, Schwarz RE, Rule W, Tian J, Xie Y, Hannan R, Nedzi L, Solberg T, Timmerman R (2015) A phase I dose-escalation trial of single-fraction stereotactic radiation therapy for liver metastases. Ann Surg Oncol 23(1): 218–224
119. Schroder FH, Hugosson J, Roobol MJ, Tammela TL, Ciatto S, Nelen V, Kwiatkowski M, Lujan M, Lilja H, Zappa M, Denis LJ, Recker F, Berenguer A, Maattanen L, Bangma CH, Aus G, Villers A, Rebillard X, van der Kwast T, Blijenberg BG, Moss SM, de Koning HJ, Auvinen A, Investigators E (2009) Screening and prostate-cancer mortality in a randomized European study. N Engl J Med 360:1320–1328
120. Kalbasi A, Li J, Berman A, Swisher-McClure S, Smaldone M, Uzzo RG, Small DS, Mitra N, Bekelman JE (2015) Dose-escalated irradiation and overall survival in men with nonmetastatic prostate cancer. JAMA Oncol 1:897–906
121. Kuban DA, Tucker SL, Dong L, Starkschall G, Huang EH, Cheung MR, Lee AK, Pollack A (2008) Long-term results of the M. D. Anderson randomized dose-escalation trial for prostate cancer. Int J Radiat Oncol Biol Phys 70:67–74
122. Zietman AL, Bae K, Slater JD, Shipley WU, Efstathiou JA, Coen JJ, Bush DA, Lunt M, Spiegel DY, Skowronski R, Jabola BR, Rossi CJ (2010) Randomized trial comparing conventional-dose with high-dose conformal radiation therapy in early-stage adenocarcinoma of the prostate: long-term results from Proton Radiation Oncology Group/American College of Radiology 95-09. J Clin Oncol 28:1106–1111
123. Brenner DJ, Hall EJ (1999) Fractionation and protraction for radiotherapy of prostate carcinoma. Int J Radiat Oncol Biol Phys 43:1095–1101
124. Brenner DJ, Martinez AA, Edmundson GK, Mitchell C, Thames HD, Armour EP (2002) Direct evidence that prostate tumors show high sensitivity to fractionation (low alpha/beta ratio), similar to late-responding normal tissue. Int J Radiat Oncol Biol Phys 52:6–13
125. Duchesne GM, Peters LJ (1999) What is the alpha/beta ratio for prostate cancer? Rationale for hypofractionated high-dose-rate brachytherapy. Int J Radiat Oncol Biol Phys 44: 747–748
126. Fowler J, Chappell R, Ritter M (2001) Is alpha/beta for prostate tumors really low? Int J Radiat Oncol Biol Phys 50:1021–1031
127. Williams SG, Taylor JM, Liu N, Tra Y, Duchesne GM, Kestin LL, Martinez A, Pratt GR, Sandler H (2007) Use of individual fraction size data from 3756 patients to directly determine the alpha/beta ratio of prostate cancer. Int J Radiat Oncol Biol Phys 68:24–33
128. Arcangeli G, Saracino B, Gomellini S, Petrongari MG, Arcangeli S, Sentinelli S, Marzi S, Landoni V, Fowler J, Strigari L (2010) A prospective phase III randomized trial of

hypofractionation versus conventional fractionation in patients with high-risk prostate cancer. Int J Radiat Oncol Biol Phys 78:11–18

129. Kuban DA, Nogueras-Gonzalez GM, Hamblin L, Lee AK, Choi S, Frank SJ, Nguyen QN, Hoffman KE, McGuire SE, Munsell MF (2010) Preliminary report of a randomized dose escalation trial for prostate cancer using hypofractionation. Int J Radiat Oncol Biol Phys 78:S58–S59

130. Kupelian PA, Willoughby TR, Reddy CA, Klein EA, Mahadevan A (2007) Hypofractionated intensity-modulated radiotherapy (70 Gy at 2.5 Gy per fraction) for localized prostate cancer: Cleveland Clinic experience. Int J Radiat Oncol Biol Phys 68:1424–1430

131. Lukka H, Hayter C, Julian JA, Warde P, Morris WJ, Gospodarowicz M, Levine M, Sathya J, Choo R, Prichard H, Brundage M, Kwan W (2005) Randomized trial comparing two fractionation schedules for patients with localized prostate cancer. J Clin Oncol 23:6132–6138

132. Pollack A, Walker G, Horwitz EM, Price R, Feigenberg S, Konski AA, Stoyanova R, Movsas B, Greenberg RE, Uzzo RG, Ma C, Buyyounouski MK (2013) Randomized trial of hypofractionated external-beam radiotherapy for prostate cancer. J Clin Oncol 31:3860–3868

133. Yeoh EE, Holloway RH, Fraser RJ, Botten RJ, Di Matteo AC, Butters J, Weerasinghe S, Abeysinghe P (2006) Hypofractionated versus conventionally fractionated radiation therapy for prostate carcinoma: updated results of a phase III randomized trial. Int J Radiat Oncol Biol Phys 66:1072–1083

134. Madsen BL, Hsi RA, Pham HT, Fowler JF, Esagui L, Corman J (2007) Stereotactic hypofractionated accurate radiotherapy of the prostate (SHARP), 33.5 Gy in five fractions for localized disease: first clinical trial results. Int J Radiat Oncol Biol Phys 67:1099–1105

135. King CR, Brooks JD, Gill H, Presti JC, JR (2012) Long-term outcomes from a prospective trial of stereotactic body radiotherapy for low-risk prostate cancer. Int J Radiat Oncol Biol Phys 82:877–882

136. Katz AJ, Santoro M, Diblasio F, Ashley R (2013) Stereotactic body radiotherapy for localized prostate cancer: disease control and quality of life at 6 years. Radiat Oncol 8:118

137. King CR, Collins S, Fuller D, Wang PC, Kupelian P, Steinberg M, Katz A (2013) Health-related quality of life after stereotactic body radiation therapy for localized prostate cancer: results from a multi-institutional consortium of prospective trials. Int J Radiat Oncol Biol Phys 87:939–945

138. King CR, Freeman D, Kaplan I, Fuller D, Bolzicco G, Collins S, Meier R, Wang J, Kupelian P, Steinberg M, Katz A (2013) Stereotactic body radiotherapy for localized prostate cancer: pooled analysis from a multi-institutional consortium of prospective phase II trials. Radiother Oncol 109:217–221

139. Boike TP, Lotan Y, Cho LC, Brindle J, Derose P, Xie XJ, Yan J, Foster R, Pistenmaa D, Perkins A, Cooley S, Timmerman R (2011) Phase I dose-escalation study of stereotactic body radiation therapy for low- and intermediate-risk prostate cancer. J Clin Oncol 29:2020–2026

140. Kim DW, Straka C, Cho LC, Timmerman RD (2014) Stereotactic body radiation therapy for prostate cancer: review of experience of a multicenter phase I/II dose-escalation study. Front Oncol 4:319

141. Kim DW, Cho LC, Straka C, Christie A, Lotan Y, Pistenmaa D, Kavanagh BD, Nanda A, Kueplian P, Brindle J, Cooley S, Perkins A, Raben D, Xie XJ, Timmerman RD (2014) Predictors of rectal tolerance observed in a dose-escalated phase 1-2 trial of stereotactic body radiation therapy for prostate cancer. Int J Radiat Oncol Biol Phys 89:509–517

142. Mariados N, Sylvester J, Shah D, Karsh L, Hudes R, Beyer D, Kurtzman S, Bogart J, Hsi RA, Kos M, Ellis R, Logsdon M, Zimberg S, Forsythe K, Zhang H, Soffen E, Francke P, Mantz C, Rossi P, Deweese T, Hamstra DA, Bosch W, Gay H, Michalski J (2015) Hydrogel spacer prospective multicenter randomized controlled pivotal trial: dosimetric and clinical effects of perirectal spacer application in men undergoing prostate image guided intensity modulated radiation therapy. Int J Radiat Oncol Biol Phys 92:971–977

143. Song DY, Herfarth KK, Uhl M, Eble MJ, Pinkawa M, van Triest B, Kalisvaart R, Weber DC, Miralbell R, Deweese TL, Ford EC (2013) A multi-institutional clinical trial of rectal dose

reduction via injected polyethylene-glycol hydrogel during intensity modulated radiation therapy for prostate cancer: analysis of dosimetric outcomes. Int J Radiat Oncol Biol Phys 87:81–87

144. Uhl M, Herfarth K, Eble MJ, Pinkawa M, van Triest B, Kalisvaart R, Weber DC, Miralbell R, Song DY, Deweese TL (2014) Absorbable hydrogel spacer use in men undergoing prostate cancer radiotherapy: 12 month toxicity and proctoscopy results of a prospective multicenter phase II trial. Radiat Oncol 9:96

145. Pirasteh A, Meyer J, Wardak Z, Yokoo T (2015) Evolving MR imaging features of poststereotactic body radiation therapy for hepatocellular carcinoma in cirrhotic livers. Association of University Radiologists 63rd annual meeting, New Orleans, LA

Chapter 9
Novel Imaging for Treatment Planning or Tumor Response

Adam Gladwish and Kathy Han

Abstract Anatomic imaging has long represented an integral part of modern radiotherapy, from planning, image-guidance to response evaluation. Functional imaging modalities now allow oncologists to supplement these anatomic images with functional maps, to elucidate the underlying biologic processes of cancer and allow delineation of both physical and biologic target volumes. Prescription of dose to this combination, commonly referred to as dose painting, represents an attractive avenue to further improve the therapeutic ratio of radiotherapy. This chapter focuses on the integration of novel imaging techniques and their role in delineating biologic radiotherapeutic targets, organized by well-known principles in radiobiology: tumor repopulation, reoxygenation, and repair. Focus is largely on clinically available imaging modalities, including positron emission tomography (PET) with various targeted radionuclides and functional magnetic resonance imaging (MRI). Other potential preclinical techniques are highlighted where relevant, particularly as they apply to promising translational concepts. Emphasis is placed on integration into treatment planning, adaptive treatment modification, and posttreatment response assessment.

Keywords Functional imaging • Image-guided radiotherapy • Dose painting • Biologic targeting • Novel imaging • MRI • PET • Magnetic resonance spectroscopy • FDG • Hypoxia imaging

Introduction

Radiotherapy is primarily a locoregional treatment modality, capable of delivering tumoricidal doses to both areas of gross disease and those at high risk of harboring microscopic spread. Therefore, by definition radiotherapy relies on the ability to

A. Gladwish • K. Han (✉)
Princess Margaret Cancer Centre, Department of Radiation Oncology, University of Toronto,
610 University Ave., Toronto, ON, Canada M5G 2M9
e-mail: adam.gladwish@sunnybrook.ca; kathy.han@rmp.uhn.on.ca

© Springer International Publishing Switzerland 2017
P.J. Tofilon, K. Camphausen (eds.), *Increasing the Therapeutic Ratio of Radiotherapy*, Cancer Drug Discovery and Development, DOI 10.1007/978-3-319-40854-5_9

accurately focus treatments to these regions, while simultaneously avoiding healthy normal tissue as much as possible. This forms the foundation of the therapeutic ratio in radiation-based treatments. Imaging is intrinsic within this process and as imaging technology has evolved, so too has modern radiotherapeutic techniques. Standard two-dimensional simulator-based planning has given way to three- and four-dimensional volume-based planning, based on improved anatomical and temporal delineation with both computed tomography (CT) and magnetic resonance imaging (MRI). Target definitions have evolved in parallel to advancing imaging techniques, and the latest International Commission on Radiation Units (ICRU) now outlines a host of anatomic-, clinical-, and geometric-based subvolumes which ultimately add together to produce the planning target volume (PTV). Furthermore, where these volumes were previously exclusively treated with homogenous doses based on predefined field borders, the aforementioned increases in imaging capability along with larger computational reserve have led to increasing use of intensity-modulated radiation therapy (IMRT) and volumetric modulated arc therapy (VMAT), whereby radiation doses can be sculpted around target volumes, further sparing the surrounding organs at risk (OARs). This increase in conformity has allowed for tumor doses to be escalated while maintaining consistent OAR doses, leading to further widening of the therapeutic window [1].

The rise of functional imaging offers promise of yet another target and perhaps a new paradigm for radiation oncologists, namely, the prescription of dose based on the intrinsic biology of the tumor being treated. This has been previously described as "dose painting" and has the theoretical advantage of being able to differentially target radiosensitive and radioresistant areas of disease, thereby maximizing the use of dose escalation to the regions that truly benefit. The concept of radiation sensitivity is most often discussed in terms of the classic tenants of radiobiology, the "4 Rs": the differential *r*epair of tumor and normal cells, the *r*edistribution of cells into more or less radiosensitive phases of the cell cycle, and the *r*epopulation and *r*eoxygenation of tumor cells between fractions (a fifth "*R*"—intrinsic radiosensitivity was introduced later to account for empirical data not explained by the other four). Advances in functional imaging provide the opportunity to directly measure and map these properties, offering a potential framework for modulated dose delivery. This chapter will review the current standard workflow of radiotherapy from treatment planning to tumor response assessment. This will provide a backbone on which to discuss various novel imaging modalities and their role in identifying and defining radiotherapeutic targets as well as characterizing post-treatment response.

Modern Radiation Therapy and Response Assessment

After the decision is made to proceed with radiotherapy, the standard workflow of modern radiotherapy typically dictates a process of treatment simulation, target/OAR delineation, radiation planning, quality assurance check, daily treatment verification, and post-treatment response assessment based on clinical exam, diagnostic imaging, and pathology where relevant (Fig. 9.1). Currently, X-ray-based imaging (helical CT, cone-beam CT scan, kV orthogonal, and MV portal imaging) represents the backbone

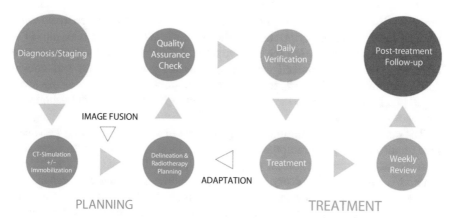

Fig. 9.1 Schematic representation of present radiotherapy workflow pathway

of this workflow. Initial simulation scans are acquired in the "treatment position," i.e., patients are scanned as they will be treated on a daily basis. These imaging datasets are then transferred to a planning system where the targets and OARs are delineated. Any adjunct information via clinical exam or other imaging modalities must be adapted to the current simulation images, sometimes objectively with image fusion and other times subjectively based on the clinical interpretation. Target volumes are defined according to the ICRU definitions, and a radiotherapy plan and dosimetric map are created based on these target volumes and pertinent OARs [2]. The plan then undergoes a quality assurance check and patients begin daily treatment. Once on treatment, the patient is set up based on the initial CT-simulation parameters and verified via some form of imaging, from 2D portal images to 3D/4D cone-beam CT scans (CBCT). After completion of treatment, the patient is seen in follow-up and evaluated with clinical exam ± imaging to determine the disease response.

To date the most impactful strategy to improve the therapeutic ratio in radiotherapy has involved improvements in the accuracy and precision of radiation delivery. This has been accomplished through improved anatomic planning images (e.g., higher-resolution CT, MRI simulators) to better delineate gross disease, advancing knowledge of patterns of relapse to better define the clinical target volume (CTV) and improved immobilization and daily image-guided imaging technologies to reduce uncertainties surrounding radiation delivery. The introduction of novel imaging modalities offers an opportunity to synergistically complement these with the ability to image and target differential tumor biology.

Dose Painting

The idea of targeting tumor subvolumes based on functional imaging is often referred to as "dose painting", a term coined by Ling and colleagues in 2005 [3]. The concept is to incorporate the quantitative output of a functional imaging modality directly into the dose prescription. This can be done as coarsely as to prescribe two tumor prescriptions, i.e., the anatomic GTV and the biologic GTV, or as finely as a prescription for each voxel scaled on the biologic parameter in question. The latter approach was first proposed by Bentzen and was coined "dose painting by numbers", referencing the popular children's coloring technique [4]. Needless to say, there are innumerable intermediaries between these two ends of the spectrum.

The concept of dose painting is integral to the process of exploiting personalized tumor biology with radiotherapy, either by local escalation or de-escalation to resistant or sensitive tissues, respectively. The realization of this technique requires a rigorous preliminary evaluation, including assessing each modality's ability to quantify a relevant oncologic parameters, how said parameters are affected by treatment, and ultimately determining a clinically relevant dose–response relationship. Furthermore, the feasibility of integration of these new modalities will require careful quality assurance testing regarding the interaction with the current radiotherapy workflow.

Functional Imaging and the Basic Radiobiology

The radiobiologic principles—4 Rs—were first described by Withers as a means of explaining the tumoricidal effects of radiotherapy [5]. Withers described the differential repair, cell cycle redistribution, repopulation of tumor cells, and reoxygenation. These concepts fit well with the empirical evidence of differential cell kill noted in standard fractionated radiotherapy and observed oxygen enhancement. Intrinsic radiosensitivity was added to this framework over a decade later by Steel et al. as a means of rationalizing the differential cell kill effects based on tumor histology [6]. Over the past 30–40 years since these concepts were introduced, the understanding of cancer biology has grown exponentially, punctuated with the translational success of molecularly targeted agents in clinical care. Nonetheless, the original 4 Rs remain a fundamental pillar of radiotherapy due to their ability to explain empiric observations, with literature consistently being published to better explain the molecular underpinnings of this success [7]. As such, the 4 Rs provide a natural and useful framework in which to discuss the integration of functional imaging within the context of radiotherapy and the potential for optimizing the therapeutic ratio (Fig. 9.2). The workflow outlined in Fig. 9.1 also illustrates the potential for integration of adjunct imaging with adaptation. The following sections will describe the role of functional imaging modalities within this framework and highlight both current clinical applications and potential for future integration of ongoing translational research. We limit the discussion to the most utilized 3 Rs, omitting redistribution due to lack of dedicated imaging.

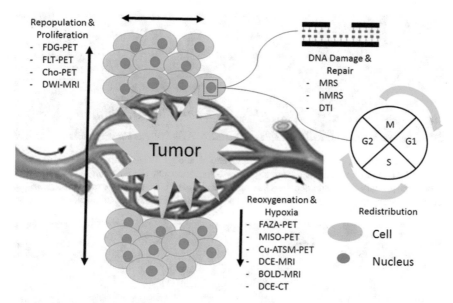

Fig. 9.2   Schematic representation of the 4 Rs of radiotherapy

Repopulation: Metabolism and Proliferation

The malignant transformation of normal tissues and the subsequent growth of new neoplasms rely on a host of molecular changes that lead to the acquisition of pro-growth capabilities, including (but not limited to) self-sufficiency in growth factors, insensitivity to antigrowth signals, limitless proliferative potential, sustained angiogenesis, and evasion of apoptosis [8]. A growing tumor is often first detected clinically (or with planned radiographic screening) as a growing mass, representing an underlying abnormal proliferation of cells. This represents the standard target of radiotherapy and is delineated in an anatomical fashion on CT or MRI. Functional imagining provides an opportunity to evaluate the underlying molecular signatures of cancer growth, to potentially aid in targeting, adaptation, and assessment of treatment response.

Glycolysis

Glycolysis is the cellular conversion of glucose to energy, a process that is upregulated in the proliferative atmosphere of malignancy. Currently, the most heavily utilized functional imaging modality in cancer care exploits this phenomenon by modifying a glucose molecule to contain a positron-emitting fluorine-18 isotope, namely, fluorodeoxyglucose (FDG). FDG-based positron-emission tomography

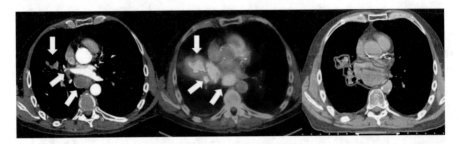

Fig. 9.3 Baseline CT (*left*), FDG-PET (*middle*), and planning CT (*right*) images of a patient with stage IIIA (T2N2) lung adenocarcinoma treated with concurrent chemoradiation. *White arrows* denote the primary tumor and nodal disease on CT and FDG-PET images; the *solid lines* delineate the radiotherapy targets, primary (red) and nodal (magenta) internal target volumes, respectively

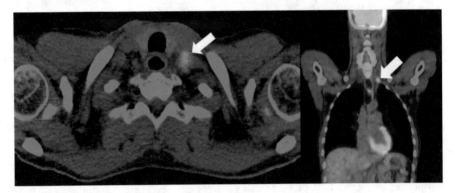

Fig. 9.4 Baseline axial and coronal FDG-PET images of a patient with squamous cell carcinoma of the upper thoracic esophagus. The FDG-PET scan identified a supraclavicular node (*white arrows*) that was subsequently included in the radiation treatment volume

(PET) is able to image the differential uptake of glucose in tumor cells over neighboring normal cells owing in part to their higher metabolic requirements. The common measurement used in PET is the standard uptake value (SUV), defined as voxel activity per dose injected per body mass. FDG-PET has been shown to be extremely powerful in identifying cancer cells, even in the absence of abnormal anatomic morphology. The combination of PET with CT has resulted in vastly improved sensitivity in detecting occult disease missed by CT, resulting in improved locoregional targeting and where appropriate omitting intensive curative treatments in patients with distant metastasis. In non-small cell lung cancer (NSCLC) (Fig. 9.3), the addition of FDG-PET to conventional staging assessment has shown a change in planned management in 20–30 % of patients, mainly in reducing the number of futile thoracotomies [9]. Similarly in esophageal cancer (Fig. 9.4), FDG-PET has been found to improve the sensitivity for detection of metastatic disease by up to 20 % over CT alone [10]. In head and neck cancers, the use of FDG-PET/CT has become common due to the high sensitivity, specificity, and accuracy for metastatic disease (>75 %) [11] and the finding that local radiotherapy plans changed from curative to palliative

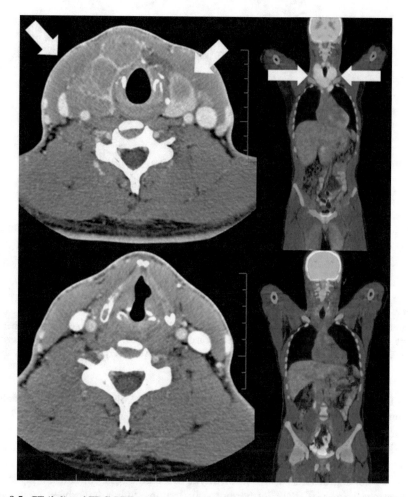

Fig. 9.5   CT (*left*) and FDG-PET (*right*) images of a patient with stage IIA$_x$ Hodgkin's lymphoma at baseline (*top*) and after the planned four cycles of combination chemotherapy and involved field radiotherapy (*bottom*). *White arrows* denote the tumor at baseline. The patient achieved complete CT and metabolic response posttreatment

intent in 13 % of patients when FDG-PET information was added [12]. FDG-PET has also had a large impact in the care of lymphoma patients, particularly those with Hodgkin's lymphoma (HL) (Fig. 9.5). Staging FDG-PET results in stage migration in ~25 % of patients with HL and a change in management in up to 15 % [13]. The standard of care for numerous malignancies now involves FDG-PET/CT in the work-up, including the lung and lymphoma to name a few.

The rise in utilization of FDG-PET as a staging investigation has led investigators to study its use as a quantitative biomarker via the SUV measurement. In an examination of patients from three prospective clinical trials evaluating chemoradiation in non-operable stage II and stage III NSCLC patients, baseline FDG-PET information

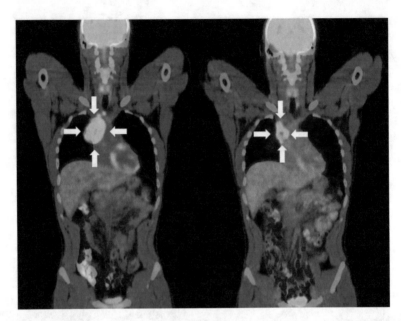

Fig. 9.6 FDG-PET scan images from baseline (*left*) and after six cycles of combination chemotherapy (*right*) of a patient with primary mediastinal diffuse large B-cell lymphoma. *White arrows* denote areas of metabolically active disease. This patient received 35 Gy in 20 fractions of involved field radiotherapy to the areas of persistent FDG uptake

was found to be predictive of local recurrence [14, 15]. Volumes generated by delineating the 70% of pretreatment SUV_{max} were well correlated with the 90% SUV_{max} recurrence volume.

Similar results have been demonstrated in cancers of the head and neck, which have shown that local recurrences are more likely to occur within FDG-avid areas and that the degree and volume of avidity is associated with both local and distant recurrence rates [16, 17]. Furthermore, analogous studies have been conducted with the addition of interim FDG-PET analysis partway through definitive head and neck radiotherapy and have demonstrated that the lack of FDG response is associated with inferior outcome [18]. Studies done in esophageal and rectal cancer are consistent, showing that the degree of metabolic response between pre- and posttreatment scans is associated with outcome [19, 20]. Adaptive PET-guided strategies have been investigated in Hodgkin's and non-Hodgkin's lymphoma alike (Fig. 9.6). In advanced-stage Hodgkin's lymphoma, treatment with six cycles of BEACOPP (escalated) followed by PET-guided radiotherapy resulted in better freedom from treatment failure and less toxicity compared to eight cycles of the same chemotherapy regimen [21]. However, interim analysis of HD10 trial showed that omitting radiotherapy in patients with stage I/stage II Hodgkin's lymphoma who attained a negative early PET scan after two cycles of chemo was associated with an increased risk of early relapse compared to standard combined modality treatment [22].

The linkage with CT has enabled PET to easily integrate into the radiotherapy workflow, and given its promise as a biomarker, the natural extension has been to utilize the combined information directly in radiotherapy planning. The obvious benefit is to identify areas that may be missed on a standard planning CT due to normal anatomic morphology but identified via FDG avidity. Not surprisingly, numerous studies have shown the alteration of final GTV volumes with the inclusion of FDG-PET information [23–26]. FDG-PET has been shown to be the most accurate modality for delineating GTV compared to MRI and CT in pharyngolaryngeal cancer when validated against surgical specimen [27]. Studies are now being conducted to evaluate the benefit of taking this biologic information further by assessing its use as a target for dose painting. As mentioned above, studies have suggested that local glycolytic activity may correlate with resistant disease and therefore a target for dose escalation. Early dose painting studies have established the feasibility of this technique for numerous sites, including the head and neck, lung, and esophagus. Madani et al. showed the safety of dose painting by numbers in a phase I study evaluating the head and neck (non-nasopharynx) of patients undergoing definitive radiotherapy [28]. They showed that a median CTV dose of 80.9 Gy was safely achievable. Similarly, Yu et al. demonstrated a sub-GTV volume based on the pretreatment $SUV_{50\%Max}$ in patients with an SCC of the esophagus could be safely escalated to 70 Gy using a simultaneous integrated boost [29]. In NSCLC, studies integrating FDG-PET into the RT planning process have shown that one can modulate the OAR to CTV dose ratio using metabolic guidance to either shrink boost volumes while keeping overall integral target doses constant (resulting in lower surrounding OAR doses) or conversely by maintaining an iso-OAR dose and dose painting nearby target subvolumes. Van Der Wel et al. showed that when using a prescription dose of 60 Gy, an FDG-PET-based plan could be implemented to reduce the mean esophagus dose from 29.8 to 23.7 Gy and the average lung dose by 2 %. Conversely, for an iso-OAR dose, the mean target dose could be increased to 71 Gy [30]. A phase II study by the Belderbos group showed that the utilization of FDG-PET in planning could be used to safely boost the mean target dose to 77 Gy [31]. Table 9.1 highlights several studies investigating the integration of FDG-PET into the radiotherapy process. For a more dedicated review, please refer to excellent summaries provided by Jelercic and Shi, respectively [23, 32]. Prospective studies are now being developed to test whether these modifications can result in meaningful clinical endpoints, including RTOG-1106 investigating whether FDG-PET-guided radiotherapy can improve local control in stage III NSCLC (RTOG-1106).

In addition to the value of metabolic imaging at baseline, the ability to compare glycolytic activity following treatment has been shown to offer independent prognostic information. In cancers of the head and neck, FDG-PET acquired 24-week post-treatment demonstrated >90 % sensitivity and specificity in locating recurrent disease and offered an 85 % rate of concurrent targeted biopsies [33]. In locally advanced esophageal cancers, Kauppi et al. demonstrated that percentage change in SUV of the primary tumor (pre- and post-neoadjuvant chemotherapy) was independently predictive of overall survival (HR 0.966 per 1 % increase, $p < 0.0001$) [34]. FDG-PET response has been correlated pathologically by Bahace et al., investigating patients with superior sulcus tumors who underwent trimodality therapy and demonstrating

Table 9.1 Summary of select studies utilizing FDG-PET in tumors treated with radiotherapy

Reference	Study type	Tumor site	N	Findings
Calais et al. [14]	Prospective	NSCLC	39	70 % SUV_{max}-threshold subvolumes at baseline correlate with 90 % SUV_{max}-threshold volume at relapse (>0.51 common volume/recurrent volume)
Bradley et al. [15]	Prospective	NSCLC	26	Integration of FDG-PET resulted in a GTV contour change in 58 % of patients, in 12 % the volume decreased due to improved ability to delineate in atelectatic lung, and 46 % the volume increased due to additional tumor detected
Roh et al. [16]	Retrospective	Hypopharynx	78	Increased metabolic tumor volume (delineated as isocontour of SUV >2.5) was associated with inferior 4-year overall survival (HR 2.66, $p=0.002$)
Due et al. [17]	Retrospective	HNSCC	520	Most recurrences occur within FDG-avid areas. Recurrence density increased with % SUV isocontour delineation and was highest for 90 % SUV_{max} ($p=0.036$)
Kilic et al. [24]	Retrospective	Rectum	20	CTV targets derived with FDG-PET/CT were significantly larger than CT alone (median CTV volume 559.73 mm³ vs. 468.43 cm³, $P=0.043$)
Nkhali et al. [26]	Retrospective (planning study)	Esophagus	10	The median GTV volume delineated at baseline and again after 37.8–42 Gy (+ concurrent cisplatin) using FDG-PET decreased from 12.9 to 5.0 cm³ ($p=0.01$), resulting in a significant reduction in the lung V_{20} (26.8–23.2 %, $p=0.006$)
Madami et al. [28]	Prospective	HNSCC	39	Phase I study showing FDG-based dose painting by numbers allowed dose escalation to a median 80.9 Gy, with no acute grade 3 toxicity and only one patient with grade 2 toxicity (mucosal ulceration). One-year local control was 87 %
Yu et al. [29]	Prospective	Esophagus	25	Dose escalation to a subvolume (50 % SUV_{max} isocontour) to 70 Gy in 2.8 Gy fractions using simultaneous integrated boost, and concurrent chemotherapy was achievable with two grade 3 toxicities (one myelosuppression, one nausea/vomiting). One-year local control was 77.4 %
van Elmpt et al. [31]	Prospective	NSCLC	20	Dose escalation to a metabolic tumor volume (50 % SUV_{max}) was achievable to ≥72 Gy in 15/20 (75 %) patients while maintaining planning OAR constraints

Abbreviations: *CTV* clinical target volume, *FDG* fluorodeoxyglucose, *GTV* gross tumor volume, *HNSCC* head and neck squamous cell carcinoma, *NSCLC* non-small cell lung cancer, *OAR* organ(s) at risk, *PET* positron emission tomography, *SUV* standardized uptake value that the maximum SUV obtained following chemoradiotherapy was correlated with the amount of remaining viable tumor cells ($R=0.55$, $p=0.007$) [35]. In squamous cell carcinomas of the cervix, Schwarz et al. showed that FDG-PET images acquired 3 months post chemoradiotherapy were predictive of the response. Twenty-three percent of patients with complete metabolic response experienced treatment failure, compared to 100% of those with progressive metabolic activity and 65% of those with partial metabolic response [36]. These results emphasize the role of FDG-PET in oncology, and particularly radiotherapy, further accentuating the importance of prospective studies integrating this information into treatment planning as discussed above.

Proliferation

The ability of tumor cells to divide and grow in a self-sustained fashion is one of the hallmarks of cancer; it has been shown that the rate of proliferation is prognostic in many cancers in many sites [37–40]. Additionally, the rate of tumor growth can increase after treatment (chemotherapy or radiotherapy), a phenomenon named "accelerated repopulation" [41]. Numerous disease sites have demonstrated a reduced rate of local control with prolonged treatment courses, highlighting the importance of this effect [42–46]. The ability to identify a tumor's specific proliferative potential at the outset of treatment and then follow dynamic changes during/ after treatment may be beneficial in modern radiotherapy.

PET

The functional imaging tracer, 3′-deoxy-3′-^{18}F-fluorothymidine (FLT), has been proposed as a noninvasive imaging biomarker for proliferation based on its biochemical pathway in dividing cells. FLT is taken up by cells and is phosphorylated by thymidine kinase-1 (TK1), trapping it within the cell (Fig. 9.7). TK1 is upregulated in S-phase and is thus an indirect measurement of cell division. FLT uptake has been shown to correlate with the gold standard in pathologic proliferative status, Ki67, in a number of cancer sites, and in and of itself has shown to be a prognostic biomarker based on treatment response [47–49]. In squamous cell cancers of the head and neck, a decrease in FLT uptake (SUV_{max} and PET-segmented GTV) during the first 2 weeks of definitive radiotherapy (± chemotherapy) was associated with better 3-year disease-free survival (88% vs. 63%, $P=0.035$, and 91% vs. 65%, $P=0.037$, respectively) [50]. The use of FLT imaging has been extensively investigated in terms of targeted growth signal modifiers, most commonly modulators of the epidermal growth factor receptor (EGFR). One study showed that early changes in FLT-PET during the first week erlotinib treatment predicted significantly longer progression-free survival (HR 0.3) in patients with NSCLC [51]. Furthermore, FLT has been shown to be a better marker of disease response than FDG-PET during radical chemoradiation, although the results are still pending on if this will translate to a difference in patient outcome in a prospective setting [52].

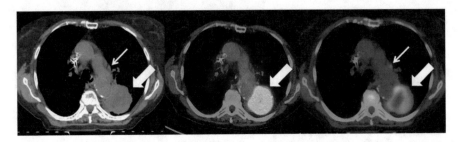

Fig. 9.7 Baseline CT (*left*), FDG-PET (*middle*), and FLT-PET (*right*) images of a patient with newly diagnosed non-small cell lung cancer. The *thick white arrow* indicates the primary tumor. The *thin white arrow* represents a mediastinal lymph node that is avid on FLT-PET scan, but not on the corresponding FDG-PET scan (courtesy of Dr. Meredith Giuliani)

Similar to FDG-PET, FLT-PET is commonly integrated with CT scanning, providing a relatively straightforward integration into the radiotherapy pathway. Planning studies investigating this integration have provided promising preliminary results. In thoracic esophageal cancers, the GTV volumes constructed using FLT-based parameters were generally 10% smaller than anatomic delineations, resulting in a 10% reduction in mean lung and heart doses ($p<0.01$) and showed higher correlation with final pathologic size [53]. Planning studies have also shown the feasibility of boosting areas of high proliferation in tumors of the oropharynx and rectum [54, 55]. A comprehensive review focused on FLT in oncology is provided by Tehrani et al. [56].

Choline is a substrate for synthesis of phosphatidylcholine, which is a major component of the cellular membrane. Choline can be tagged with a carbon-11 or fluorine-18 positron-emitting radionuclide for use in PET scanning (Cho-PET). With cellular turnover elevated in malignancies, accumulation of choline can be demonstrated in areas of active disease. Cho-PET has been most heavily investigated in prostate cancer and has shown improved sensitivity and specificity for both regional and distant disease detection over conventional staging modalities [57]. Cho-PET has also been investigated in regard to identifying dominant tumor nodules within an intact prostate, possibly for local dose escalation strategies. Currently the standard imaging for this task is multi-parametric MRI (mpMRI). However, a meta-analysis by Chan et al. showed that while Cho-PET alone was roughly equivalent to mpMRI in identifying a dominant nodule, the combination of both had improved sensitivity and specificity over either alone [58]. Planning studies using Cho-PET for defining subvolumes for dose escalation up to 90 Gy have shown gains in estimated tumor control probability (TCP) without exceeding OAR tolerances [59, 60]. Pinkawa et al. implemented this technique up to 80 Gy and showed no adverse effects on toxicity or quality of life [61]. The utilization of Cho-PET has been more widely accepted in the setting of recurrent disease and now represents the standard of care in many countries, including the United States, for restaging prior to definitive salvage treatment [62]. There is single institution data supporting the feasibility of Cho-PET-directed salvage treatment up to 74 Gy; however larger series and longer-term outcomes are needed [63]. Table 9.2 provides a summary of relevant literature pertaining to radiotherapy and proliferative imaging modalities.

Table 9.2 Summary of select studies utilizing FLT and choline PET in tumors treated with radiotherapy

Reference	Tracer	Study type	Tumor site	N	Findings
Hoeben et al. [50]	FLT	Retrospective	HNSCC	48	A relative change in tumor $SUV_{max} \geq 45\%$ from baseline to after 1.5 weeks of treatment (median 14 Gy, range 10–24 Gy) was associated with improved disease-free survival (88% vs. 63%, $p=0.035$)
Everitt et al. [52]	FLT	Prospective	NSCLC	20	Visual analysis of both FLT and FDG PET after 2 weeks of CRT (compared to baseline) showed that 52% of patients had a partial metabolic response, while 76% had a partial proliferative response, suggesting earlier tumor cell proliferation is affected more rapidly than metabolism
Troost et al. [55]	FLT	Prospective	HNSCC	10	A significant decrease in SUV_{max} was seen during radiotherapy (compared to baseline), greatest after 2 weeks of treatment (20 Gy), but continuing through 4 (40 Gy) weeks of treatment (7.6 vs. 3.1 vs. 1.7, $p=0.0001$ and 0.001, respectively)
Chang et al. [59]	Cho	Prospective (planning study)	Prostate	8	A SIB to 90 Gy to a subvolume defined by 70% SUV_{max} threshold resulted in a higher TCP across all patients (mean increase 37%, $p<0.001$) with no significant change in NTCP rectum and bladder
Pinkawa et al. [61]	Cho	Prospective	Prostate	67	Delivery of a SIB to 80 Gy to a subvolume defined by a tumor-to-background ratio >2 did not result in significantly increased acute or late bladder/bowel toxicity or decreased QoL (median 2 and 19 months post-RT) compared to a similar cohort not treated with SIB

Cho choline, *CRT* chemoradiotherapy, *FDG* fluorodeoxyglucose, *FLT* 3′-deoxy-3′-[18F]-fluorothymidine, *HNSCC* head and neck squamous cell carcinoma, *NSCLC* non-small cell lung cancer, *NTCP* normal tissue complication probability, *PET* positron emission tomography, *QoL* quality of life, *RT* radiotherapy, *SIB* simultaneous integrated boost, *SUV* standardized uptake value, *TCP* tumor control probability

Diffusion-Weighted MRI

MR diffusion imaging is an imaging sequence based on the thermally driven random motion of water molecules (Brownian motion). By applying strong gradient pulses, local diffusivity can be measured, and regions can vary depending on the local microenvironment. Generally, higher cellular density equates to lower diffusivity [64]. The metric generally used to quantify this diffusivity within a given volume element is referred to as the apparent diffusion coefficient (ADC), given in units of area/time. The term "apparent" is used because true diffusion is affected by innumerable variables which cannot be individually quantified in-situ (i.e., intravoxel motion, microvascular perfusion, physical obstacles within the cell, etc). Lower ADC values represent more restricted diffusion (Fig. 9.8); it has been reported across numerous sites that regions of malignancy have lower ADC values than surrounding healthy tissue [65–68]. Intuitively, regions of increased proliferation lead to areas of increased cellularity; and ADC has also been shown to correlate with Ki67 in both bladder and breast cancer [69, 70]. Furthermore, areas of reduced ADC have been shown to be associated with higher grades of breast, bladder, endometrial, and prostate cancer [69, 71–73]. The use of DWI in the identification of high-grade prostate cancer has been particularly useful and relevant for management decisions and now features prominently in the prostate imaging reporting and data system (PI-RADS) classification system for MRI evaluation of prostate cancer [74]. In a recent review by Futterer et al., DWI was able to provide a negative predictive value of up to 98 % for the presence of greater than Gleason 6 prostate cancer [75]. Baseline ADC values have also been shown to be biomarkers of disease-free survival in patients undergoing radical chemoradiation for squamous cell carcinomas of the cervix. A retrospective study by

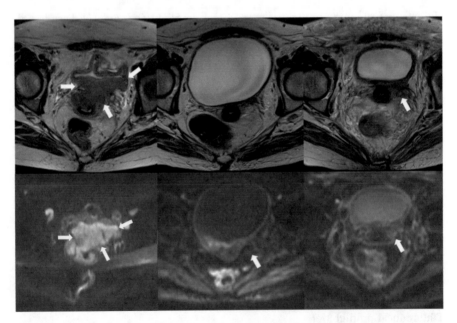

Fig. 9.8 Axial MRI images acquired pretreatment (*left*), 3 months after completion of chemoradiation (*mid*) and at the time of recurrence 1 year post-chemoradiation (*right*) in a woman who presented with stage IVA cervical squamous cell carcinoma. Along the top are T2-weighted images, and below are the corresponding diffusion-weighted images ($b=800$ s/mm^2). *White arrows* denote initial disease and the area of recurrence. Note the persistent restricted diffusion even at time of radiographic complete response posttreatment

Micco et al. demonstrated that a higher pretreatment mean tumor ADC was associated with better disease-free and overall survival in patients treated with chemoradiation on univariate analysis (HR 0.56, $p=0.007$; HR 0.46, $p=0.02$) [76]. Similar findings were reported by other groups investigating cervical cancer [77, 78]. In postoperative recurrences of cervical cancer, a tumor ADC$>0.95 \times 10^{-3}$ mm^2/s was predictive of a lack of complete response to chemoradiation in bulky lesions (sensitivity 85.7%; specificity 100%, $p=0.05$) [79]. In rectal cancer, a systemic review showed that pretreatment ADC was predictive of pCR following neoadjuvant chemoradiation with a negative predictive value of 90% and a specificity of 68% [80].

Much like FLT imaging, DWI-MRI has shown promise in measuring the dynamic changes of malignancies throughout and after treatment, offering an in vivo barometer of treatment effect. The hypothesis is that treatment-induced cell death will result in lower cellular density, reducing the restrictions to intercellular water diffusion and therefore increasing local ADC. Unlike single pretreatment measurements, increasing ΔADC with treatment (ADC$_{post}$–ADC$_{pre}$) has consistently shown positive associations with outcome. A work by Yu et al. demonstrated that patients treated with stereotactic radiotherapy for hepatocellular carcinoma with an increment of $\geq$20% in ADC value (6 months vs. pretreatment) had significantly better local progression-free survival at 1 year [81]. Greater increases in tumor ADC early (mostly 1–3 weeks) during RT ± concurrent chemotherapy have been associated with better response in many cancers: high-grade glioma [82], head and neck squamous cell carcinoma [83], nasopharynx cancer [84], liver tumor (hepatocellular carcinoma, liver metastases, cholangiocarcinoma) [85], rectal cancer [86–88], and cervix cancer [89–91]. In particular, a meta-analysis done by Fu et al. demonstrated a significant association between ΔADC and the status of residual tumor postchemoradiation in locally advanced cervical cancer patients ($p<0.001$), suggesting its utility in monitoring treatment response [92]. There is currently limited work investigating the real-time integration of DWI-MRI directly into radiotherapy planning, but preliminary work does show promise [93–95]. Table 9.3 provides a representative summary of evidence investigating DWI-MRI in conjunction with radiotherapy.

Summary

A trait common to many malignancies is the increase in cellular proliferation, which can manifest as local increases in glycolysis and cellular density. Novel functional imaging modalities have probed each of these facets directly, including quantifying FDG uptake with PET, assessing cellular density with DWI-MRI, and directly estimating local proliferation rates with FLT-PET. Each of these modalities has been shown to be useful in oncologic imaging and have been investigated to improve staging. Each is increasingly showing promise as a quantitative peri-treatment biomarker for treatment response and/or long-term outcome. Retrospective studies have shown benefit with integration into radiotherapy planning/dose painting, and larger prospective trials are now ongoing.

Table 9.3 Representative summary of literature investigating DWI-MRI utility in radiotherapy

Reference	Study type	Tumor site	Timing of DWI	N	Findings
Micco et al. [76]	Retrospective	Cervix	Pretreatment	49	Decreased baseline mean tumor ADC was associated with inferior DFS and OS on univariate analysis (HR 0.56, $p=0.007$, and HR 0.46, $p=0.02$, respectively)
Nakamura et al. [77]	Retrospective	Cervix	Pretreatment	80	Decreased baseline mean tumor ADC was associated with inferior DFS on multivariate analysis (HR 4.11, $p=0.013$)
Chopra et al. [79]	Prospective	Cervix (recurrent)	Pretreatment	20	Mean tumor ADC $>1.0 \times 10^{-3}$ mm^2/s was predictive of partial response to CRT (sensitivity 85.7%; specificity 100%, AUC$=0.96$, $p=0.05$). Of nine partial responders, three had residual disease spatially corresponding to baseline area of restricted diffusion
Joye et al. [80]	Meta-analysis	Rectal	Pre- and posttreatment	226	A decreased baseline tumor ADC and increased ΔADC (pre–post was predictive of pCR following neoadjuvant chemoradiation-NPV 90%, PPV 35%; and NPV 94%, PPV 46%, respectively)
Yu et al. [81]	Retrospective	HCC	Pre- and posttreatment	48	ΔADC [(pre–post)/pre]>20% was associated with better 1-year local control (100% vs. 75.8%, $p=0.02$). Post-treatment scans were taken 3–5 months following SBRT (15–20 Gy/3 fractions)
Hamstra et al. [82]	Prospective	High-grade glioma	Pre-, mid-, and posttreatment	60	Patients with an increase in ADC in >4.7% of voxels within the GTV after 3 weeks of RT (30 ± 4 Gy) had longer median survival (52.6 months vs. 10.9 months, $p<0.003$)
Galban et al. [83]	Prospective	HNSCC	Pre- and mid-treatment	15	The mean whole tumor ADC after 3 weeks of CRT was significantly higher in patients with radiographic CR than in those with PR (0.0016 mm^2/s vs. 0.0014 mm^2/s, $p<0.05$)
Chen et al. [84]	Prospective	Nasopharynx	Pre-, mid-, and posttreatment	31	ΔADC (mid-pre and post-pre) of both primary tumor and metastatic lymph nodes was significantly higher in patients with CR than those with residual disease ($p \leq 0.05$)
Fu et al. [92]	Meta-analysis	Cervix	Pre- and posttreatment	577	Post-treatment ADC was significantly higher than pretreatment ADC in patients treated with CRT (standardized mean difference 2.95 mm^2/s, 95% CI 2.19–3.72, $p<0.001$)

ADC apparent diffusion coefficient, *CRT* chemoradiotherapy, *HCC* hepatocellular carcinoma, *HNSCC* head and neck squamous cell carcinoma, *OS* overall survival, *pCR* pathological complete response, *SBRT* stereotactic body radiotherapy

Reoxygenation: Hypoxia and Vascularization

Hypoxia refers to the phenomenon where cells are deprived of oxygen, which is essential for a variety of cellular functions. A prolonged hypoxic environment leads to changes in cellular metabolism and genomic expression that can result in alterations of glycolysis and DNA repair. Tumor hypoxia is often a result of the rapid proliferation and abnormal vasculature associated with malignant growth. The chaotic and unorganized growth of cancer creates an unpredictable variation of oxygenation among and within tumors. Hypoxic tumors are more resistant to treatment and are associated with poor clinical outcome [96, 97]. There is strong prospective evidence that modification of hypoxia itself leads to improved tumor control [98–100]. With regard to radiotherapy, in particular, the lack of oxygen disrupts one of the major radiobiologic methods of cell killing—free radicals. The deposition of high-energy photons leads to local ionization; the resultant free radicals directly inflict DNA damage. This damage can become permanent with the fixation of nearby oxygen to become stable organic peroxides. In the absence of oxygen, this damage can be repaired more effectively. The gold standard for measuring hypoxia is polarographic electrodes, which can measure oxygen tension directly in the tissue [101, 102]. However, this method requires the invasive introduction of an electrode into the tissue itself; therefore, it is not feasible in many cancer sites. The ability to detect hypoxia noninvasively by imaging enables not only better quantification of tumor heterogeneity but also a potential biologic target for radiotherapy.

PET

A number of positron-emitting tracers have been evaluated for imaging hypoxia. The most prominent probes are nitroimidazole-based, a compound that was first shown by Chapman to remain trapped within hypoxic cells [103]. Among the nitroimidazole-based probes, the most investigated are fluoromisonidazole (FMISO), diacetyl-bis-N4-methylthiosemicarbazone (Cu^{60} or Cu^{64}-ATSM), and fluoroazomycin arabinoside (FAZA) (Fig. 9.9). These probes have shown promise as not only a reliable biomarker of hypoxia but also an association with outcome across many tumor types. Pre-treatment PET imaging of tumor hypoxia in patients with head and neck, lung, brain, and cervical cancers has been shown to correlate with disease-/progression-free survival [104–107], cancer-specific survival [108, 109], and overall survival [110–113] following (chemo)radiation. A meta-analysis by Horsman across multiple tumor types and a variety of tracers showed that hypoxic tumors were more likely to have poor response to radiotherapy (OR 0.27, 95 % CI, 0.18–0.39) [114].

Although a meta-analysis showed that hypoxia-modifying therapies improved locoregional control (HR 0.77; 95 % CI 0.71–0.86) and overall survival (HR 0.87; 95 % CI 0.80–0.95), they have not been adopted in clinical practice because of practical limitations and toxicities [100]. Initial studies looked at ameliorating the hypoxic environment directly via improving oxygenation (carbogen + nicotinamide), hypoxic

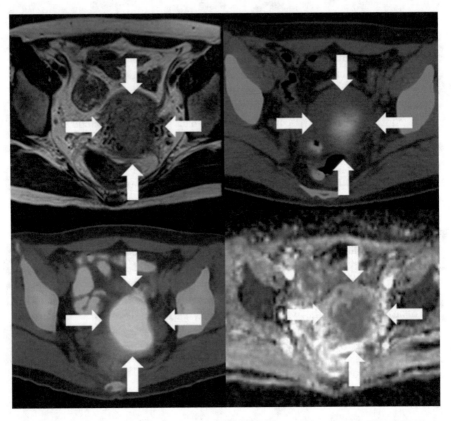

Fig. 9.9 Baseline axial T2 MRI (*left upper*), FAZA-PET/CT (*right upper*), FDG-PET (*left lower*), and ADC map (*right lower*) images of a patient with stage IIIB cervix squamous cell carcinoma. *White arrows* indicate the primary tumor. Note the tumor shows focal FAZA uptake, strong FDG uptake, and restricted diffusion

radiosensitizers (e.g., nimorazole), or direct hypoxic cytotoxins (e.g., tirapazamine). These strategies are not specific to the spatial distribution of hypoxia. Radiotherapy allows for integrated and personalized hypoxia targeting via dose painting. Several dosimetric studies highlighted the feasibility of this approach without excess dose to the OAR. Planning studies in carcinomas of the head and neck using FAZA-PET have shown the ability to dose escalate hypoxic regions in a simultaneous boost up to 86 Gy, without significant effect on existing OAR dose constraints. Specifically, Servagi-Vernat et al. showed that this adaptive FAZA-based dose painting is feasible with FAZA-PET imaging at three time points (baseline, post 7 and 12 fractions), offering the ability to target hypoxic regions dynamically over time [115]. Similarly, dose escalation to hypoxic regions identified by FMISO-PET beyond 80 Gy is feasible without excessive increase of dose to the OARs [116, 117].

An important limitation of dose painting based on hypoxic PET signals is the temporal instability of hypoxia. Radiotherapy based on pretreatment scans inherently assumes a robust target throughout treatment. Various studies have suggested that this may not be the case in regard to hypoxia, and specifically both acute and chronic hypoxia can be important in radiation resistance. Work by Lin et al. investigated this prospectively in a group of head and neck cancer patients who had consecutive pre-treatment FMISO-PET scans 3 days apart. They found that the mean D95 for the hypoxic GTV was an average of 7 Gy lower (range 3–12 Gy) when the initial plan was applied to the second scan [118]. Bollineni et al. performed serial FAZA-PET imaging in patients with HNSCC and NSCLC and found four cases: (1) increasing hypoxia, (2) decreasing hypoxia, (3) stable hypoxia, and (4) stable non-hypoxia with patients falling into any one of these categories [119]. Further work on the reproducibility, temporal variability, and adapting radiotherapy to hypoxic subvolumes identified by hypoxia tracers is required.

In addition to its *prognostic* value, PET imaging with FAZA can also monitor and/or predict response to hypoxia-targeted therapy. Xenograft studies showed that FAZA tumor uptake declined by 55–70% 1–3 days after administration of BAY 87-2243, a preclinical inhibitor of mitochondrial complex I that decreases tumor hypoxia and sensitizes tumor to radiation [106, 120]. Another xenograft study showed FAZA uptake to predict response to hypoxic cytotoxin tirapazamine and radiation [121]. Table 9.4 provides a representative review of the literature of PET-based hypoxia imaging in conjunction with radiotherapy, and further description of the use of PET-based hypoxia imaging can be found in excellent reviews by Padhani and Fleming [122, 123].

MRI

Several specific MRI sequences have been shown to correlate with tumor hypoxia. Dynamic contrast-enhanced MRI (DCE-MRI) is the most clinically utilized of these. DCE-MRI is a surrogate measurement for hypoxia, as it directly measures vasculature and local disruptions to blood flow. The main principle is to acquire a baseline non-contrast T1-weighted image as a reference set. A gadolinium-based contrast agent is then injected at a known rate and a second set of T1-weighted images is acquired. The contrast is readily seen as an increase in signal and the dynamic change in signal can be quantified. Based on the signal seen outside the vasculature, a parameter called K^{trans}, which represents the "leakiness" of the local vasculature, is modeled. Tumors often have poorly organized and quasi-functional vasculature which can be quantified using DCE-MRI. DCE-MRI has been found to be correlated with oxygen levels measured by polarographic electrodes in cervical cancer [124, 125]. In prostate cancer, hypoxia-inducible factor 2α (HIF-2), a known hypoxia pathway, has been shown to be negatively correlated with the 5th percentile K^{trans} in a histologic comparative study [126]. Similarly, negative correlations with K^{trans} were shown with hypoxic and radioresistant xenografts of cervical carcinoma and primary glioma [127, 128]. Halle et al. combined DCE-MRI data with gene expression profiles of biopsies from patients with cervical cancer treated with definitive chemoradiation [129]. They first identified a DCE parameter called A_{Brix} that had the strongest association with progression-free survival in these patients (in which tumors with

Table 9.4 Summary of select PET-based hypoxia imaging studies in tumors treated with radiotherapy

Reference	Tracer	Study type	Tumor site	N	Findings
Mortensen et al. [104]	FAZA	Prospective	HNSCC	40	Significant difference in 2-year DFS between patients with hypoxic tumor at baseline (T/M ≥1.4) vs. non-hypoxic tumor (60 % vs. 93 %, respectively)
Zips et al. [107]	FMISO	Prospective	HNSCC	25	Greater hypoxic volume and tumor-to-background ratio after 1 and 2 weeks of RT were associated with inferior local PFS
Dehdashti et al. [108]	Cu60-ATSM	Prospective	Cervix	38	Significant difference in 3-year PFS between patients with hypoxic tumor (T/M>3.5) vs. normoxic tumor (28 % vs. 71 %, respectively)
Kikuchi et al. [109]	FMISO	Prospective	HNSCC	17	Patients with hypoxic tumors (SUV$_{max}$ ≥ 2.3 or T/M ≥ 1.3) pre-RT had lower local control rates
Spence et al. [113]	FMISO	Prospective	GBM	22	Increasing hypoxic subvolumes of tumor (number of voxels with T/B>1.2) and maximum T/B value were each independently associated with inferior OS following CRT (log HR 0.05; 1.57, respectively; $p<0.05$)
Servagi-Vernat et al. [115]	FAZA	Retrospective (planning study)	HNSCC	12	Hypoxic subvolumes within the GTV (SUV$_{tumor}$ >3σ * SUV$_{muscle}$) could be safely boosted to 86 Gy without violating OAR tolerances
Chang et al. [116]	FMISO	Retrospective (planning study)	HNSCC	8	A mean increase in TCP of 20 % could be achieved by targeting hypoxic subvolumes (T/M>1.5) to 84 Gy (compared to 70 Gy plan). The 84 Gy plan increased the mean parotid and mandible NTCP by 18 % and 25 %, respectively, although the differences were not statistically significant
Henriques de Figueiredo et al. [117]	FMISO	Retrospective (planning study)	HNSCC	10	Dose escalation to a hypoxic target volume (automatic segmentation based on adaptive Bayesian method) (79.8 Gy from 70 Gy standard plan) led to a mean increase in TCP of 18.1 % with a mean increase in paroid NTCP of 4.6 %

Cu60-ATSM diacetyl-bis-N4-methylthiosemicarbazone, *DFS* disease-free survival, *FAZA* fluorazomycin arabinoside, *FMISO* fluoromisonidazole, *GBM* glioblastoma multiforme, *HNSCC* head and neck squamous cell carcinoma, *NSCLC* non-small cell lung cancer, *NTCP* normal tissue complication probability, *PFS* progression-free survival, *RT* radiotherapy, *SIB* simultaneous integrated boost, *T/B* tumor-to-blood ratio, *TCP* tumor control probability, *T/M* tumor-to-muscle ratio, *SUV* standardized uptake value low A_{Brix} appeared to be most aggressive) [129]. They then found that low A_{Brix} was associated with the upregulation of hypoxia response genes and HIF1α protein and constructed a DCE-MRI signature with the most important genes reflected by A_{Brix}. This DCE-MRI hypoxia gene signature was independently associated with progression-free survival and locoregional control (RR 2.5, 95% CI 1.3–4.8, and RR 3.7, 95% CI 1.2–11.8) [129]. Integration of DCE-MRI into the radiotherapy workflow is becoming more feasible with the increasing availability of MRI and specifically MRI simulators within radiotherapy departments. In cervical cancer, the quantity of low-enhancement (i.e., poorly vascularized, likely hypoxic) tumor regions predicted subsequent tumor recurrence [130] and persistently low perfusion from the pre-RT through mid-RT phase independently correlated with inferior local control and disease-free and overall survival [131]. This suggests a potential role for biologic targeting and possible dose escalation; however, prospective studies are warranted. Early planning studies in prostate cancer have demonstrated the feasibility of an integrated boosts to DCE-defined targets to 90 Gy [132]. This has led to several phase 2 studies demonstrating that this strategy can be implemented safely, and now we await the results of a recently completed phase 3 randomized controlled trials investigating the impact on clinical outcome [133, 134].

Another functional MRI technique aimed at measuring in vivo oxygenation is blood–oxygen-level-dependent contrast imaging (BOLD-MRI). Initially developed as a tool for functional brain imaging, this technique is based on the varying magnetic susceptibility of hemoglobin due to oxygenation status. An advantage of this technique is the lack of contrast required for quantification. It was found to correctly predict treatment response to hypoxia-modifying agents in various rodent models [135, 136]. Pathologic correlative studies showed that BOLD-MRI parameters are correlated with HIF-1α staining in both invasive breast cancer and high-grade glioma [137, 138]. Similarly, in prostate cancer, BOLD-MRI findings correlated hypoxia measurements using polarographic electrodes [139]. Investigations of BOLD-MRI directly within the radiotherapy workflow have not yet been done and remain an intriguing avenue for research.

Similar to PET-based hypoxia imaging, temporal uncertainties are present in MRI-based modalities. A planning study by Sovik et al. on canine sarcomas showed that plan adaptation based on hypoxic subvolumes defined by DCE-MRI improved the tumor control probability by 20%, if replanned twice a week as compared to a single baseline acquisition [140]. Dedicated studies investigating the temporal uncertainties of tumor hypoxia imaged via BOLD-MRI are required. A recent review of MRI-based hypoxia imaging in cancer is provided by Matsuo [141].

CT

Analogous to DCE-MRI is perfusion-based computed tomography, DCE-CT. Based on a similar acquisition but with iodinated rather than gadolinium-based contrast media, DCE-CT quantifies comparable modeling parameters. Again these parameters are linked to tumor vasculature and have been shown to be a useful surrogate for hypoxia. In NSCLC, DCE-CT derived tumoral blood volume is negatively correlated with histologically based hypoxia via pimonidazole staining [142]. Similarly, in head and neck cancers, tumor hypoxia is correlated with DCE-CT parameters, although not as strongly as with DCE-MRI [143]. Prospective studies investigating the role of anti-angiogenic therapy in head and neck cancers have demonstrated a decline in tumor blood flow and CT enhancement with DCE-CT post-treatment [144]. In high-grade glioma, serial postoperative DCE-CT in patients treated with combined chemoradiation demonstrated a negative correlation between tumor blood flow and blood volume in the residual tumor with survival [145]. As with PET-CT, DCE-CT presents a promising candidate for integration into the radiotherapy workflow, perhaps even more so given the ability to obtain scans directly on a standard CT simulator (with appropriate post-acquisition processing). Future dosimetric and clinical studies integrating DCE-CT are needed. Review articles highlighting the role of DCE-CT in radiotherapy are provided by van Elmpt and Astner et al. [146, 147].

Summary

Hypoxia has been well established as a negative predictive feature in oncology and specifically has been associated with radioresistance. The identification and quantification of tumor hypoxia offers a chance to customize treatment and/or subsequent clinical follow-up. Radiographic biomarkers offer the ability to quantify hypoxia in sites not amenable to direct measurement and also allow measurements in a fully geometric and temporal manner. The integration of these imaging modalities into the radiotherapy workflow has the potential to facilitate hypoxia-directed dose painting, adaptation, and personalized follow-up. Further prospective work is required to fully elucidate the clinical benefit of such a strategy.

Repair

Radiotherapy inflicts DNA damage, and ultimately cell killing, by a process of breaking base-pair linkages via ionization. The cellular response to this assault is to initiate DNA repair via one of several pathways (e.g., homologous repair, nonhomologous end joining, base excision repair, etc.) [148]. Due to the scale, the repair itself cannot be directly visualized; however, surrogates have been developed to provide macroscopic insight into this process. The obvious goal of radiotherapy is to minimize tumor repair and maximize normal healthy tissue repair, and the most direct route is by shaping target and avoidance doses, respectively. The potential for measuring repair in vivo represents an intriguing adjunct to this strategy. Not only does it represent an independent marker for delineation, as often the repair mechanisms differ between tumor and normal tissues, but there is potential for measuring the local repair efficiency within each, enabling targeting of high repair regions of tumor and avoiding poorly repairing healthy structures [149]. Doubling down in this manner presents an intriguing tactic for widening the therapeutic window.

Magnetic Resonance Spectroscopy

Magnetic resonance spectroscopy (MRS) is a noninvasive technique to measure metabolite concentrations in the tissue. The principal difference between MRS and anatomic MR measurements is that the signal obtained from hydrogen precession (influenced by neighboring protons) is used to quantify chemical shifts rather than provide contrast information. Another key aspect is to ensure water/fat suppression as these signals would otherwise dominate the observed spectrum. By comparing an acquired shift spectrum against a library of characteristic spectra, various compounds can be identified and their relative concentrations quantified. The most common metabolites that are characterized by MRS are choline (Cho), a component of cellular membranes (increased levels suggest increased cellular turnover), creatine (decreased levels suggest necrosis/cell death), glucose, N-acetyl-aspartate (NAA, a prominent neuronal metabolite reduced in areas of neuronal destruction), and lactate (increased in areas of hypoxia). The most investigated sites utilizing MRS for radiotherapeutic applications are the brain and prostate.

Various studies investigating MRS in gliomas have linked a Cho/NAA ratio >2 (both pre- and postoperatively) with worse outcome [150, 151]. This suggests a potential target for dose escalation, and subsequent planning studies have demonstrated dosimetric feasibility in targeting subvolumes with elevated Cho/NAA ratios up to 72 Gy [152]. A single arm, prospective phase II study of stereotactic boost (15–24 Gy) to regions with an elevated Cho/NAA>2 (plus standard conformal radiotherapy to 60 Gy) has shown acceptable toxicity and a 6.2-month improvement in median survival versus historical controls, but phase III studies are needed [153]. Furthermore, following completion of adjuvant treatment, a secondary problem of distinguishing residual glioma versus benign regions of necrosis and tissue repair is prevalent. This phenomenon, called pseudoprogression, occurs in ~30% of patients [154]. Studies have shown MRS as a promising tool in this area, with an elevated Cho/nCho (nCho represents the Cho in the contralateral brain) or Cho/NAA ratio both demonstrating a high specificity for true tumor progression [155, 156]. In a meta-analysis by Zhang et al. evaluating a total of 455 patients with high-grade glioma, an elevated Cho/Cr ratio had a sensitivity and specificity each of 83% (95% CI 0.77–0.89 and 0.74–0.90, respectively) for classifying tumor progression [157].

In prostate cells, citrate represents an important metabolite that plays a critical role in metabolism together with zinc ions. High concentrations of citrate are unique to glandular areas of the prostate, which are highest in the peripheral zone. Cancerous prostate cells dedifferentiate and lose the ability to accumulate and secrete citrate, and energy pathways subsequently alter. Elevated citrate/Cho or citrate/Cr ratios have been shown to be associated with prostate cancer [158]. Targeted biopsies utilizing MRS and MRI guidance have shown a sensitivity, specificity, and accuracy of 100%, 70.6%, and 79.2%, respectively (95% CI 61.6–100.0, 46.9–86.7, and 57.9–92.9, respectively), in a population of men with a rising PSA and previously negative biopsy [159]. Furthermore, a ratio of choline + creatine + spermine to citrate showed a positive correlation (Spearman's coefficient 0.77, $p < 0.001$) with Gleason score, therefore suggesting an ability to preferentially identify areas of increased aggressiveness [160]. Naturally, this led to planning studies investigating the feasibility of MRS-guided dose escalation, which proved possible up to 90 Gy with EBRT and up to 130% (~40 Gy) with brachytherapy boost [161, 162]. Limited focal targeting of a dominant intraprostatic lesion, defined by T2W and MRS to 82 Gy and de-escalation of remaining prostate dose to 74 Gy, resulted in a significant rise in TCP (80.1% vs. 75.3%, $p < 0.001$) and reduction in rectal normal tissue complication probability (3.84% vs. 9.7%, $p = 0.04$) [163]. Prospective studies evaluating the clinical effect of these strategies are lacking.

In addition to standard MRS, hyperpolarized MRS (hMRS) via dynamic nuclear polarization allows for molecules other than hydrogen to be imaged. This can offer advantages in signal-to-noise ratio (as hydrogen is ubiquitous in the body) as well as offer imaging of otherwise low-density areas such as the lungs. One area of interest specific to radiotherapy is the evaluation of radiation-induced lung injury or radiation pneumonitis (RP). Lung doses are often the limiting factor for treatment plans of thoracic based malignancies, particularly lung cancer. This limits the prospects of dose escalation. Carbon-13 is a suitable candidate for hyperpolarization and has been tagged to pyruvate, which converts to lactate, bicarbonate, and alanine upon metabolism. Animal models showed that elevated lactate levels based on C-13 hMRS were associated with RP and were detectable as little as 5 days post-conformal radiotherapy, suggesting a role for early detection and treatment modification in a patient population [164]. Work in hyperpolarized gases (helium-3 and xenon-129) has shown promise as inhaled contrast agents for hMRS, allowing highly detailed ventilation scans, useful for accurately describing a number of lung diseases [165]. Planning studies have suggested that integration of ^{3}He-based hMRS can reduce the volume of ventilated lung that is irradiated, potentially reducing the risk of RP by up to 10% versus a standard plan [166], and the potential clinical benefit is being assessed in an ongoing randomized controlled trial [167]. A recent review by Nguyen et al. examines the potential role of MRS in modern image-guided radiotherapy [168].

Limitations of spectroscopy are generally related to poor spatial resolution, exacerbated by volume averaging between adjacent voxels. This is accentuated particularly in the era of ever-improving anatomical imaging. Furthermore, inhomogeneities within the magnetic field can result in differences in metabolite quantification, which makes standardization among centers and between individual patients difficult and can limit generalizable protocols.

Diffusion Tensor Imaging

Diffusion tensor imaging (DTI) is a form of DWI that was discussed earlier, but in DTI the directional diffusion is also measured. DWI assesses the Brownian motion of water molecules and quantifies their ability to disperse within a given space. DTI measures this on a directional basis, determining if some paths are more restricted than others. Imagine a garden hose, where water is quite free to "diffuse" longitudinally through the tube, but that flow is significantly attenuated axially by the rubber casing. DTI has been most utilized in brain imaging where neurons are akin to the garden hose in the previous example [169]. Typically a series of DWI images are taken along six different gradient orientations, and diffusion can then be quantified in terms of a vector field rather than a single scalar quantity. Generally, increases in axial diffusivity and decreases in longitudinal diffusivity (e.g., a leak in the hose) are suggestive of neuronal injury or demyelination regardless of mechanism [170]. In radiotherapy, changes in anisotropic diffusion have been noted after radical treatment for gliomas and also retrospectively in pediatric patients who underwent whole brain radiotherapy. These changes have been correlated with decline in neurocognitive tests, compared to pretreatment or healthy controls, suggesting permanent neuronal damage [171, 172]. The ability to distinguish individual nerve tracts and identify those compromised by tumor suggests a method of improved tumor delineation and also a means of identifying eloquent, intact neuronal pathways. A planning study in 13 glioblastoma multiforme patients by Berberat et al. showed a mean reduction in CTV volume of 50 % ($p<0.005$) was achieved using DTI-based delineations as compared to T2-weighted imaging alone [173]. Prospective implementation of neuronal pathway imaging has been utilized in radiosurgical series, demonstrating low rates of neurologic complication in the treatment of arterial-venous malformations and an improvement of motor dysfunction as compared to the absence of DTI imaging [174, 175]. The integration of DTI into areas outside the brain is lacking, but the rise in spinal stereotactic treatments offers an intriguing potential application.

Summary

Improving the healthy tissue repair profile is critical to minimizing radiation toxicity and thereby widening the therapeutic ratio. The surest way of implementing this goal is to decrease the radiotherapy delivered to normal tissue and particularly highly functional subunits of healthy tissue. The implementation of MRS, hMRS, and DTI has shown promise of not only providing functional information and assisting accurate delineation of tumor invasion but also for directly imaging the function of surrounding anatomy. This has been most developed in the area of brain imaging via neuronal mapping (DTI) and lung through ventilation/perfusion mapping via hMRS. Future work will entail prospective patient data to support improvement of the therapeutic ratio and extension into other body sites.

Technical Considerations

The integration of functional imaging technology into the radiotherapy workflow offers not only additional information to guide treatment planning but also the potential of a new paradigm in radiation oncology practice. However, there exist a number of technical and practical limitations in each of these new imaging modalities; these will require a thorough understanding and characterization prior to full realization of this goal. Many of these limitations apply to all of the techniques described in this chapter and will be reviewed together here.

Simulation

The current radiotherapy workflow as discussed at the beginning of this chapter is based on CT simulation, whereby the patient is positioned on a flat table top and immobilized in the treatment position. This allows for the planning image to represent the daily treatment reality, offering a reproducible environment to derive safety margins. CT simulation is generally fast, on the order of seconds or minutes for four-dimensional acquisitions. Functional imaging modalities described in this chapter often require additional hardware (PET/MRI) that may or may not accommodate treatment immobilization and/or positioning. Both PET and functional MRI often require lengthy scan times depending on the intended image set(s), typically between 20 and 60 min [23, 95]. During this time patients can move, shift, or cough, resulting in degraded image accuracy. These sources of uncertainty must be accounted for in radiotherapy planning to ensure appropriate tumor coverage, particularly when curative doses are intended. Commonly, these uncertainties are incorporated via additional safety margins within the PTV. This results in larger treatment volumes, more irradiated healthy tissue, and therefore increased toxicity, opposite the therapeutic goals. Developments are being made in these areas, with radiotherapy centers increasingly acquiring dedicated imaging equipment (modified to accommodate patient positioning/immobilization) and optimizing image acquisition techniques to reduce scan times [176–178].

Resolution and Registration

Current anatomical CT and MRI scans allow for high-resolution acquisitions, up to 1–2 mm^3 when required, to enable high-precision anatomical delineation and radiation planning. Many of the functional imaging modalities can only acquire images with much coarser pixilation to maintain an adequate signal-to-noise ratio. Not only does this make it difficult to register images, the volume averaging effect can also blur functional features at a tumor's edge. This can be even more pronounced at tissue interfaces. How one interprets a high-resolution anatomic scan together with a lower resolution but perhaps more biologically relevant image remains uncertain. In addition to spatial resolution, the issue of temporal resolution also exists. There is much literature to suggest that metabolism, proliferation, hypoxia, and repair are not static processes and can change significantly during the course of treatment [119, 179, 180]. When is the right time to image and is a single baseline scan all that is required, or should plans be adapted during treatment? If a biologic feature is targeted, over what time frame is that volume relevant? These are questions that will require further study to adequately address. Relevant reviews addressing these issues for glycolytic and hypoxia-based PET modalities as they relate to the radiotherapy workflow are provided by Scripes and Thorwarth [181, 182]. These issues are further accentuated when merging or fusing multiple imaging modalities together into a single viewable series; where in addition to resolution, deformation becomes prevalent. This can happen between scans on different modalities and also within a single modality throughout time. Whether the tissue is expanding, shrinking, or simply changing shape, the effect on target volumes, both anatomic and biologic, and how they relate to a planned dose distribution will be critical for integrative and adaptive radiotherapy. There is much work focusing on deformable registration algorithms both for intra- and inter-imaging modality, but wide clinical implementation and verification is still incomplete [183–185].

A related issue to resolution is spatial/geometric distortion. While generally not an issue for CT- or PET-based imaging modalities, this can be a large problem in MRI. Distortions in MRI are generally related to inhomogeneities in the main magnetic field and nonlinearities in localizing gradient pulses. These distortions can be intrinsic to scanner-specific field generation, in which case they can usually be modeled and overcome, or by insertion of a nonuniform object into the magnetic field—which is unavoidable as the goal is to have patients within the scanner. As these artifacts are unique to each shape, they can be more difficult to systematically address. In diagnostic radiology, these distortions may not represent a significant issue, as description and identification of disease may depend less on robust spatial integrity; however in targeted radiotherapy, precision and accuracy are of the utmost importance. There are ongoing efforts to develop more robust MRI sequences specifically to address this problem, as well as MRI phantoms to verify spatial accuracy [186, 187]; however, the default radiotherapy reaction is as before to increase safety margins, which again is ultimately counterproductive.

Verification

A key aspect in reducing uncertainties (and therefore volumes) in radiotherapy is the treatment verification process, where daily setup is compared to and adjusted according to treatment planning scans. The precision of this task is directly related to the PTV margin utilized in patient planning. Currently the radiotherapy workflow is organized around CT-based planning and daily verification via orthogonal

X-rays, megavoltage portal films, or volumetric cone-beam CT scans. This practice is relatively robust as image comparison among X-ray-based modalities is straightforward. Introduction of functional imaging modalities, particularly MRI based, represents a new challenge for daily verification. The most utilized approach is to verify registration between planning scan and the adjunct planning images, leaving daily verification solely X-ray based. As discussed above, this approach has several shortcomings and the alternative is again to increase the PTV margin. Ongoing work toward MRI-based verification scans in MRI-linac systems offers perhaps a better solution to this problem [188–190].

Summary

Functional imaging and the capability to target and optimize treatment plans according to biology in addition to anatomy represent an exciting new area in radiation oncology. However, a number of technical challenges must be considered before true integration can take place. Questions remain on when the optimal time is to obtain biologic imaging (and whether this needs to be repeated during treatment), how to incorporate radiotherapy immobilization, how precise image registration is (± deformation), and how to verify daily treatment position. With ongoing development of new imaging modalities and new radiotherapy delivery platforms, these questions will hopefully be addressed.

Conclusion

Since its inception, radiation oncology has been an image-guided treatment modality. Advances in imaging technology have allowed for the direct visualization and quantification of biologic processes critical to therapy response. This chapter has outlined and summarized a variety of these techniques including PET (with a variety of tracers), diffusion- and contrast-based MRI (and CT), and spectroscopy, organized by three of the classic tenants of radiobiology: *r*epopulation, *r*eoxygenation, and *r*epair. The ability to better delineate and target tumors according to their biologic underpinnings and specifically how they enhance or compromise interactions with radiotherapy will allow further personalization of patient care. Retrospective and ongoing prospective studies investigating these interactions have shown promising results in terms of tumor control and treatment toxicity. The long-term viability of this strategy will depend on the maturation of these and future studies, as well as overcoming current technical limitations, including spatial-temporal resolution and workflow integration. With ongoing effort, the goal of multimodality-based radiotherapy is achievable and can potentially provide a fulcrum to further tilt the therapeutic ratio in the patients' favor.

References

1. Nakamura K et al (2014) Recent advances in radiation oncology: intensity-modulated radiotherapy, a clinical perspective. Int J Clin Oncol 19(4):564–569
2. Hodapp N (2012) The ICRU Report 83: prescribing, recording and reporting photon-beam intensity-modulated radiation therapy (IMRT). Strahlenther Onkol 188(1):97–99
3. Ling CC, Li XA (2005) Over the next decade the success of radiation treatment planning will be judged by the immediate biological response of tumor cells rather than by surrogate measures such as dose maximization and uniformity. Med Phys 32(7):2189–2192
4. Bentzen SM (2005) Theragnostic imaging for radiation oncology: dose-painting by numbers. Lancet Oncol 6(2):112–117
5. Withers HR (1985) Biologic basis for altered fractionation schemes. Cancer 55(Suppl 9): 2086–2095
6. Steel GG (1996) From targets to genes: a brief history of radiosensitivity. Phys Med Biol 41(2):205–222
7. Harrington K, Jankowska P, Hingorani M (2007) Molecular biology for the radiation oncologist: the 5Rs of radiobiology meet the hallmarks of cancer. Clin Oncol (R Coll Radiol) 19(8): 561–571
8. Hanahan D, Weinberg RA (2000) The hallmarks of cancer. Cell 100(1):57–70
9. Fischer BM, Lassen U, Hojgaard L (2011) PET-CT in preoperative staging of lung cancer. N Engl J Med 364(10):980–981
10. Schmidt T et al (2015) Value of functional imaging by PET in esophageal cancer. J Natl Compr Canc Netw 13(2):239–247
11. Ng SH et al (2008) Distant metastases and synchronous second primary tumors in patients with newly diagnosed oropharyngeal and hypopharyngeal carcinomas: evaluation of (18) F-FDG PET and extended-field multi-detector row CT. Neuroradiology 50(11):969–979
12. Abramyuk A et al (2013) Modification of staging and treatment of head and neck cancer by FDG-PET/CT prior to radiotherapy. Strahlenther Onkol 189(3):197–201
13. Gallamini A, Borra A (2014) Role of PET in lymphoma. Curr Treat Options Oncol 15(2): 248–261
14. Calais J et al (2015) Areas of high 18F-FDG uptake on preradiotherapy PET/CT identify preferential sites of local relapse after chemoradiotherapy for non-small cell lung cancer. J Nucl Med 56(2):196–203
15. Bradley J et al (2004) Impact of FDG-PET on radiation therapy volume delineation in non-small-cell lung cancer. Int J Radiat Oncol Biol Phys 59(1):78–86
16. Roh JL et al (2014) Clinical significance of pretreatment metabolic tumor volume and total lesion glycolysis in hypopharyngeal squamous cell carcinomas. J Surg Oncol 110(7): 869–875
17. Due AK et al (2014) Recurrences after intensity modulated radiotherapy for head and neck squamous cell carcinoma more likely to originate from regions with high baseline [18F]-FDG uptake. Radiother Oncol 111(3):360–365
18. Hoeben BA et al (2013) Molecular PET imaging for biology-guided adaptive radiotherapy of head and neck cancer. Acta Oncol 52(7):1257–1271
19. van Stiphout RG et al (2014) Nomogram predicting response after chemoradiotherapy in rectal cancer using sequential PETCT imaging: a multicentric prospective study with external validation. Radiother Oncol 113(2):215–222
20. Schollaert P et al (2014) A systematic review of the predictive value of (18)FDG-PET in esophageal and esophagogastric junction cancer after neoadjuvant chemoradiation on the survival outcome stratification. J Gastrointest Surg 18(5):894–905
21. Engert A et al (2012) Reduced-intensity chemotherapy and PET-guided radiotherapy in patients with advanced stage Hodgkin's lymphoma (HD15 trial): a randomised, open-label, phase 3 non-inferiority trial. Lancet 379(9828):1791–1799

22. Raemaekers JM et al (2014) Omitting radiotherapy in early positron emission tomography-negative stage I/II Hodgkin lymphoma is associated with an increased risk of early relapse: clinical results of the preplanned interim analysis of the randomized EORTC/LYSA/FIL H10 trial. J Clin Oncol 32(12):1188–1194
23. Jelercic S, Rajer M (2015) The role of PET-CT in radiotherapy planning of solid tumours. Radiol Oncol 49(1):1–9
24. Kilic D et al (2015) Is there any impact of PET/CT on radiotherapy planning in rectal cancer patients undergoing preoperative IMRT? Turk J Med Sci 45(1):129–135
25. Vojtisek R et al (2014) The impact of PET/CT scanning on the size of target volumes, radiation exposure of organs at risk, TCP and NTCP, in the radiotherapy planning of non-small cell lung cancer. Rep Pract Oncol Radiother 19(3):182–190
26. Nkhali L et al (2015) FDG-PET/CT during concomitant chemo radiotherapy for esophageal cancer: reducing target volumes to deliver higher radiotherapy doses. Acta Oncol 54(6): 909–915
27. Daisne JF et al (2004) Tumor volume in pharyngolaryngeal squamous cell carcinoma: comparison at CT, MR imaging, and FDG PET and validation with surgical specimen. Radiology 233(1):93–100
28. Madani I et al (2011) Maximum tolerated dose in a phase I trial on adaptive dose painting by numbers for head and neck cancer. Radiother Oncol 101(3):351–355
29. Yu W et al (2015) Safety of dose escalation by simultaneous integrated boosting radiation dose within the primary tumor guided by (18)FDG-PET/CT for esophageal cancer. Radiother Oncol 114(2):195–200
30. van Der Wel A et al (2005) Increased therapeutic ratio by 18FDG-PET CT planning in patients with clinical CT stage N2-N3M0 non-small-cell lung cancer: a modeling study. Int J Radiat Oncol Biol Phys 61(3):649–655
31. van Elmpt W et al (2012) The PET-boost randomised phase II dose-escalation trial in non-small cell lung cancer. Radiother Oncol 104(1):67–71
32. Shi X et al (2014) PET/CT imaging-guided dose painting in radiation therapy. Cancer Lett 355(2):169–175
33. Mukundan H et al (2014) MRI and PET-CT: comparison in post-treatment evaluation of head and neck squamous cell carcinomas. Med J Armed Forces India 70(2):111–115
34. Kauppi JT et al (2012) Locally advanced esophageal adenocarcinoma: response to neoadjuvant chemotherapy and survival predicted by ([18F])FDG-PET/CT. Acta Oncol 51(5):636–644
35. Bahce I et al (2014) Metabolic activity measured by FDG PET predicts pathological response in locally advanced superior sulcus NSCLC. Lung Cancer 85(2):205–212
36. Schwarz JK et al (2012) Metabolic response on post-therapy FDG-PET predicts patterns of failure after radiotherapy for cervical cancer. Int J Radiat Oncol Biol Phys 83(1):185–190
37. Pathmanathan N, Balleine RL (2013) Ki67 and proliferation in breast cancer. J Clin Pathol 66(6):512–516
38. Wang XW, Zhang YJ (2014) Targeting mTOR network in colorectal cancer therapy. World J Gastroenterol 20(15):4178–4188
39. Ruschoff J et al (1996) Prognostic significance of molecular biological and immunohistological parameters in gastrointestinal carcinomas. Recent Results Cancer Res 142:73–88
40. Skalova A, Leivo I (1996) Cell proliferation in salivary gland tumors. Gen Diagn Pathol 142(1):7–16
41. Kim JJ, Tannock IF (2005) Repopulation of cancer cells during therapy: an important cause of treatment failure. Nat Rev Cancer 5(7):516–525
42. Janssen S et al (2009) Anal cancer treated with radio-chemotherapy: correlation between length of treatment interruption and outcome. Int J Colorectal Dis 24(12):1421–1428
43. Duncan W et al (1996) Adverse effect of treatment gaps in the outcome of radiotherapy for laryngeal cancer. Radiother Oncol 41(3):203–207
44. Moonen L et al (1998) Muscle-invasive bladder cancer treated with external beam radiation: influence of total dose, overall treatment time, and treatment interruption on local control. Int J Radiat Oncol Biol Phys 42(3):525–530

45. Fyles A et al (1992) The effect of treatment duration in the local control of cervix cancer. Radiother Oncol 25(4):273–279
46. Robertson C et al (1998) Similar decreases in local tumor control are calculated for treatment protraction and for interruptions in the radiotherapy of carcinoma of the larynx in four centers. Int J Radiat Oncol Biol Phys 40(2):319–329
47. Nakajo M et al (2014) Correlations of (18)F-fluorothymidine uptake with pathological tumour size, Ki-67 and thymidine kinase 1 expressions in primary and metastatic lymph node colorectal cancer foci. Eur Radiol 24(12):3199–3209
48. Yamamoto Y et al (2012) Correlation of 18F-FLT uptake with tumor grade and Ki-67 immunohistochemistry in patients with newly diagnosed and recurrent gliomas. J Nucl Med 53(12):1911–1915
49. Woolf DK et al (2014) Evaluation of FLT-PET-CT as an imaging biomarker of proliferation in primary breast cancer. Br J Cancer 110(12):2847–2854
50. Hoeben BA et al (2013) 18F-FLT PET during radiotherapy or chemoradiotherapy in head and neck squamous cell carcinoma is an early predictor of outcome. J Nucl Med 54(4):532–540
51. Zander T et al (2011) Early prediction of nonprogression in advanced non-small-cell lung cancer treated with erlotinib by using [(18)F]fluorodeoxyglucose and [(18)F]fluorothymidine positron emission tomography. J Clin Oncol 29(13):1701–1708
52. Everitt SJ et al (2014) Differential 18F-FDG and 18F-FLT uptake on serial PET/CT imaging before and during definitive chemoradiation for non-small cell lung cancer. J Nucl Med 55(7):1069–1074
53. Zhang G et al (2015) Gradient-based delineation of the primary GTV on FLT PET in squamous cell cancer of the thoracic esophagus and impact on radiotherapy planning. Radiat Oncol 10(1):11
54. Patel DA et al (2007) Impact of integrated PET/CT on variability of target volume delineation in rectal cancer. Technol Cancer Res Treat 6(1):31–36
55. Troost EG et al (2010) 18F-FLT PET/CT for early response monitoring and dose escalation in oropharyngeal tumors. J Nucl Med 51(6):866–874
56. Tehrani OS, Shields AF (2013) PET imaging of proliferation with pyrimidines. J Nucl Med 54(6):903–912
57. Contractor K et al (2011) Use of [11C]choline PET-CT as a noninvasive method for detecting pelvic lymph node status from prostate cancer and relationship with choline kinase expression. Clin Cancer Res 17(24):7673–7683
58. Chan J et al (2015) Is choline PET useful for identifying intraprostatic tumour lesions? A literature review. Nucl Med Commun
59. Chang JH et al (2012) Intensity modulated radiation therapy dose painting for localized prostate cancer using (1)(1)C-choline positron emission tomography scans. Int J Radiat Oncol Biol Phys 83(5):e691–e696
60. Niyazi M et al (2010) Choline PET based dose-painting in prostate cancer—modelling of dose effects. Radiat Oncol 5:23
61. Pinkawa M et al (2012) Dose-escalation using intensity-modulated radiotherapy for prostate cancer—evaluation of quality of life with and without (18)F-choline PET-CT detected simultaneous integrated boost. Radiat Oncol 7:14
62. Goldstein J et al (2014) Does choline PET/CT change the management of prostate cancer patients with biochemical failure? Am J Clin Oncol
63. Alongi F et al (2014) 11C choline PET guided salvage radiotherapy with volumetric modulation arc therapy and hypofractionation for recurrent prostate cancer after HIFU failure: preliminary results of tolerability and acute toxicity. Technol Cancer Res Treat 13(5):395–401
64. Hamstra DA, Rehemtulla A, Ross BD (2007) Diffusion magnetic resonance imaging: a biomarker for treatment response in oncology. J Clin Oncol 25(26):4104–4109
65. Thoeny HC, De Keyzer F, King AD (2012) Diffusion-weighted MR imaging in the head and neck. Radiology 263(1):19–32
66. Thoeny HC, Forstner R, De Keyzer F (2012) Genitourinary applications of diffusion-weighted MR imaging in the pelvis. Radiology 263(2):326–342

67. Petralia G, Thoeny HC (2010) DW-MRI of the urogenital tract: applications in oncology. Cancer Imaging 10(Spec no A):S112–S123
68. Mascalchi M et al (2005) Diffusion-weighted MR of the brain: methodology and clinical application. Radiol Med 109(3):155–197
69. Sevcenco S et al (2014) Quantitative apparent diffusion coefficient measurements obtained by 3-Tesla MRI are correlated with biomarkers of bladder cancer proliferative activity. PLoS One 9(9), e106866
70. Cipolla V et al (2014) Correlation between 3T apparent diffusion coefficient values and grading of invasive breast carcinoma. Eur J Radiol 83(12):2144–2150
71. Kim EJ et al (2015) Histogram analysis of apparent diffusion coefficient at 3.0t: correlation with prognostic factors and subtypes of invasive ductal carcinoma. J Magn Reson Imaging
72. Donati OF et al (2014) Prostate cancer aggressiveness: assessment with whole-lesion histogram analysis of the apparent diffusion coefficient. Radiology 271(1):143–152
73. Woo S et al (2014) Histogram analysis of apparent diffusion coefficient map of diffusion-weighted MRI in endometrial cancer: a preliminary correlation study with histological grade. Acta Radiol 55(10):1270–1277
74. Rothke M et al (2013) PI-RADS classification: structured reporting for MRI of the prostate. Röfo 185(3):253–261
75. Futterer JJ et al (2015) Can clinically significant prostate cancer be detected with multiparametric magnetic resonance imaging? A systematic review of the literature. Eur Urol 68(6): 1045–1053
76. Micco M et al (2014) Combined pre-treatment MRI and 18F-FDG PET/CT parameters as prognostic biomarkers in patients with cervical cancer. Eur J Radiol 83(7):1169–1176
77. Nakamura K et al (2012) The mean apparent diffusion coefficient value (ADCmean) on primary cervical cancer is a predictive marker for disease recurrence. Gynecol Oncol 127(3): 478–483
78. Kuang F et al (2013) The value of apparent diffusion coefficient in the assessment of cervical cancer. Eur Radiol 23(4):1050–1058
79. Chopra S et al (2012) Evaluation of diffusion-weighted imaging as a predictive marker for tumor response in patients undergoing chemoradiation for postoperative recurrences of cervical cancer. J Cancer Res Ther 8(1):68–73
80. Joye I et al (2014) The role of diffusion-weighted MRI and (18)F-FDG PET/CT in the prediction of pathologic complete response after radiochemotherapy for rectal cancer: a systematic review. Radiother Oncol 113(2):158–165
81. Yu JI et al (2014) The role of diffusion-weighted magnetic resonance imaging in the treatment response evaluation of hepatocellular carcinoma patients treated with radiation therapy. Int J Radiat Oncol Biol Phys 89(4):814–821
82. Hamstra DA et al (2008) Functional diffusion map as an early imaging biomarker for high-grade glioma: correlation with conventional radiologic response and overall survival. J Clin Oncol 26(20):3387–3394
83. Galban CJ et al (2009) A feasibility study of parametric response map analysis of diffusion-weighted magnetic resonance imaging scans of head and neck cancer patients for providing early detection of therapeutic efficacy. Transl Oncol 2(3):184–190
84. Chen Y et al (2014) Diffusion-weighted magnetic resonance imaging for early response assessment of chemoradiotherapy in patients with nasopharyngeal carcinoma. Magn Reson Imaging 32(6):630–637
85. Eccles CL et al (2009) Change in diffusion weighted MRI during liver cancer radiotherapy: preliminary observations. Acta Oncol 48(7):1034–1043
86. Sun YS et al (2010) Locally advanced rectal carcinoma treated with preoperative chemotherapy and radiation therapy: preliminary analysis of diffusion-weighted MR imaging for early detection of tumor histopathologic downstaging. Radiology 254(1):170–178
87. Kim SH et al (2011) Apparent diffusion coefficient for evaluating tumour response to neoadjuvant chemoradiation therapy for locally advanced rectal cancer. Eur Radiol 21(5):987–995

88. Cai G et al (2013) Diffusion-weighted magnetic resonance imaging for predicting the response of rectal cancer to neoadjuvant concurrent chemoradiation. World J Gastroenterol 19(33):5520–5527

89. Harry VN et al (2008) Diffusion-weighted magnetic resonance imaging in the early detection of response to chemoradiation in cervical cancer. Gynecol Oncol 111(2):213–220

90. Kim HS et al (2013) Evaluation of therapeutic response to concurrent chemoradiotherapy in patients with cervical cancer using diffusion-weighted MR imaging. J Magn Reson Imaging 37(1):187–193

91. Fu C et al (2012) The value of diffusion-weighted magnetic resonance imaging in assessing the response of locally advanced cervical cancer to neoadjuvant chemotherapy. Int J Gynecol Cancer 22(6):1037–1043

92. Fu ZZ et al (2015) Value of apparent diffusion coefficient (ADC) in assessing radiotherapy and chemotherapy success in cervical cancer. Magn Reson Imaging 33(5):516–524

93. Liney GP et al (2015) Quantitative evaluation of diffusion-weighted imaging techniques for the purposes of radiotherapy planning in the prostate. Br J Radiol 88(1049):20150034

94. Regini F et al (2014) Rectal tumour volume (GTV) delineation using T2-weighted and diffusion-weighted MRI: implications for radiotherapy planning. Eur J Radiol 83(5):768–772

95. Tsien C, Cao Y, Chenevert T (2014) Clinical applications for diffusion magnetic resonance imaging in radiotherapy. Semin Radiat Oncol 24(3):218–226

96. Walsh JC et al (2014) The clinical importance of assessing tumor hypoxia: relationship of tumor hypoxia to prognosis and therapeutic opportunities. Antioxid Redox Signal 21(10):1516–1554

97. Peitzsch C et al (2014) Hypoxia as a biomarker for radioresistant cancer stem cells. Int J Radiat Biol 90(8):636–652

98. Vaupel P, Mayer A (2007) Hypoxia in cancer: significance and impact on clinical outcome. Cancer Metastasis Rev 26(2):225–239

99. Overgaard J (2011) Hypoxic modification of radiotherapy in squamous cell carcinoma of the head and neck—a systematic review and meta-analysis. Radiother Oncol 100(1):22–32

100. Overgaard J (2007) Hypoxic radiosensitization: adored and ignored. J Clin Oncol 25(26): 4066–4074

101. Brizel DM et al (1996) Radiation therapy and hyperthermia improve the oxygenation of human soft tissue sarcomas. Cancer Res 56(23):5347–5350

102. Fyles AW et al (1998) Cervix cancer oxygenation measured following external radiation therapy. Int J Radiat Oncol Biol Phys 42(4):751–753

103. Chapman JD (1979) Hypoxic sensitizers—implications for radiation therapy. N Engl J Med 301(26):1429–1432

104. Mortensen LS et al (2012) FAZA PET/CT hypoxia imaging in patients with squamous cell carcinoma of the head and neck treated with radiotherapy: results from the DAHANCA 24 trial. Radiother Oncol 105(1):14–20

105. Thorwarth D et al (2005) Kinetic analysis of dynamic 18F-fluoromisonidazole PET correlates with radiation treatment outcome in head-and-neck cancer. BMC Cancer 5:152

106. Chang E et al (2014) 18F-FAZA PET imaging response tracks the reoxygenation of tumors in mice upon treatment with the mitochondrial complex I inhibitor BAY 87-2243. Clin Cancer Res 21(2):335–346

107. Zips D et al (2012) Exploratory prospective trial of hypoxia-specific PET imaging during radiochemotherapy in patients with locally advanced head-and-neck cancer. Radiother Oncol 105(1):21–28

108. Dehdashti F et al (2008) Assessing tumor hypoxia in cervical cancer by PET with 60Cu-labeled diacetyl-bis(N4-methylthiosemicarbazone). J Nucl Med 49(2):201–205

109. Kikuchi M et al (2011) 18F-fluoromisonidazole positron emission tomography before treatment is a predictor of radiotherapy outcome and survival prognosis in patients with head and neck squamous cell carcinoma. Ann Nucl Med 25(9):625–633

110. Vercellino L et al (2012) Hypoxia imaging of uterine cervix carcinoma with (18)F-FETNIM PET/CT. Clin Nucl Med 37(11):1065–1068

111. Li L et al (2010) Comparison of 18F-Fluoroerythronitroimidazole and 18F-fluorodeoxyglucose positron emission tomography and prognostic value in locally advanced non-small-cell lung cancer. Clin Lung Cancer 11(5):335–340
112. Rajendran JG et al (2006) Tumor hypoxia imaging with [F-18] fluoromisonidazole positron emission tomography in head and neck cancer. Clin Cancer Res 12(18):5435–5441
113. Spence AM et al (2008) Regional hypoxia in glioblastoma multiforme quantified with [18F] fluoromisonidazole positron emission tomography before radiotherapy: correlation with time to progression and survival. Clin Cancer Res 14(9):2623–2630
114. Horsman MR et al (2012) Imaging hypoxia to improve radiotherapy outcome. Nat Rev Clin Oncol 9(12):674–687
115. Servagi-Vernat S et al (2015) Hypoxia-guided adaptive radiation dose escalation in head and neck carcinoma: a planning study. Acta Oncol 54(7):1008–1016
116. Chang JH et al (2013) Hypoxia-targeted radiotherapy dose painting for head and neck cancer using (18)F-FMISO PET: a biological modeling study. Acta Oncol 52(8):1723–1729
117. Henriques de Figueiredo B et al (2015) Hypoxia imaging with [18F]-FMISO-PET for guided dose escalation with intensity-modulated radiotherapy in head-and-neck cancers. Strahlenther Onkol 191(3):217–224
118. Lin Z et al (2008) The influence of changes in tumor hypoxia on dose-painting treatment plans based on 18F-FMISO positron emission tomography. Int J Radiat Oncol Biol Phys 70(4):1219–1228
119. Bollineni VR et al (2014) Dynamics of tumor hypoxia assessed by 18F-FAZA PET/CT in head and neck and lung cancer patients during chemoradiation: possible implications for radiotherapy treatment planning strategies. Radiother Oncol 113(2):198–203
120. Helbig L et al (2014) BAY 87-2243, a novel inhibitor of hypoxia-induced gene activation, improves local tumor control after fractionated irradiation in a schedule-dependent manner in head and neck human xenografts. Radiat Oncol 9:207
121. Beck R et al (2007) Pretreatment 18F-FAZA PET predicts success of hypoxia-directed radio-chemotherapy using tirapazamine. J Nucl Med 48(6):973–980
122. Padhani A (2006) PET imaging of tumour hypoxia. Cancer Imaging 6:S117–S121
123. Fleming IN et al (2015) Imaging tumour hypoxia with positron emission tomography. Br J Cancer 112(2):238–250
124. Cooper RA et al (2000) Tumour oxygenation levels correlate with dynamic contrast-enhanced magnetic resonance imaging parameters in carcinoma of the cervix. Radiother Oncol 57(1): 53–59
125. Mayr NA et al (1996) Tumor perfusion studies using fast magnetic resonance imaging technique in advanced cervical cancer: a new noninvasive predictive assay. Int J Radiat Oncol Biol Phys 36(3):623–633
126. Borren A et al (2013) Expression of hypoxia-inducible factor-1alpha and -2alpha in whole-mount prostate histology: relation with dynamic contrast-enhanced MRI and Gleason score. Oncol Rep 29(6):2249–2254
127. Ellingsen C et al (2014) DCE-MRI of the hypoxic fraction, radioresponsiveness, and metastatic propensity of cervical carcinoma xenografts. Radiother Oncol 110(2):335–341
128. Linnik IV et al (2014) Noninvasive tumor hypoxia measurement using magnetic resonance imaging in murine U87 glioma xenografts and in patients with glioblastoma. Magn Reson Med 71(5):1854–1862
129. Halle C et al (2012) Hypoxia-induced gene expression in chemoradioresistant cervical cancer revealed by dynamic contrast-enhanced MRI. Cancer Res 72(20):5285–5295
130. Mayr NA et al (2000) Pixel analysis of MR perfusion imaging in predicting radiation therapy outcome in cervical cancer. J Magn Reson Imaging 12(6):1027–1033
131. Mayr NA et al (2010) Longitudinal changes in tumor perfusion pattern during the radiation therapy course and its clinical impact in cervical cancer. Int J Radiat Oncol Biol Phys 77(2):502–508

132. van Lin EN et al (2006) IMRT boost dose planning on dominant intraprostatic lesions: gold marker-based three-dimensional fusion of CT with dynamic contrast-enhanced and 1H-spectroscopic MRI. Int J Radiat Oncol Biol Phys 65(1):291–303
133. Garibaldi E et al (2016) Clinical and technical feasibility of ultra-boost irradiation in Dominant Intraprostatic Lesion by Tomotherapy: preliminary experience and revision of literature. Panminerva Med 58(1):16–22
134. Lips IM et al (2011) Single blind randomized phase III trial to investigate the benefit of a focal lesion ablative microboost in prostate cancer (FLAME-trial): study protocol for a randomized controlled trial. Trials 12:255
135. Hallac RR et al (2014) Correlations of noninvasive BOLD and TOLD MRI with pO2 and relevance to tumor radiation response. Magn Reson Med 71(5):1863–1873
136. Al-Hallaq HA et al (2000) MRI measurements correctly predict the relative effects of tumor oxygenating agents on hypoxic fraction in rodent BA1112 tumors. Int J Radiat Oncol Biol Phys 47(2):481–488
137. Toth V et al (2013) MR-based hypoxia measures in human glioma. J Neurooncol 115(2): 197–207
138. Liu M et al (2013) BOLD-MRI of breast invasive ductal carcinoma: correlation of R2* value and the expression of HIF-1alpha. Eur Radiol 23(12):3221–3227
139. Chopra S et al (2009) Comparing oxygen-sensitive MRI (BOLD R2*) with oxygen electrode measurements: a pilot study in men with prostate cancer. Int J Radiat Biol 85(9):805–813
140. Sovik A et al (2007) Radiotherapy adapted to spatial and temporal variability in tumor hypoxia. Int J Radiat Oncol Biol Phys 68(5):1496–1504
141. Matsuo M et al (2014) Magnetic resonance imaging of the tumor microenvironment in radiotherapy: perfusion, hypoxia, and metabolism. Semin Radiat Oncol 24(3):210–217
142. Mandeville HC et al (2012) Operable non-small cell lung cancer: correlation of volumetric helical dynamic contrast-enhanced CT parameters with immunohistochemical markers of tumor hypoxia. Radiology 264(2):581–589
143. Newbold K et al (2009) An exploratory study into the role of dynamic contrast-enhanced magnetic resonance imaging or perfusion computed tomography for detection of intratumoral hypoxia in head-and-neck cancer. Int J Radiat Oncol Biol Phys 74(1):29–37
144. Nyflot MJ et al (2015) Phase 1 trial of bevacizumab with concurrent chemoradiation therapy for squamous cell carcinoma of the head and neck with exploratory functional imaging of tumor hypoxia, proliferation, and perfusion. Int J Radiat Oncol Biol Phys 91(5):942–951
145. Yeung TP et al (2015) Survival prediction in high-grade gliomas using CT perfusion imaging. J Neurooncol 123(1):93–102
146. van Elmpt W et al (2014) Imaging techniques for tumour delineation and heterogeneity quantification of lung cancer: overview of current possibilities. J Thorac Dis 6(4):319–327
147. Astner ST et al (2010) Imaging of tumor physiology: impacts on clinical radiation oncology. Exp Oncol 32(3):149–152
148. Shibata A, Jeggo PA (2014) DNA double-strand break repair in a cellular context. Clin Oncol (R Coll Radiol) 26(5):243–249
149. Tamulevicius P, Wang M, Iliakis G (2007) Homology-directed repair is required for the development of radioresistance during S phase: interplay between double-strand break repair and checkpoint response. Radiat Res 167(1):1–11
150. Crawford FW et al (2009) Relationship of pre-surgery metabolic and physiological MR imaging parameters to survival for patients with untreated GBM. J Neurooncol 91(3):337–351
151. Saraswathy S et al (2009) Evaluation of MR markers that predict survival in patients with newly diagnosed GBM prior to adjuvant therapy. J Neurooncol 91(1):69–81
152. Ken S et al (2013) Integration method of 3D MR spectroscopy into treatment planning system for glioblastoma IMRT dose painting with integrated simultaneous boost. Radiat Oncol 8:1
153. Einstein DB et al (2012) Phase II trial of radiosurgery to magnetic resonance spectroscopy-defined high-risk tumor volumes in patients with glioblastoma multiforme. Int J Radiat Oncol Biol Phys 84(3):668–674

154. Jahangiri A, Aghi MK (2012) Pseudoprogression and treatment effect. Neurosurg Clin N Am 23(2):277–287, viii–ix
155. Huang J et al (2011) Differentiation between intra-axial metastatic tumor progression and radiation injury following fractionated radiation therapy or stereotactic radiosurgery using MR spectroscopy, perfusion MR imaging or volume progression modeling. Magn Reson Imaging 29(7):993–1001
156. Elias AE et al (2011) MR spectroscopy using normalized and non-normalized metabolite ratios for differentiating recurrent brain tumor from radiation injury. Acad Radiol 18(9):1101–1108
157. Zhang H et al (2014) Role of magnetic resonance spectroscopy for the differentiation of recurrent glioma from radiation necrosis: a systematic review and meta-analysis. Eur J Radiol 83(12):2181–2189
158. Mueller-Lisse UG, Scherr MK (2007) Proton MR spectroscopy of the prostate. Eur J Radiol 63(3):351–360
159. Yuen JS et al (2004) Endorectal magnetic resonance imaging and spectroscopy for the detection of tumor foci in men with prior negative transrectal ultrasound prostate biopsy. J Urol 171(4):1482–1486
160. Selnaes KM et al (2013) Spatially matched in vivo and ex vivo MR metabolic profiles of prostate cancer—investigation of a correlation with Gleason score. NMR Biomed 26(5): 600–606
161. DiBiase SJ et al (2002) Magnetic resonance spectroscopic imaging-guided brachytherapy for localized prostate cancer. Int J Radiat Oncol Biol Phys 52(2):429–438
162. Pickett B et al (1999) Static field intensity modulation to treat a dominant intra-prostatic lesion to 90 Gy compared to seven field 3-dimensional radiotherapy. Int J Radiat Oncol Biol Phys 44(4):921–929
163. Riches SF et al (2014) Effect on therapeutic ratio of planning a boosted radiotherapy dose to the dominant intraprostatic tumour lesion within the prostate based on multifunctional MR parameters. Br J Radiol 87(1037):20130813
164. Thind K et al (2014) Mapping metabolic changes associated with early Radiation Induced Lung Injury post conformal radiotherapy using hyperpolarized (1)(3)C-pyruvate Magnetic Resonance Spectroscopic Imaging. Radiother Oncol 110(2):317–322
165. Kauczor HU et al (1996) Normal and abnormal pulmonary ventilation: visualization at hyperpolarized He-3 MR imaging. Radiology 201(2):564–568
166. Hodge CW et al (2010) On the use of hyperpolarized helium MRI for conformal avoidance lung radiotherapy. Med Dosim 35(4):297–303
167. Hoover DA et al (2014) Functional lung avoidance for individualized radiotherapy (FLAIR): study protocol for a randomized, double-blind clinical trial. BMC Cancer 14:934
168. Nguyen ML et al (2014) The potential role of magnetic resonance spectroscopy in image-guided radiotherapy. Front Oncol 4:91
169. Le Bihan D et al (2001) Diffusion tensor imaging: concepts and applications. J Magn Reson Imaging 13(4):534–546
170. Stebbins GT, Murphy CM (2009) Diffusion tensor imaging in Alzheimer's disease and mild cognitive impairment. Behav Neurol 21(1):39–49
171. Chapman CH et al (2012) Diffusion tensor imaging of normal-appearing white matter as biomarker for radiation-induced late delayed cognitive decline. Int J Radiat Oncol Biol Phys 82(5):2033–2040
172. Edelmann MN et al (2014) Diffusion tensor imaging and neurocognition in survivors of childhood acute lymphoblastic leukaemia. Brain 137(Pt 11):2973–2983
173. Berberat J et al (2014) Diffusion tensor imaging for target volume definition in glioblastoma multiforme. Strahlenther Onkol 190(10):939–943
174. Koga T et al (2012) Outcomes of diffusion tensor tractography-integrated stereotactic radiosurgery. Int J Radiat Oncol Biol Phys 82(2):799–802
175. Koga T et al (2012) Integration of corticospinal tractography reduces motor complications after radiosurgery. Int J Radiat Oncol Biol Phys 83(1):129–133

176. Hanvey S, Glegg M, Foster J (2009) Magnetic resonance imaging for radiotherapy planning of brain cancer patients using immobilization and surface coils. Phys Med Biol 54(18):5381–5394

177. Ahmed M et al (2010) The value of magnetic resonance imaging in target volume delineation of base of tongue tumours—a study using flexible surface coils. Radiother Oncol 94(2):161–167

178. Houweling AC et al (2010) Magnetic resonance imaging at 3.0T for submandibular gland sparing radiotherapy. Radiother Oncol 97(2):239–243

179. Houweling AC et al (2013) FDG-PET and diffusion-weighted MRI in head-and-neck cancer patients: implications for dose painting. Radiother Oncol 106(2):250–254

180. Decker G et al (2014) Intensity-modulated radiotherapy of the prostate: dynamic ADC monitoring by DWI at 3.0 T. Radiother Oncol 113(1):115–120

181. Scripes PG, Yaparpalvi R (2012) Technical aspects of positron emission tomography/computed tomography in radiotherapy treatment planning. Semin Nucl Med 42(5):283–288

182. Thorwarth D, Alber M (2010) Implementation of hypoxia imaging into treatment planning and delivery. Radiother Oncol 97(2):172–175

183. Yu G et al (2015) Accelerated gradient-based free form deformable registration for online adaptive radiotherapy. Phys Med Biol 60(7):2765–2783

184. Leibfarth S et al (2013) A strategy for multimodal deformable image registration to integrate PET/MR into radiotherapy treatment planning. Acta Oncol 52(7):1353–1359

185. Niu CJ et al (2012) A novel technique to enable experimental validation of deformable dose accumulation. Med Phys 39(2):765–776

186. Torfeh T et al (2015) Development and validation of a novel large field of view phantom and a software module for the quality assurance of geometric distortion in magnetic resonance imaging. Magn Reson Imaging 33(7):939–949

187. Haack S et al (2014) Correction of diffusion-weighted magnetic resonance imaging for brachytherapy of locally advanced cervical cancer. Acta Oncol 53(8):1073–1078

188. Keall PJ, Barton M, Crozier S (2014) The Australian magnetic resonance imaging-linac program. Semin Radiat Oncol 24(3):203–206

189. Lagendijk JJ, Raaymakers BW, van Vulpen M (2014) The magnetic resonance imaging-linac system. Semin Radiat Oncol 24(3):207–209

190. Jaffray DA et al (2014) A facility for magnetic resonance-guided radiation therapy. Semin Radiat Oncol 24(3):193–195

Chapter 10
Increasing the Therapeutic Efficacy of Radiotherapy Using Nanoparticles

Ajlan Al Zaki, David Cormode, Andrew Tsourkas, and Jay F. Dorsey

Abstract Nanoparticles have garnered significant interest in recent decades for both biomedical imaging and therapeutic applications. The ability to finely tune their sizes and morphologies and modify their surface properties to enable cell-specific receptor targeting for tumor localization and prolonged circulation and the potential of low or reduced toxicity make them attractive agents in both cancer imaging and therapy. Recent studies have shown that nanoparticles in combination with radiation therapy can lead to an increase in the number of DNA double-stranded breaks compared with radiation alone and improve cancer survival in mouse models. With recent advances in imaging modalities as well as new radiation therapy technologies, targeted radiation therapy with nanoparticles is actively being pursued as a strategy to increase the effectiveness of radiation-induced cancer cell death while minimizing damage to normal tissues. This chapter will highlight the past and current developments of nanomedicines used to increase the therapeutic ratio of radiotherapy for in vitro models and in vivo models, the mechanisms of radiation enhancement and interaction of ionizing radiation with nanoparticles, and explore the potential for future integration into clinical radiotherapy practice.

Keywords Nanoparticles • Radiosensitizer • Radiotherapy • Imaging • Targeted radiation therapy

A. Al Zaki
George Washington University, School of Medicine and Health Sciences,
Washington, DC 20052, USA
e-mail: ajlan@gwu.edu

D. Cormode • J.F. Dorsey (✉)
Department of Radiation Oncology, Perelman School of Medicine, University of
Pennsylvania, Philadelphia, PA 19104, USA
e-mail: JayD@uphs.upenn.edu

A. Tsourkas
Department of Bioengineering, University of Pennsylvania, Philadelphia, PA 19104, USA
e-mail: atsourk@seas.upenn.edu

© Springer International Publishing Switzerland 2017
P.J. Tofilon, K. Camphausen (eds.), *Increasing the Therapeutic
Ratio of Radiotherapy*, Cancer Drug Discovery and Development,
DOI 10.1007/978-3-319-40854-5_10

Overview of Nanoparticles

Nanoparticles are generally defined as objects on the scale of 1–200 nm in diameter. Due to several inherent advantages, they are being investigated extensively for their potential use in the prevention, diagnosis, and treatment of disease. This technology may have the potential to impact medicine, improve quality of life, lower healthcare costs, and ultimately improve patient outcomes [1]. Additional formulations are being introduced into the clinic for many applications including drug delivery [2], immunization [3, 4], image-guided surgery [5, 6], and imaging [7, 8]. With the growing number of nanoparticle formulations and the variety of materials used, the number of distinct nanoplatforms is too numerous to count. Some of the more commonly used nanoparticles include gold nanoparticles (AuNPs) due to their relative ease of synthesis and tunability as well as unique physicochemical properties, superparamagnetic iron oxide nanoparticles (SPIONs) which possess electromagnetic properties that can be utilized for contrast imaging and magnetic therapy, and polymer-based nanoplatforms. Polymer nanoparticles include liposomal formulations, biodegradable polyethylene glycol block polycaprolactone/polylactic acid (PEG-PCL/PLA) micellar nanocarriers, and polymersomes that can be developed to house therapeutic/imaging agents depending on their hydrophilic and hydrophobic properties [9, 10].

Nanoparticles can be synthesized using different materials ranging from inorganic heavy metals with solid cores to amphiphilic polymers with soft shell components. Their shapes and sizes can be finely tuned, and their surfaces can be modified with ligands to help impart stealthiness and deter opsonization by antibodies and complement proteins, thereby increasing circulation times. They can be designed to carry high therapeutic payloads to increase drug accumulation at disease sites while minimizing off-target toxicities, possess unique properties that respond to extracellular microenvironments to improve cellular uptake and drug release, respond to external stimuli such as electromagnetic radiation to help increase site-specific cellular damage or improve image contrast, and easily integrate both therapeutic and diagnostic functionalities enabling both disease detection and treatment within a single administration. The surface coating of the nanoparticles can also influence the interaction of nanoformulations with their extracellular environment as well as specific cell types.

Strategies of nanoparticle targeting can either be classified as passive targeting or active targeting. Passive targeting of nanoparticle formulations is the preferential, but nonspecific, accumulation at a disease site, mediated by the pharmacokinetics of the nanoparticle and the characteristics of the diseased tissue (i.e., without the use of a targeting ligand). The most well-known example of passive targeting is the enhanced permeability and retention effect, which occurs in tumors. As a tumor grows, it will eventually reach a size where metabolic requirements exceed the capability of the existing nearby vascular supply [11]. Consequently, the tumor will respond by secreting factors to promote the process of angiogenesis resulting in the formation of new blood vessels that facilitate continued growth. Many of these rapidly forming blood vessels are poorly formed, possessing large gaps between endothelial cells, and have non-intact basement membranes, resulting in an increased permeability to structures in the nano-size range [12]. In addition, these actively growing tumors typically have impaired and disorganized lymphatic vessels, causing poor lymphatic drainage which results in the retention of material in the tumor interstitium [11]. This phenomenon of leaky blood vessels and ineffective lymphatic drainage is known as the enhanced permeability and retention (EPR) effect and is the major factor contributing to nanoparticle accumulation in malignancies for diagnostic and therapeutic applications.

Typically many passes through the circulation are necessary in order for an adequate amount of nanoparticles to extravasate at the tumor site for successful imaging and therapy. Therefore, a key design feature for successful passive delivery is a nanoparticle with prolonged in vivo circulation times. However, a major obstacle to passive tumor delivery is clearance by the reticuloendothelial system (RES), also commonly known as the mononuclear phagocyte system, which efficiently clears nanoparticulate material from the systemic circulation [13–15]. As a result, for maximal tumor accumulation, nanoparticle formulations must be designed with minimal removal by the RES. Many parameters of a nanoparticle (e.g., size, shape, surface charge, hydrophilicity, and specific coating material) can influence the nanoparticle's interaction with blood and cellular components, thereby affecting blood pool residence times and hence tumor accumulation [16].

The hydrodynamic diameter of a nanoparticle has a strong influence on circulation time and passive nanoparticle tumor penetration [16]. Nanoparticles smaller than 5 nm in diameter are rapidly filtered via the kidneys and excreted in the urine; therefore, their circulation time is very short and their tumor accumulation is low. The size range where nanoparticle blood clearance is minimized, in order to maximize passive delivery by EPR, is in the size range of 5–200 nm. For nanoparticle sizes exceeding roughly 200 nm, extravasation through capillary fenestrations becomes impaired (depending on the tumor type, some tumors have larger or small endothelial fenestrae). In addition, particles of larger size, i.e., >400 nm, are comparable in diameter to capillaries in the lungs and liver and are therefore cleared quickly by these organs, preventing tumor uptake [17].

Surface charge is another important characteristic that affects nanoparticle circulation time and passive tumor delivery by EPR. Previous studies have shown that particles possessing a neutral or mildly negative surface charge exhibit the most favorable circulation profiles and, therefore, optimal tumor accumulation. Particles with strongly negative surface charges interact unfavorably with the RES decreasing circulation time, whereas particles with a positive charge interact electrostatically with the cell membrane and are primarily localized at the site of injection [18].

Finally, the surface coating of the nanoparticle also influences nanoparticle circulation time. Since many groups have demonstrated that incorporation of polyethylene glycol (PEG) into the surface of nanoparticles helps avoid opsonization and prolong circulation times [19, 20], nanoparticle PEGylation is a very popular method to impart in vivo stealth properties [21].

In contrast to passive targeting, active targeting is a nanoparticle delivery strategy whereby the surface of the nanoparticle is modified with targeting ligands to specific receptors or biomarkers such as the folate or the HER2/NEU receptor within the tumor. These strategies achieve tumor delivery via specific interactions with either cancer cells or their microenvironment. Examples of targeting ligands used for such purposes include antibodies, proteins, peptides, aptamers, sugars, and small molecules. However, successful active targeting is still frequently dependent on initial efficient extravasation of the nanoparticles through the permeable tumor endothelium. Therefore, the nanoparticle's physicochemical properties, which influence blood circulation and passive delivery by the EPR effect, are also applicable for designing actively targeted nanoparticles. A consequence of this is that covering the entire surface of a nanoparticle with targeting ligands does not result in optimal targeting, since the stealth properties of the nanoparticle are compromised. Optimal ratios of ligands to surface area need to be determined for individual formulations, but in general occupying 20–40 % of the surface with ligands results in the best targeting [22].

Upon successful penetration of nanoparticles into tumor sites, actively targeted agents possess several key advantages compared to passive targeting strategies. While completely passive targeting is dependent on poor lymphatic drainage in order to achieve nanoparticle retention at the tumor site, active targeting can result in greater tumor retention due to specific binding to receptors. In addition, in some cases, the nanoparticle can undergo receptor-mediated internalization and enhance drug delivery to tumor cells as opposed to other cells within the tumor microenvironment such as macrophages that are capable of phagocytosing nanoparticles, thereby reducing delivery to cancer cells [23]. Thus, actively targeted nanoparticles can accumulate at higher concentrations and deliver their payload within cells compared to passively targeted formulations, which are more easily washed out of the tumor interstitial compartment.

Over the past few decades, the combination of nanoparticles with radiotherapy has been a topic of considerable interest (Fig. 10.1). The chemical composition of nanoparticles can be tailored such that they have different mechanisms of interaction between ionizing radiation and nanoparticles. Consequently, studies have been performed to increase the therapeutic efficacy in conventional radiation therapy by using nanoparticles with high atomic numbers (Z) as radiation sensitizers that can increase the emission of secondary electrons via their strong photoelectric and Compton effects [25]. Others have looked into the design of nanoparticle drug carriers in which triggered release of chemotherapeutic agents can be controlled by the application of an external radiation beam [26]. Finally, some reports use ionizing radiation to activate nanoparticles that induce cytotoxicity through alternative mechanisms such as phototherapy [27]. This chapter will highlight the most common application of nanoparticles in radiation therapy and their ability to increase the radiobiological effectiveness (RBE).

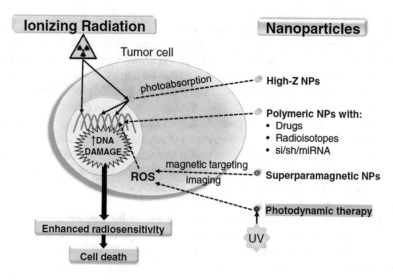

Fig. 10.1 A schematic depiction of the interaction of nanoparticles with ionizing radiation [24]. With permission from J.W. Bergs et al.

Safety and Potential Toxicity of Nanoparticles

For the successful clinical translation of nanoparticles, as with any medicine, thorough and careful evaluation of both the safety and pharmacokinetics of the agent is needed. Analysis of nanomaterial toxicity can be done using either in vitro or in vivo methods. The in vitro approach is by far the most commonly used as results can be determined rapidly at a low cost without the use of animals and can provide some insight into the biocompatibility of a nanoplatform. Some commonly accepted methods include the MTT assay for mitochondrial function, the clonogenic assays for cell proliferation and colony studies, and the lactate dehydrogenase assay for evaluating the integrity of the cell membrane, as well as using immunohistochemistry markers for measuring apoptosis and necrosis. While these methods are effective for providing some guidance of potential toxicity profiles, the in vivo interaction of nanoparticles with complex and dynamic biological systems cannot be predicted with substantial accuracy. Therefore, in vivo testing of nanoparticles is often done to determine the pharmacokinetic and pharmacodynamic profile and to understand their biocompatibility and safety. Methods for in vivo evaluation include determining organ biodistribution using multiple time points, blood sample collections for the analysis of circulation half-lives and liver enzymes, changes in appetite or weight, inflammatory cytokines, and histological tissue sectioning for microscopic examination to organ-specific toxicity. Additionally, blood chemistry analytes exist for the evaluation of specific organ toxicity such alanine aminotransferase (ALT), aspartate aminotransferase (AST), alkaline phosphatase, and total bilirubin for the evaluation of the hepatobiliary system and potential hemolysis.

When designing a nanomedicine for clinical translation, careful consideration of the factors and components that are responsible for the generation of toxicity are in order to maximize the chances of creating a safe agent. For example, silver is generally considered nontoxic when used on a large scale but can be toxic when used on a nanoscale [28]. Furthermore, the pharmacokinetic and pharmacodynamic profiles may provide a basis for potential fates and effects within the human body. For example, particles that are removed by the RES have the potential to cause toxicity and damage in those tissues involved in the clearance of the nanoparticles (liver, spleen, bone marrow). Therefore, the safety of nanoparticles will depend on many parameters including the chemical composition of the nanoformulation, size, shape, reactivity, stability, surface coating, and charge. One must therefore take into account all these properties when evaluating the safety and biocompatibility of nanoparticles.

The general rule of thumb for limiting the potential for nanoparticle toxicity as it relates to nanoparticle size is that they are inversely proportional to one another. This is because nanoparticles become more reactive as they become smaller, and their surface area to volume ratio increases. In addition to size, the nanoparticle shape and surface charge can also contribute to nanoparticle-induced toxicity. Studies have shown that the shape of nanoformulations dictates resulting interactions with biological systems including diffusion, translocation across cell membranes, and biodistribution [29]. For instance, a study evaluating cellular uptake of nanoparticles has shown that spherical AuNPs have a higher uptake in cells compared to gold nanorods [30]. With respect to surface charge, particles with a net negative surface charge tended to be less toxic than those with a positive surface charge, since cell membranes are negatively charged and positively charged particles are taken up by cells more readily. This concept can be exploited to help improve nanoparticle transportation into cancer cells. In one example, nanoparticle surfaces can be linked with a neutral compound that can become positively charged within low-pH microenvironments of certain tumors enabling local intracellular delivery of payload [31]. Surface coating is another important characteristic to consider since it can affect nanoparticle surface charge, hydrophilicity, hydrophobicity, protein adsorption, circulation half-lives, and interaction with specific cell types [32]. The final aspect to take into consideration is nanoparticle stability. This is relevant since nanoparticles can break down in the harsh, acidic environment of lysosomes increasing the concentration of toxic ions within cells, resulting in the buildup of reactive oxygen species [33]. The main mechanisms through which nanoparticles have the potential to exert a toxic effect on biological structures include the generation of free radicals and reactive oxygen species [34], or altering the binding stability and catalytic activity of protein structures, which can ultimately result in the induction of inflammation, genotoxicity, cytotoxicity, and developmental abnormalities [35].

While these nanoparticle characteristics are useful for predicting the potential for toxicity, a clear-cut correlation may not always exist across different nanoparticle platforms and other materials. For example, iron nanoparticles are generally regarded as safe and have been approved by the Food and Drug Administration for the treatment of anemia and contrast-enhanced MRI imaging [36, 37]. On the other hand, it was found that inclusion of safe iron oxides in emulsions made from edible oils resulted in nanoparticles that could produce toxicity, since the iron oxides catalyzed the oxidation of the oils to produce toxic substances [38]. Similarly, gadolinium used clinically as an MRI contrast agent is well tolerated; however, in patients with compromised kidney function gadolinium, exposure can result in nephrogenic systemic fibrosis [39]. Gold is considered to be very safe. In fact, gold has been used in medical practice throughout history and continues today as a treatment for rheumatoid arthritis [23]. Accordingly, when 12.5 nm AuNPs were administered intraperitoneally into mice every day for 8 days, no evidence of toxicity was observed in any of the studies performed, including survival, behavior, animal weight, organ morphology, blood biochemistry, and tissue histology [40]. In addition studies utilizing 1.9 nm and 0.8 nm AuNPs did not suggest any toxicity in mice [41]. In another study, a toxicological analysis of mice evaluating the intravenous injection of 0.9 nm and 5 nm up to 3 months showed no signs of illness and revealed blood chemistry values within normal limits [42]. Numerous other studies also support the assertion that AuNPs are not toxic to cells [43–48].

Nanoparticles in Radiation Therapy

Since current irradiation strategies may fail to kill all cancer cells within an irradiated volume, it may be beneficial to selectively enhance radiation at the cellular level. Consequently, many approaches have been developed to enhance the radiation effects specifically within tumors. A radiosensitizer is an agent or drug that increases the cytotoxic susceptibility of cancer cells to radiation therapy. Ideally a radiosensitizer would act specifically on tumor cells while sparing normal tissues, have favorable pharmacokinetic profiles for tumor accumulation prior or during radiation therapy, and be nontoxic. A variety of approaches have been implemented to increase radiation response to help decrease cellular resistance to ionizing radiation while minimizing toxicity to normal tissues. These include oxygen imitators [49–51], thymine analogues [52], inhibitors of cellular repair and cellular processes [53–56], thiol scavengers [52], and nanoparticles [25]. Among these, nanoparticles are favorable because they are able to increase tumor penetration, reduce required radiation doses thereby minimizing adverse effects compared to conventional radiosensitizers, and have been shown to be a promising strategy for increasing the efficiency of radiation therapy [57]. Studies have shown that nanoparticle carriers formed from poly(lactic-co-glycolic acid) PLGA, a biodegradable polymer that can be easily hydrolyzed into the metabolites lactic acid and glycolic acid, containing paclitaxel and etanidazole are able increase radiation sensitivity in tumor cell lines compared to free drug alone or nanoparticles containing only one of the agents [58]. Furthermore, nanoparticles have been used to encapsulate the poorly water-soluble radiosensitizer docetaxel to circumvent the undesirable side effects associated with administration of free drug [59]. Another polymeric nanoparticle that has shown to be a more effective radiation sensitizer in vivo compared to free drug alone is Genexol-PM, a polymeric micelle containing paclitaxel used for the treatment of non-small cell lung cancer [60]. However, the most extensively studied nanoparticles for radiation enhancement are those with high Z numbers. For example, gold [61], gadolinium [62], bismuth [63], titanium [64], hafnium [65], germanium [66], and platinum [67] have been evaluated for their radiosensitization capabilities. This is because high Z materials have a higher probability of emitting auger electrons and photoelectrons producing highly oxidizing free radical molecules that cause cellular death. Of all the high Z material nanoparticles, AuNPs have been the most thoroughly evaluated. The next section will focus primarily on radiation therapy involving nanoformulations containing AuNP.

Mechanisms of Interaction of Radiation with Nanoparticles

The primary objective of radiation therapy is to deprive cancer cells of their mitotic potential and ultimately promote cancer cell death. The main interaction of X-rays in cells is by Compton scattering, producing secondary high-energy electrons that exert their effects on biological structures. In the cell, DNA is the desired biological target of ionizing radiation. There are two mechanisms by which radiation can interact with DNA. The first is known as direct action where ionizing radiation interacts directly with DNA to cause damage. The second is known as indirect action where ionizing radiation interacts with the surrounding water molecules, generating free radicals, notably hydroxyl radicals [68], which cause lethal damage to cellular DNA. Hydroxyl radicals are generated either directly by the oxidation of water by ionizing radiation or indirectly by the formation of secondary partially reactive oxygen species (ROS). ROS include superoxide ($O2^-$), hydrogen peroxide (H_2O_2), and hydroxyl radicals ($OH^=$). The damage caused can include DNA strand breaks that are initiated by the removal of a deoxyribose hydrogen atom by the activated hydroxyl radical [69]. Excessive damage to cells exposed to radiation can lead to either double-strand breaks (DSB) or single-strand breaks (SSB). DSBs are the not the most common type of radiation-induced damage but are regarded as the most serious and potentially lethal. At this stage, some cells will arrest their cell cycle to repair the damage. If the damage is beyond repair then the cell will undergo apoptosis. Alternatively, some cancer cells with mutations in cell cycle checkpoints can continue to proliferate following radiation exposure. However, the majority of these cells will undergo cell death during mitosis as a result of sustained DNA damage and chromosomal defects. The postmitotic or reproductive mode of cell death is considered to be the most prevalent mechanism in cells exposed to ionizing radiation [70–72]. The apoptotic signaling pathway can be initiated in various cellular compartments that include the plasma membrane, cytoplasm, and nucleus [73]. In the plasma membrane, ionizing radiation can promote lipid-oxidative damage through interactions with radiation-induced free radicals resulting in altered ion channels, a buildup in arachidonic acid, and the production of ceramide which is involved in mediating cellular death. Cell death occurs via free radical molecules eliciting cumulative un-repairable lipid-oxidative damage [75].

The mechanism of nanoparticle enhancement, in X-ray therapy, is dependent on the energy of incident ionizing photons and different interactions between the photons and nanoparticles. The three fundamental mechanisms of radiation enhancement are the photoelectric effect, Compton scattering, and pair production. The photoelectric effect is the predominant mechanism of radiosensitization of high atomic number (Z) elements, for photons with energies in the range of 10–500 keV [76]. The cross section of the photoelectric effect varies with the atomic number approximately proportional to Z^3, meaning that higher Z atoms will have a larger absorption cross section. The photoelectric effect is also dependent on the energy of the photon, with a maximum cross section when the photon energy is equal to the binding energy of orbital electrons. This effect decreases sharply as energy is increased and varies as E^{-3}. For example, the binding energies of electrons bound to gold are 79 keV for the inner shells, 13 keV, and 3 keV for outer shells, while those of soft tissue are on the order of 1 keV or lower resulting from the lower atomic number of organic matter. Therefore, gold would absorb significantly more energy than soft tissue in the kilovoltage energy range. When photons with energies in these ranges interact with AuNPs, they can produce electrons, characteristic X-rays of gold atoms, or Auger electrons. Once an atom absorbs a photon, an electron may be emitted resulting in an ionized atom.

When photons of energy greater than the binding energy of an inner shell electron collide, that electron is ejected leaving behind a vacancy in an orbital electron shell. As a result, outer electrons in a higher-energy state fill the vacancy in the lower-energy orbital. This process is accompanied by either a fluorescent photon or an Auger electron ejected from an outer shell with an energy equal to the difference between the two orbital shells. If multiple shells exist within an atom, then further Auger electrons can be generated as outer shell electrons fill in the vacancies. This phenomenon is known as the Auger cascade. The number of Auger electrons emitted is directly proportional to the atomic number. Therefore, high Z atoms are expected to generate more Auger electrons than elements with lower atomic numbers [77]. The range of these emitted electrons has been calculated to be around tens of nanometers depositing their energy along their path and distributing radiation throughout the system [77]. Furthermore, the Auger electron "shower" can produce highly positively charged ions, causing local Coulomb force fields that can disrupt nearby cellular structures.

The enhancement of radiation with high Z material was first realized when DNA damage was detected in lymphocytes isolated from patients receiving iodinated contrast agents for X-ray imaging [78]. Since then many other studies have demonstrated that radiation therapy in combination with iodine suppresses tumor growth and improves survival in animal models [79]. Another interesting approach was the incorporation of iodine into cellular DNA yielding a threefold improvement in in vitro radiosensitization [80]. However, this strategy is not as effective if insufficient levels of thymine are substituted with iododeoxyuridine. Although the mechanisms of radiation enhancement of gold nanoparticles are not completely understood, it is currently believed that the interaction of X-rays with high Z atoms induces the release of photoelectrons and Auger electrons [76] (Fig. 10.2).

Given that gold has a higher Z number (79 vs 53), it is likely that gold as a radiosensitizer would be much more effective than iodine. When photon ener-

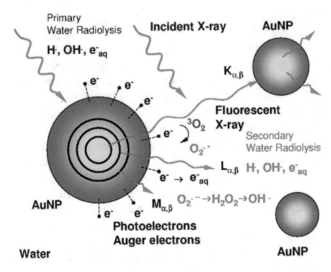

Fig. 10.2 Schematic depiction of increased generation of reactive oxygen species by the emission of photoelectrons and Auger electrons from AuNPs in the presence of ionizing radiation [74]

gies are greater than 500 keV, Compton effects begin to dominate. The Compton effect is the incoherent or inelastic scattering between an X-ray photon and an electron of an atom. In this interaction, only a part of the energy is transferred to the electron. The resulting emitted electron is known as a Compton electron, leaving behind an ionized atom or molecule. In contrast to photoelectric interactions where most photoelectrons are inner electrons, Compton interactions increase for loosely bound electrons. So most of the Compton electrons are valence electrons. In contrast to Auger electrons, Compton electrons are capable of traveling several hundred microns. For incident photons with energies higher than 1.02 MeV, a process known as pair production dominates where the photon is absorbed by the nucleus with the production of a positron and electron pairs. The probability of pair production increases with the atomic number as Z^2 and linearly with the energy of incident photons. The interaction of charged particles is more complex; however, some studies have speculated that proton-AuNP interactions lead to the increased production of low-energy delta-ray electrons producing a high degree of lethal damage within the cells, thus lowering the surviving fraction of cells [81].

While most nanoparticle radiosensitization has primarily been attributed to their photon absorption capabilities, recent studies highlight that a significant biological component may be responsible for radiosensitization. In the absence of radiation, nanoparticles have been reported to induce ROS that cause oxidative DNA damage [82]. In addition, nanomaterials have been shown to cause alterations in the cell cycle with an increase in cells at the G2/M phase [83]. In a recent study by Kang et al., the nuclear targeting of AuNPs was shown to cause cytokinesis arrest leading to the failure of complete cell division and apoptosis [84]. Although experimental evidence may suggest the involvement of biological components in radiosensitization, the exact mechanisms are still not clearly understood.

In Vitro Radiosensitization Using AuNPs

By far the majority of in vitro and in vivo studies analyzing AuNP-mediated radioenhancement rely on passively targeted nanoparticles. One of the earliest studies using gold for radioenhancement was performed by Regulla and colleagues [85]. In this study, enhanced radiation effects were observed in mouse embryo fibroblasts that were exposed to gold surfaces compared to those exposed to polymethyl methacrylate. Secondary electrons were found to travel a range of approximately 10 μm. Following this study, numerous other experimental studies using AuNPs over both orthovoltage (200–500 keV) and megavoltage (>100 keV) ranges have been described. The results of these reports are difficult to compare directly since they were performed using many parameters such as size, shape, surface coating, concentration, radiation type and energy, and origin of cell lines (Table 10.1 adapted from Butterworth et al.). In an attempt to address these issues, Brun and coworkers investigated AuNP radiation enhancement by systematically altering AuNP concentrations, AuNP diameter, and incident X-ray energy (range 14.8–70 keV). They determined that the conditions with the most radiation enhancement were those using larger sized AuNPs, high gold concentration, and 50 keV photons providing dose enhancement factors of 6 [98]. In a separate study, 1.9 nm AuNPs enhanced the response of bovine aortic endothelial cell damage inflicted by X-ray irradiation, with a dose enhancement factor up to 24.6 [91]. While optimal sizes for AuNP radiation therapy may be inconclusive, it is generally accepted that radiation-induced DNA damage will increase with increasing concentrations of AuNPs [99]. In vitro experiments using brachytherapy sources and AuNPs have also been reported and initially demonstrated an increased biological effect with irradiation with values up to 130 % greater than without AuNPs [100].

Most photoelectrons, Auger electrons, and other secondary electrons have low energies and a short range in tissues (nm to μm) delivering lethal doses in their immediate surroundings [101]. The possibility of having AuNPs target specific cancer cells may increase the production of secondary electrons within the vicinity of DNA molecules, especially if they involve cellular internalization [102]. Chattopadhyay et al. was one of the first to validate this hypothesis by synthesizing trastuzumab-PEG-AuNPs [97]. Briefly, SK-BR-3 cells were irradiated after treatment with either phosphate-buffered saline, PEG-AuNPs, or trastuzumab-PEG-AuNPs. The DNA DSBs as measured by γ-H2AX foci increased 5.1 and 3.3 times for targeted AuNPs compared to cells treated with PBS or PEG-AuNPs, respectively. AuNPs modified with either cysteamine or thioglucose have been shown to have differential accumulation in cancer cells. While cysteamine-modified AuNPs

Table 10.1 Summary of in vitro radiosensitization experiments using AuNPs

Author	Size (nm)	Concentration	Surface coating	Cell model	Energy source	DEF	SER
Geng et al. [86]	14	5 nM	Glucose	SK-OV-3	90 kVp	1.002	1.3
					6 MV	1.00009	1.2
Jain et al. [87]	1.9	12 µM	Thiol	DU-145	160 kVp	1.05	<1.41
				MDA-231 MB	6 MV	1.0005	<1.29
				L132	15 MV	1.0005	1.16
					6 MeV e⁻	1	<1.12
					16 MeV e⁻	1	1.35
Chithrani et al. [79]	14	1 nM	Citrate	HeLa	220 kVp	1.09	1.17–
	74				6 MV e⁻	1.0008	1.16
	50				662 keV	1.0006	
Liu et al. [88]	6.1	>1 mM	PEG	CT-26	6 keV e⁻	1	2
				EMT-6	160 kVp	1.02	1.1
					6 MV	1.002	1
Butterworth et al. [89]	1.9	2.4 µM	Thiol	DU-145	160 kVp	1.01	<1
		0.24 µM		MDA-231 MB			
				AG0-1522			
				Astro			
				L132		1.01	<1.67
				T98G		1.01	<1.97
				MCF-7		1.01	<1.04
				PC-3		1.01	<1
						1.01	<1.91
						1.01	<1.41
						1.01	<1.07
						1.01	1.3
Kong et al. [90]	10.8	15 nM	Glucose	MCF-7	200 kVp	1.01	1.3
					662 keV	1.00008	1.6
			Cysteamine	MCF-10A	1.2 MV	1.00001	
Rahman et al. [91]	1.9	<1 mM	Thiol	BAEC	80 kV	6.6	20
					150 kV	5.2	1.4
					6 MV e⁻	1	2.9
					12 MV e⁻	1	3.7
Roa et al. [83]	10.8	15 nM	Glucose	DU-145	662 keV	1.00008	>1.5
Zhang et al. [92]	30	15 nM	Glucose-TGS	DU-145	200 kVp	1.0083	>1.3
						1.0083	>1.5
Chang et al. [93]	13	11 nM	Citrate	B16F10	6 MV e⁻	1	1

(continued)

Table 10.1 (continued)

Author	Size (nm)	Concentration	Surface coating	Cell model	Energy source	DEF	SER
Chien et al. [94]	20	<2 mM	Citrate	CT-26	6 MV e⁻	1	1.19
Zhang et al. [95]	4.8	0.095–3 mM	Citrate	K562	2–10 kR gamma		
	12.1						
	27.3						
	46.6						
Liu et al. [96]	4.7	500 µM	PEG	CT-26	6 MV		1.3–1.6
Chattopadhyay et al. [97]	30	0.3 nM	Trastuzumab-PEG	SK-BR-3	300 kVp		5.1
Brun et al. [98]	8.1	1–5 nM	Citrate	Plasmid DNA	30 kV		<3.3
	20.2				80 kV		
	37.5				80 kV		
	74				100 kV		
	91.7				120 kV		
					150 kV		

SER surface enhancement ratio, *DEF* dose enhancement factor

were preferentially limited to the cell membrane of MCF-7 breast cancer cells, glucose-AuNPs are internalized and distributed throughout the cytoplasm [86, 90]. Furthermore, glucose-AuNPs exhibited enhanced irradiation (200 kVp)-induced cell death compared to cysteamine-AuNPs and irradiation alone. Finally, in an independent study, the radiotoxicity of proton therapy with AuNP internalization was increased by approximately 15–20 % compared to proton therapy without AuNPs [81]. However, the meaning of these results is not clear, as targeted AuNPs were not compared to nontargeted AuNPs.

In Vivo Radiosensitization Using AuNPs

In 2004, Hainfeld et al. performed the first animal study evaluating enhanced tumor radiosensitization via AuNPs. Using 1.9 nm AuNPs in combination with 250 kVp X-rays (30 Gy), overall tumor-xenograft mouse survival was 86 % versus 20 % for radiation alone and 0 % for gold only [103]. Since then AuNP radiosensitization has been demonstrated in vivo with murine mammary ductal carcinoma [104], murine squamous cell carcinomas [103], human sarcoma cells [105], and cervical carcinoma (see Table 10.2) [111]. In a study by Zhang and colleagues, in vivo radiosensitization was studied using four different sizes of PEG-AuNPs, and demonstrated that while all sizes can decrease tumor volumes after gamma radiation (5 Gy), the smallest (4.8 nm) and largest (46.6 nm) particles tested had weaker sensitization effects than 12.1 and 27.3 nm [109]. However, in a recent study by Zhang et al.,

Table 10.2 Summary of in vivo radiosensitization experiments using AuNPs

Author	Size (nm)	AuNP dose (g kg⁻¹)	Surface coating	Cell model	Source energy	Dose (Gy)	Predicted DE
Hainfeld et al. [106]	1.9	0–2.7	Thiol	SCCVII	68 kV	30	1.84
					157 kV		1.315
Hebert et al. [104]	5	0–0.675	DTDTPA-Gd	MCF7-L1	150 kV	10	1.01
Chang et al. [93]	13	0–0.036	Citrate	B16F10	MV e⁻	25	1.01
Hainfeld et al. [103]	1.9	0–2.7	Thiol	EMT-6	250 kV	26–30	1.56
Joh et al. [105]	12.4	0–1.25	PEG	HT1080	175 kV	6 Gy	1.16
				U20S			1.07
Joh et al. [107] PLOS	12	0–1.25	PEG	U251	175 kV	20 Gy	1.3
Kim et al. [108]	14	0–0.3	Citrate	CT26	Proton 40 MV	10–41 Gy	
Zhang et al. [109]	4.8	0–4	PEG	U14	Gamma rays	5 Gy	1.41
	12.1						1.65
	27.3						1.58
	46.6						1.42
Chattopadhyay et al. [97]	30		Herceptin	MDA-MB-361	100 kV	11 Gy	
Atkinson et al. [110]		n/a	n/a		n/a	6 Gy	
Zhang et al. [111]	1.5	0.01	GSH	U14	662 kV	5 Gy	
			BSH				
Al Zaki et al. [112]	75	0–0.65	PEG	HT1080	175 kV	6 Gy	1.2
McQuade et al. [113]	100	0–0.4	PEG	HT1080	175 kV	6 Gy	1.32
Sun et al. [114]	75	0–0.3	PEG	U251	150 kV	4 Gy	
Vilchis-Juarez et al. [115]	20		RGD,¹⁷⁷Lu	C6			
Miladi et al. [116]	2		DTDTPA-GD₅₀	Osteosarcoma 9LGS	Gamma rays 662 kV	25 Gy 20 Gy	

DE dose enhancement

glutathione-coated AuNPs with sizes less than 2 nm have the ability to accumulate preferentially within subcutaneous tumor-bearing mice providing strong radioenhancement for cancer therapy [111]. More recently, Joh et al. showed that PEG-AuNPs and radiation therapy can enhance DNA damage and tumor cell destruction and improve survival in mice with orthotopic glioblastoma multiforme tumors [107]. Intriguingly, they also showed that ionizing radiation could compromise tumor vasculature significantly increasing the accumulation of AuNPs within brain tumor-bearing mice. All of these strategies mentioned are examples of passive tumor targeting of AuNPs that are reliant on the EPR effect. To our knowledge, a study conducted by Chattopadhyay and coworkers is the only one that has assessed the in vivo radioenhancement effects of targeted AuNPs, using a tumor-specific HER-2-targeted nanoplatform [101]. However, the benefits of having targeted AuNPs versus untargeted were not conclusive as there were no in vivo comparisons made, and AuNPs were administered via intratumoral injections.

Very few in vivo studies have been carried out using MV photon energy beams that are commonly used in radiotherapy. However, some emerging studies are suggestive of the clinical potential of AuNPs in improving outcomes of radiotherapy. Using 6 MV electrons with 13 nm AuNPs, tumor growth was significantly retarded, and survival was prolonged compared to radiation alone in mice with melanoma flank tumors [93]. Increased tumor sensitization with AuNPs has also been demonstrated using proton therapy [108]. Proton beam irradiations of 45 MeV (10–41 Gy) were delivered to subcutaneous colon carcinoma tumors in mice after receiving a single dose of 100–300 mg/kg of AuNPs, which led to a 58–100 % 1 year survival versus 11–13 % in proton only irradiation.

Theranostic Agents

There has been a growing trend to integrate both diagnostic and therapeutic agents within a single formulation at the nanoscale level; an approach known as theranostics. The benefit of this combination will enable both disease detection and treatment within a single procedure. Direct visualization of nanoparticle distribution within the tumor can provide guidance for treatment localization, monitor disease progression, and aid in the prediction of therapeutic outcome. Crucial information such as this could invariably be useful for physicians to provide their patients with personalized treatment strategies that help minimize off-target toxicity and improve clinical outcomes. While still at the preclinical stage, a number of studies have demonstrated the use of theranostic nanoformulations for imaging and radiation therapy enhancement. Gadolinium and gold nanoparticles can be used as multimodal agents. Their high Z material improves the efficacy of radiation therapy and can be used as contrast agents for magnetic resonance imaging (MRI) and computed tomography (CT), respectively. A multifunctional micellar nanocarrier was prepared by encapsulating both AuNP for radiosensitization and SPIONs for contrast-enhanced imaging (Fig. 10.3). MRI imaging suggested that the heterogeneity of tumor permeability and initial response to radiation therapy was predicted based on the extent of contrast enhancement within the tumor (Fig. 10.4) [113]. Similarly, via the use of gadolinium-based ultra-rigid platforms (USRPs), lung tumors were detected noninvasively using ultrashort echo time magnetic resonance imaging (Fig. 10.5) and improved the mean survival time compared to mice receiving radiation therapy alone (Fig. 10.6) [117]. In another example, a theranostic agent was prepared using magnetic Fe_3O_4 and silver nanocomposites for simultaneous cancer

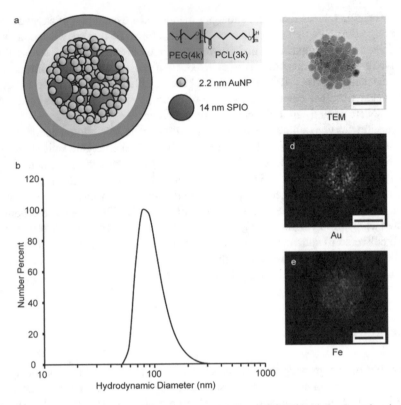

Fig. 10.3 (**a**) Schematic depiction of a gold nanoparticle and SPION-loaded polymeric micelles (GSMs). These particles are administered intravenously into tumor-bearing mice. Once particles accumulate within tumors, they provide T_2-weighted contrast-enhanced MRI imaging for localizing external beam radiation therapy. (**b**) Dynamic light scattering measurements of GSMs. (**c**) Electron micrograph of GSMs. (**d**, **e**) Energy-dispersive spectroscopy analysis on GSMs with Au and Fe signals detected, respectively

therapy and diagnosis of nasopharyngeal carcinoma [118]. These nanocomposites were conjugated to an epidermal growth factor receptor antibody resulting in an enhancement in radiotoxicity by a factor of 2.26.

While these examples show promise for theranostic agents in cancer therapy, further investigation is warranted. Currently, combining both imaging and therapeutic functionalities significantly increases the cost and complexity of nanoparticle preparation, which adds concerns for commercial viability, altered pharmacokinetics, reduced drug loading capacity, and regulatory hurdles for clinical translation. The incorporation of high sensitivity and quantifiable positron emission tomography (PET) imaging agents onto the surfaces of existing FDA-approved nanoplatforms might be a promising alternative approach to improve nanoparticle biodistribution and antitumor efficacy.

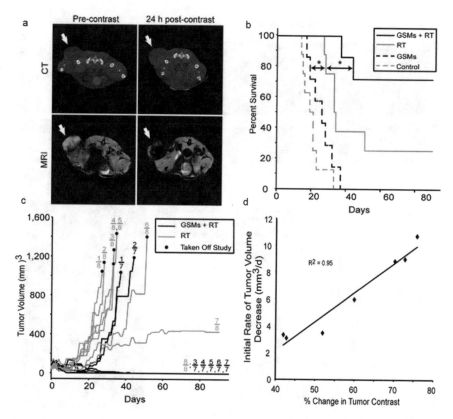

Fig. 10.4 (**a**) CT (*top*) and MR (*bottom*) imaging of HT1080 flank tumor-bearing mice 24 h postinjection of GSMs. Tumor contrast is enhanced on MR imaging. (**b**) Kaplan-Meier survival curve in HT1080 tumor-bearing mice receiving no treatment (*n*=8), radiation therapy only (*n*=8), GSMs only (*n*=7), or radiation therapy 24 h post-intravenous injection of GSMs (*n*=7). The radiation dose used was 6 Gy at 150 kVp (**c**) Plot of average tumor volumes in mice taken over following treatment with GSMs and radiation therapy or radiation therapy alone. (**d**) Graph of initial rate of tumor volume decrease against the percent change in tumor contrast for mice receiving GSMs plus radiation therapy

Future/Clinical Translation

With the rapid development and progress of the field of nanotechnology for bio-medical applications, there has been wide evaluation of their use for enhanced diagnosis and therapeutic effect in existing treatment modalities. During the past decade, many nanoformulations have been developed as anticancer agents that exert their cytotoxic effects by enhancing the efficacy of radiation therapy. Of the published studies, most have focused on nanoparticles composed of high Z elements like gold, bismuth, and gadolinium. While these approaches have proven successful in preclinical studies, the exact mechanisms of radiosensitization are not yet clearly understood. Therefore, additional studies are needed to

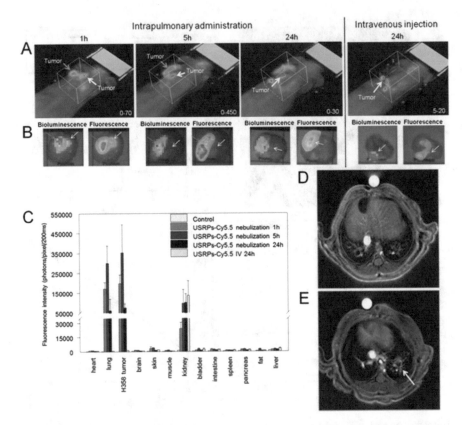

Fig. 10.5 In vivo imaging of H358-Luc orthotopic lung tumor imaging. (**a**) Fluorescence imaging of USRPs-CY5.5. (**b**) Bioluminescence and fluorescence showing the colocalization between H358-Luc tumors and fluorescent USRPs. (**c**) Organ biodistribution of USRPs following intrapulmonary administration. (**d, e**) MR imaging of lung tumors pre- and postadministration of USRPs

help elucidate the biological effects exerted by the addition of nanoparticles and therefore direct improved nanoformulation design. Since the majority of studies conducted have focused on irradiation using kilovoltage energies that are limited to superficial tumors and brachytherapy in a clinical setting, the extent of radiosensitization when nanoparticles are exposed to the more clinically utilized megavoltage energies is required. Furthermore, relevant animal models are needed to more accurately mimic clinical disease to determine the potential of nanoparticles for radiosensitization.

Although radiation enhancement has proven to be successful using a variety of nanoparticle formulations, the number of clinical trials using nanoparticles as radiosensitizers is still limited. Current barriers must be overcome that hinder translation of nanoparticles to the clinic. These include the difficulty associated with selection of the optimal nanoplatform, improvement of ligand conjugation efficiencies and technologies, as well as the development of synthetic strategies for nanoparticle

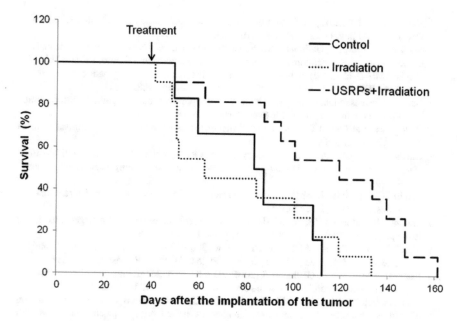

Fig. 10.6 Survival curve of H358-Luc lung tumor-bearing mice without treatment ($n=6$), treated using a single irradiation only ($n=11$), and irradiated 24 h after intrapulmonary administration of USRPs ($n=11$). Irradiations were performed at 10 Gy

scale-up that follow good manufacturing process with fewer steps, high consistency, and lower costs [119].

Despite these hurdles for clinical translation, some nanotechnology platforms have made it to clinical trials for testing in radiation therapy and are currently being investigated. Phase I clinical trials of hafnium oxide nanoparticles (NBTXR3) were well tolerated and revealed a favorable safety profile with promising signs of antitumor activity. Hafnium oxide nanoparticles (NBTXR3) are currently undergoing phase II/III clinical trials (NCT02379845) after demonstrating efficacy and safety in patients with soft tissue sarcomas in phase I studies [24]. With further advancements in nanoparticle production, purification, and conjugation techniques combined with findings from ongoing and future studies, the number of nanoplatforms that will be translated to clinical studies is expected to increase.

References

1. Pautler M, Brenner S (2010) Nanomedicine: promises and challenges for the future of public health. Int J Nanomedicine 5:803–809
2. Barenholz Y (2012) Doxil(R)–the first FDA-approved nano-drug: lessons learned. J Control Release 160:117–134

3. Kanekiyo M et al (2013) Self-assembling influenza nanoparticle vaccines elicit broadly neutralizing H1N1 antibodies. Nature 499:102–106
4. des Rieux A, Fievez V, Garinot M, Schneider YJ, Preat V (2006) Nanoparticles as potential oral delivery systems of proteins and vaccines: a mechanistic approach. J Control Release 116:1–27
5. Kircher MF et al (2012) A brain tumor molecular imaging strategy using a new triple-modality MRI-photoacoustic-Raman nanoparticle. Nat Med 18:829–834
6. Jiang S, Gnanasammandhan MK, Zhang Y (2010) Optical imaging-guided cancer therapy with fluorescent nanoparticles. J R Soc Interface 7:3–18
7. Reddy GR et al (2006) Vascular targeted nanoparticles for imaging and treatment of brain tumors. Clin Cancer Res 12:6677–6686
8. Cheng Z, Al Zaki A, Hui JZ, Muzykantov VR, Tsourkas A (2012) Multifunctional nanoparticles: cost versus benefit of adding targeting and imaging capabilities. Science 338:903–910
9. Torchilin VP (2002) PEG-based micelles as carriers of contrast agents for different imaging modalities. Adv Drug Deliv Rev 54:235–252
10. Prabhu RH, Patravale VB, Joshi MD (2015) Polymeric nanoparticles for targeted treatment in oncology: current insights. Int J Nanomedicine 10:1001–1018
11. Maeda H, Wu J, Sawa T, Matsumura Y, Hori K (2000) Tumor vascular permeability and the EPR effect in macromolecular therapeutics: a review. J Control Release 65:271–284
12. Konerding MA, Fait E, Gaumann A (2001) 3D microvascular architecture of pre-cancerous lesions and invasive carcinomas of the colon. Br J Cancer 84:1354–1362
13. Balasubramanian SK, Jittiwat J, Manikandan J, Ong CN, Yu LE, Ong WY (2010) Biodistribution of gold nanoparticles and gene expression changes in the liver and spleen after intravenous administration in rats. Biomaterials 31(8):2034–2042
14. Cho WS, Cho M, Jeong J, Choi M, Cho HY, Han BS, Kim SH, Kim HO, Lim YT, Chung BH (2009) Acute toxicity and pharmacokinetics of 13 nm-sized PEG-coated gold nanoparticles. Toxicol Appl Pharmacol 236(1):16–24
15. Niidome T, Yamagata M, Okamoto Y, Akiyama Y, Takahashi H, Kawano T, Katayama Y, Niidome Y (2006) PEG-modified gold nanorods with a stealth character for in vivo applications. J Control Release 114(3):343–347
16. Frank A, Pridgen E, Molnar LK, Farokhzad OC (2008) Factors affecting the clearance and biodistribution of polymeric nanoparticles. Mol Pharm 5(4):505–515
17. Blanco E, Shen H, Ferrari M (2015) Nanoparticle size, shape and surface charge dictate biodistribution among the different organs including the lungs, liver, spleen and kidneys. Nat Biotechnol 33:941–951
18. He C, Hu Y, Yin L, Tang C, Yin C (2010) Effects of particle size and surface charge on cellular uptake and biodistribution of polymeric nanoparticles. Biomaterials 31(13):3657–3666
19. Lemarchand C, Gref R, Couvreur P (2004) Polysaccharide-decorated nanoparticles. Eur J Pharm Biopharm 58:327–341
20. Lemarchand C, Gref R, Passirani C, Garcion E, Petri B, Muller R, Costantini D, Couvreur P (2006) Influence of polysaccharide coating on the interactions of nanoparticles with biological systems. Biomaterials 27:108–118
21. Koo OM, Rubinstein I, Onyuksel H (2005) Role of nanotechnology in targeted drug delivery and imaging: a concise review. Nanomedicine 1:193–212
22. Elias DR, Poloukhtine A, Popik V, Tsourkas A (2013) Effect of ligand density, receptor density, and nanoparticle size on cell targeting. Nanomedicine 9(2):194–201
23. Xu S, Olenyuk BZ, Okamato CT, Hamm-Alvarez SF (2013) Targeting receptor-mediated endocytic pathways with nanoparticles: rationale and advances. Adv Drug Deliv Rev 65(1):121–138
24. Bergs JWJ, Wacker MG, Hehlgans S, Piiper A, Multhoff G, Rodel C, Rodel F (2015) The role of recent nanotechnology in enhancing the efficacy of radiation therapy. Biochim Biophys Acta 1856(1):130–143
25. Retif P, Pinel S, Toussaint M, Frochot C, Chouikrat R, Bastogne T, Barberi-Heyob M (2015) Nanoparticles for radiation therapy enhancement: the key parameters. Theranostics 5(9):1030–1044

26. Starkewolf ZB, Miyachi L, Wong J, Guo T (2013) X-ray triggered release of doxorubicin from nanoparticle drug carriers for cancer therapy. Chem Commun 49:2545–2547
27. Chen W, Zhang J (2006) Using nanoparticles to enable simultaneous radiation and photodynamic therapies for cancer treatment. J Nanosci Nanotechnol 6(4):1159–1166
28. AshaRani PV, Kah Mun GL, Hande MP, Valiyaveettil S (2009) Cytotoxicity and genotoxicity of silver nanoparticles in human cells. ACS Nano 3(2):279–290
29. Chithrani BD, Ghazani AA, Chan WCW (2006) Determining the size and shape dependence of gold nanoparticle uptake into mammalian cells. Nano Lett 6(4):662–668
30. Arnida, Janat-Amsbury MM, Ray A, Peterson CM, Ghandehari H (2011) Geometry and surface characteristics of gold nanoparticles influence their biodistribution and uptake by macrophages. Eur J Pharm Biopharm 77(3):417–423
31. Cheng Z, Al Zaki A, Hui JZ, Muzykantov VR, Tsourkas A (2012) Multifunctional nanoparticles: cost versus benefit of adding targeting and imaging capabilities. Science 338(6109):903–910
32. Albanese A, Tang PS, Chan WCW (2012) The effect of nanoparticle size, shape, and surface chemistry on biological systems. Annu Rev Biomed Eng 14:1–16
33. Petros RA, DeSimone JD (2010) Strategies in the design of nanoparticles for therapeutic applications. Nature 9:615–627
34. Fu PP, Xia Q, Hwang HM, Ray PC, Yu H (2014) Mechanisms of nanotoxicity: generation of reactive oxygen species. J Food Drug Anal 22(1):64–75
35. Park MV, Neigh AM, Vermeulen JP, de la Fonteyene LJ, Verharen HW, Briede JJ, van Loveren H, de Jong WH (2011) The effect of particle size on the cytotoxicity, inflammation, developmental toxicity and genotoxicity of silver nanoparticles. Biomaterials 32(36):9810–9817
36. Schwenk MH (2010) Ferumoxytol: A new intravenous iron preparation for the treatment of iron deficiency anemia in patients with chronic kidney disease. Pharmacotherapy 30(1):70–79
37. Thomas R, Park IK, Jeong YY (2013) Magnetic iron oxide nanoparticles for multimodal imaging and therapy of cancer. Int J Mol Sci 14(8):15910–15930
38. van Tilborg GAF, Cormode DP, Jarzyna PA, van der Toorn A, van der Pol SMA, van Bloois L, Fayad ZA, Storm G, Mulder WJM, de Vries HE, Dijkhuizen RM (2012) Nanoclusters of iron oxide: effect of core composition on structure, biocompatibility and cell labeling efficacy. Bioconjug Chem 23:941–950
39. Tommaro A, Narcisi A, Tuchinda P, Sina B (2015) Nephrogenic systemic fibrosis following gadolinium administration. Cuitis 96(1):E23–E25
40. Lasagna-Reeves C, Gonzalez-Romero D, Barria MA, Olmedo I, Clos A, Sadagopa Ramanujam VM, Urayama A, Vergara L, Kogan MJ, Soto C (2010) Bioaccumulation and toxicity of gold nanoparticles after repeated administration in mice. Biochem Biophys Res Commun 393(4):649–655
41. Hainfeld JF, Dilmanian FA, Slatkin DN, Smilowitz HM (2008) Radiotherapy enhancement with gold nanoparticles. J Pharm Pharmacol 60(8):977–985
42. Al Zaki A, Hui JZ, Higbee E, Tsourkas A (2015) Biodistribution, clearance, and toxicology of polymeric micelles loaded with 0.9 or 5 nm gold nanoparticles. J Biomed Nanotechnol 11(10):1836–1846
43. Chen PC, Mwakwari SC, Oyelere AK (2008) Gold nanoparticles: from nanomedicine to nanosensing. Nanotechnol Sci Appl 1:45–66
44. Connor EE, Mwamuka J, Gole A, Murphy CJ, Wyatt MD (2005) Gold nanoparticles are taken up by human cells but do not cause acute cytotoxicity. Small 1(3):325–327
45. Lewinski N, Colvin V, Drezek R (2008) Cytotoxicity of nanoparticles. Small 4(1):26–49
46. Pan Y, Neuss S, Leifert A, Fischler M, Wen F, Simon U, Schmid G, Brandau W, Jahnen-Dechent W (2007) Size-dependent cytotoxicity of gold nanoparticles. Small 3(11):1941–1949
47. Shukla R, Bansal V, Chaudhary M, Basu A, Bhonde RR, Sastry M (2005) Biocompatibility of gold nanoparticles and their endocytotic fate inside the cellular compartment: a microscopic overview. Langmuir 21(23):10644–10654
48. Tkachenko AG, Xie H, Coleman D, Glomm W, Ryan J, Anderson MF, Franzen S, Feldheim DL (2003) Multifunctional gold nanoparticle-peptide complexes for nuclear targeting. J Am Chem Soc 125(16):4700–4701

49. Chassagne D, Charreau I, Sancho-Garnier H, Eschwege F, Malaise EP (1992) First analysis of tumor regression for the European randomized trial of etanidazole combined with radiotherapy in head and neck carcinomas. Int J Radiat Oncol Biol Phys 22:581–584

50. Murayama C et al (1993) Radiosensitization by a new potent nucleoside analog: 1-(1′,3′,4′-trihydroxy-2′-butoxy)methyl-2-nitroimidazole(RP-343). Int J Radiat Oncol Biol Phys 26:433–443

51. Murayama C et al (1989) Radiosensitization by a new nucleoside analogue: 1-[2-hydroxy-1-(hydroxymethyl)ethoxy]methyl-2-nitroimidazole (RP-170). Int J Radiat Oncol Biol Phys 17:575–581

52. Wardman P (2007) Chemical radiosensitizers for use in radiotherapy. Clin Oncol (R Coll Radiol) 19:397–417

53. Kvols LK (2005) Radiation sensitizers: a selective review of molecules targeting DNA and non-DNA targets. J Nucl Med 46(Suppl 1):187S–190S

54. Servidei T et al (2001) The novel trinuclear platinum complex BBR3464 induces a cellular response different from cisplatin. Eur J Cancer 37:930–938

55. Richmond RC (1984) Toxic variability and radiation sensitization by dichlorodiammineplatinum(II) complexes in Salmonella typhimurium cells. Radiat Res 99:596–608

56. Amorino GP, Freeman ML, Carbone DP, Lebwohl DE, Choy H (1999) Radiopotentiation by the oral platinum agent, JM216: role of repair inhibition. Int J Radiat Oncol Biol Phys 44:399–405

57. Dorsey JF, Sun L, Joh DY, Witztum A, Al Zaki A, Kao GD, Alonso-Basanta M, Avery S, Tsourkas A, Hahn SM (2013) Gold nanoparticles in radiation research: potential applications for imaging and radiosensitization. Transl Cancer Res 2(4):280–291

58. Jin C, Bai L, Wu H, Tian F, Guo G (2007) Radiosensitization of paclitaxel, etanidazole and paclitaxel + etanidazole nanoparticles on hypoxic human tumor cells in vitro. Biomaterials 28(25):3723–3730

59. Werner ME, Copp JA, Karve S et al (2011) Folate-targeted polymeric nanoparticle formulation of docetaxel is an effective molecularly targeted radiosensitizer with efficacy dependent on the timing of radiotherapy. ACS Nano 5:8990–8998

60. Werner ME, Cummings ND, Sethi M et al (2013) Preclinical evaluation of Genexol-PM, a nanoparticle formulation of paclitaxel, as a novel radiosensitizer for the treatment of non-small cell lung cancer. Int J Radiat Oncol Biol Phys 86:463–468

61. Jeremic B, Aguerri AR, Filipovic N (2013) Radiosensitization by gold nanoparticles. Clin Transl Oncol 15:593–601

62. Young SW, Qing F, Harriman A et al (1996) Gadolinium(III) texaphyrin: a tumor selective radiation sensitizer that is detectable by MRI. Proc Natl Acad Sci U S A 93:6610–6615

63. Yao MH, Ma M, Chen Y, Jia XQ, Xu G, Xu HX, Chen HR, Wu R (2014) Multifunctional BiS23/PLGA nanocapsule for combined HIFU/radiation therapy. Biomaterials 35(28):8197–8205

64. Mirjolet C, Papa AL, Crehange G, Raguin O, Seignez C, Paul C, Truc G, Maingon P, Millot N (2013) The radiosensitization effect of titanate nanotubes as a new tool in radiation therapy for glioblastoma: a proof-of-concept. Radiother Oncol 108(1):136–142

65. Maggiorella L, Barouch G, Devaux C, Pottier A, Deutsch E, Bourhis J, Borghi E, Levy L (2012) Nanoscale radiotherapy with hafnium oxide nanoparticles. Future Oncol 8(9):1167–1181

66. Lin MH, Hsu TS, Yang PM, Tsai MY, Perng TP, Lin LY (2009) Comparison of organic and inorganic germanium compounds in cellular radiosensitivity and preparation of germanium nanoparticles as a radiosensitizer. Int J Radiat Biol 85:214–226

67. Porcel E, Liehn S, Remita H, Usami N, Kobayashi K, Furusawa Y et al (2010) Platinum nanoparticles: a promising material for future cancer therapy? Nanotechnology 21:85103

68. Riley PA (1994) Free radicals in biology: oxidative stress and the effects of ionizing radiation. Int J Radiat Biol 65:27–33

69. Balasubramanian B, Pogozelski WK, Tullius TD (1998) DNA strand breaking by the hydroxyl radical is governed by the accessible surface areas of the hydrogen atoms of the DNA backbone. Proc Natl Acad Sci U S A 95:9738–9743

70. Steel GG, McMillan TJ, Peacock JH (1989) The 5Rs of radiobiology. Int J Radiat Biol 56:1045–1048
71. Radford IR, Broadhurst S (1986) Enhanced induction by X-irradiation of DNA double-strand breakage in mitotic as compared with S-phase V79 cells. Int J Radiat Biol Relat Stud Phys Chem Med 49:909–914
72. Bedford JS (1991) Sublethal damage, potentially lethal damage, and chromosomal aberrations in mammalian cells exposed to ionizing radiations. Int J Radiat Oncol Biol Phys 21:1457–1469
73. Bredesen DE (2000) Apoptosis: overview and signal transduction pathways. J Neurotrauma 17:801–810
74. Misawa M, Takahashi J (2011) Generation of reactive oxygen species induced by gold nanoparticles under X-ray and UV irradiations. Nanomedicine 7:604–614
75. Giusti AM, Raimondi M, Ravagnan G, Sapora O, Parasassi T (1998) Human cell membrane oxidative damage induced by single and fractionated doses of ionizing radiation: a fluorescence spectroscopy study. Int J Radiat Biol 74:595–605
76. Mesbahi A (2010) A review on gold nanoparticles radiosensitization effect in radiation therapy of cancer. Rep Prac Oncol Radiother 15:176–180
77. Kobayashi K, Usami N, Porcel E, Lacombe S, Le Sech C (2010) Enhancement of radiation effect by heavy elements. Mutat Res 704:123–131
78. Adams FH, Norman A, Mello RS, Bass D (1977) Effect of radiation and contrast media on chromosomes. Preliminary report. Radiology 124:823–826
79. Chithrani DB et al (2010) Gold nanoparticles as radiation sensitizers in cancer therapy. Radiat Res 173:719–728
80. Nath R, Bongiorni P, Rockwell S (1990) Iododeoxyuridine radiosensitization by low- and high-energy photons for brachytherapy dose rates. Radiat Res 124:249–258
81. Polf JC et al (2011) Enhanced relative biological effectiveness of proton radiotherapy in tumor cells with internalized gold nanoparticles. Appl Phys Lett 98:193702
82. Butterworth KT, McMahon SJ, Currell FJ, Prise KM (2012) Physical basis and biological mechanisms of gold nanoparticle radiosensitization. Nanoscale 4:4830–4838
83. Roa W et al (2009) Gold nanoparticle sensitize radiotherapy of prostate cancer cells by regulation of the cell cycle. Nanotechnology 20:375101
84. Kang B, Mackey MA, El-Sayed MA (2010) Nuclear targeting of gold nanoparticles in cancer cells induces DNA damage, causing cytokinesis arrest and apoptosis. J Am Chem Soc 132:1517–1519
85. Regulla DF, Hieber LB, Seidenbusch M (1998) Physical and biological interface dose effects in tissue due to X-ray-induced release of secondary radiation from metallic gold surfaces. Radiat Res 150:92–100
86. Geng F et al (2011) Thio-glucose bound gold nanoparticles enhance radio-cytotoxic targeting of ovarian cancer. Nanotechnology 22:285101
87. Jain S et al (2011) Cell-specific radiosensitization by gold nanoparticles at megavoltage radiation energies. Int J Radiat Oncol Biol Phys 79:531–539
88. Liu CJ et al (2010) Enhancement of cell radiation sensitivity by pegylated gold nanoparticles. Phys Med Biol 55:931–945
89. Butterworth KT et al (2010) Evaluation of cytotoxicity and radiation enhancement using 1.9 nm gold particles: potential application for cancer therapy. Nanotechnology 21:295101
90. Kong T et al (2008) Enhancement of radiation cytotoxicity in breast-cancer cells by localized attachment of gold nanoparticles. Small 4:1537–1543
91. Rahman WN et al (2009) Enhancement of radiation effects by gold nanoparticles for superficial radiation therapy. Nanomedicine 5:136–142
92. Zhang X et al (2008) Enhanced radiation sensitivity in prostate cancer by gold-nanoparticles. Clin Invest Med 31:E160–E167
93. Chang MY et al (2008) Increased apoptotic potential and dose-enhancing effect of gold nanoparticles in combination with single-dose clinical electron beams on tumor-bearing mice. Cancer Sci 99:1479–1484

94. Chien, C.C. et al. (2006) Synchrotron radiation instrumentation. Ninth international conference on synchrotron radiation instrumentation. vol 879
95. Zhang XD et al (2009) Irradiation stability and cytotoxicity of gold nanoparticles for radiotherapy. Int J Nanomedicine 4:165–173
96. Liu CJ et al (2008) Enhanced x-ray irradiation-induced cancer cell damage by gold nanoparticles treated by a new synthesis method of polyethylene glycol modification. Nanotechnology 19:295104
97. Chattopadhyay N et al (2010) Design and characterization of HER-2-targeted gold nanoparticles for enhanced X-radiation treatment of locally advanced breast cancer. Mol Pharm 7:2194–2206
98. Brun E, Sanche L, Sicard-Roselli C (2009) Parameters governing gold nanoparticle X-ray radiosensitization of DNA in solution. Colloids Surf B Biointerfaces 72:128–134
99. Zheng Y, Hunting DJ, Ayotte P, Sanche L (2008) Radiosensitization of DNA by gold nanoparticles irradiated with high-energy electrons. Radiat Res 169:19–27
100. Ngwa W et al (2013) In vitro radiosensitization by gold nanoparticles during continuous low-dose-rate gamma irradiation with I-125 brachytherapy seeds. Nanomedicine 9:25–27
101. Chattopadhyay N et al (2013) Molecularly targeted gold nanoparticles enhance the radiation response of breast cancer cells and tumor xenografts to X-radiation. Breast Cancer Res Treat 137:81–91
102. Hossain M, Su M (2012) Nanoparticle location and material dependent dose enhancement in X-ray radiation therapy. J Phys Chem C Nanomater Interfaces 116:23047–23052
103. Hainfeld JF, Slatkin DN, Smilowitz HM (2004) The use of gold nanoparticles to enhance radiotherapy in mice. Phys Med Biol 49:N309–N315
104. Hebert EM, Debouttiere PJ, Lepage M, Sanche L, Hunting DJ (2010) Preferential tumour accumulation of gold nanoparticles, visualised by Magnetic Resonance Imaging: radiosensitisation studies in vivo and in vitro. Int J Radiat Biol 86:692–700
105. Joh DY et al (2013) Theranostic gold nanoparticles modified for durable systemic circulation effectively and safely enhance the radiation therapy of human sarcoma cells and tumors. Transl Oncol 6:722–731
106. Hainfeld JF et al (2010) Gold nanoparticles enhance the radiation therapy of a murine squamous cell carcinoma. Phys Med Biol 55:3045–3059
107. Joh DY et al (2013) Selective targeting of brain tumors with gold nanoparticle-induced radiosensitization. PLoS One 8, e62425
108. Kim JK et al (2012) Enhanced proton treatment in mouse tumors through proton irradiated nanoradiator effects on metallic nanoparticles. Phys Med Biol 57:8309–8323
109. Zhang XD et al (2012) Size-dependent radiosensitization of PEG-coated gold nanoparticles for cancer radiation therapy. Biomaterials 33:6408–6419
110. Atkinson RL et al (2010) Thermal enhancement with optically activated gold nanoshells sensitizes breast cancer stem cells to radiation therapy. Sci Transl Med 2:55ra79
111. Zhang XD et al (2014) Enhanced tumor accumulation of sub-2 nm gold nanoclusters for cancer radiation therapy. Adv Healthc Mater 3:133–141
112. Al Zaki A, Joh D, Cheng Z, de Barros AL, Kao GD, Dorsey JF, Tsourkas A (2014) Gold-loaded polymeric micelles for computed tomography–guided radiation therapy treatment and radiosensitization. ACS Nano 8(1):104–112
113. McQuade C, Al Zaki A, Desai Y, Vido M, Sakhuja T, Cheng Z, Hickey R, Joh D, Park S-J, Kao GD, Dorsey JF, Tsourkas A (2015) A multi-functional nanoplatform for imaging, radiotherapy, and the prediction of therapeutic response. Small 11(7):834–843
114. Sun L, Joh DY, Al Zaki A, Stangl M, Murty S, Davis JJ, Baumann BC, Alonso-Basanta M, Kao GD, Tsourkas A, Dorsey JF (2015) Theranostic application of mixed gold and superparamagnetic iron oxide nanoparticle micelles in glioblastoma multiforme. J Biomed Nanotechnol 11:1–10
115. Vilchis-Juarez A, Ferro-Flores G, Santos-Cuevas C, Morales-Avila E, Ocampo-Garcia B, Diaz-Nieto L, Luna-Gutierrez M, Jimenez-Mancilla N, Pedraza-Lopez M, Gomez-Olivan L (2014) Molecular targeting radiotherapy with cyclo-RGDfK(C) peptides conjugated to 177Lu-labeled gold nanoparticles in tumor bearing mice. J Biomed Nanotechnol 10:395–404

116. Miladi I, Alric C, Dufort S, Mowat P, Dutour A, Mandon C, Laurent G, Bräuer-Krisch E, Herath N, Coll JL, Dutreix M, Lux F, Bazzi R, Billotey C, Janier M, Perriat P, Le Duc G, Roux S, Tillement O (2014) The in vivo radiosensitizing effect of gold nanoparticles based MRI contrast agents. Small 10(6):1116–1124
117. Dufort S, Bianchi A, Henry M, Lux F, Le Duc G, Josserand V, Louis C, Perriat P, Cremillieux Y, Tillement O, Coll JL (2015) Nebulized gadolinium-based nanoparticles: A theranostic approach for lung tumor imaging and radiosensitization. Small 11(2):215–221
118. Zhao D, Sun X, Tong J, Ma J, Bu X, Xu R, Fan R (2012) A novel multifunctional nanocomposite C225-conjugated Fe3O4/Ag enhances the sensitivity of nasopharyngeal carcinoma cells to radiotherapy. Acta Biochim Biophys Sin (Shanghai) 44(8):678–684
119. Aillon KL, Xie Y, El-Gendy N, Berkland CJ, Forrest ML (2009) Effects of nanomaterial physicochemical properties on in vivo toxicity. Adv Drug Deliv Rev 61:457–466

Index

© Springer International Publishing Switzerland 2017
P.J. Tofilon, K. Camphausen (eds.), *Increasing the Therapeutic
Ratio of Radiotherapy*, Cancer Drug Discovery and Development,
DOI 10.1007/978-3-319-40854-5

Printed in the United States
By Bookmasters